SHELL-SHOCKED BRITISH ARMY VETERANS IN IRELAND, 1918–39

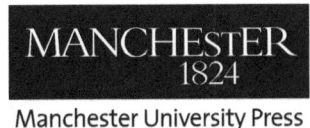

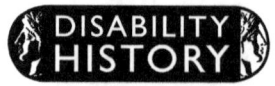

Series editors
Dr Julie Anderson, Professor Walton O. Schalick, III

This series published by Manchester University Press responds to the growing interest in disability as a discipline worthy of historical research. The series has a broad international historical remit, encompassing issues that include class, race, gender, age, war, medical treatment, professionalisation, environments, work, institutions and cultural and social aspects of disablement including representations of disabled people in literature, film, art and the media.

Already published
Deafness, community and culture in Britain: Leisure and cohesion, 1945–1995
Martin Atherton
Rethinking modern prostheses in Anglo-American commodity cultures, 1820–1939
Claire L. Jones (ed.)
Destigmatising mental illness? Professional politics and public education in Britain, 1870–1970
Vicky Long
Intellectual disability: A conceptual history, 1200–1900
Patrick McDonagh, C. F. Goodey and Tim Stainton (eds)
Fools and idiots? Intellectual disability in the Middle Ages
Irina Metzler
Framing the moron: The social construction of feeble-mindedness in the American eugenic era
Gerald V. O'Brien
Recycling the disabled: Army, medicine, and modernity in WWI Germany
Heather R. Perry
Disability in the Industrial Revolution: Physical impairment in British coalmining, 1780–1880
David M. Turner and Daniel Blackie
Worth saving: Disabled children during the Second World War
Sue Wheatcroft

SHELL-SHOCKED BRITISH ARMY VETERANS IN IRELAND, 1918–39

A DIFFICULT HOMECOMING

Michael Robinson

Manchester University Press

Copyright © Michael Robinson 2020

The right of Michael Robinson to be identified as the author of this work has been asserted by him in accordance with the Copyright, Designs and Patents Act 1988.

Published by Manchester University Press
Oxford Road, Manchester M13 9PL
www.manchesteruniversitypress.co.uk

British Library Cataloguing-in-Publication Data
A catalogue record for this book is available from the British Library

ISBN 978 1 5261 4005 0 hardback
ISBN 978 1 5261 6249 6 paperback

First published 2020

The publisher has no responsibility for the persistence or accuracy of URLs for any external or third-party internet websites referred to in this book, and does not guarantee that any content on such websites is, or will remain, accurate or appropriate.

Typeset
by Toppan Best-set Premedia Limited

In loving memory of George Leslie Tate.

Contents

List of tables	*page* viii
List of figures	ix
Series editors' foreword	xi
Acknowledgements	xii
A note on language and anonymisation	xiii
List of abbreviations	xiv
Introduction	1
1 'A definitive neurasthenic temperament'? The Irish Tommy and veteran	22
2 Neurasthenic pensioners in revolutionary Ireland	63
3 Neurasthenic pensioners in the Irish Free State and Northern Ireland	100
4 The war hospital in Ireland	148
5 The Service Patient scheme in Ireland	185
Conclusion	227
Select bibliography	233
Index	248

List of tables

1	Pension scale and payment in accordance with neurasthenic pensioners' condition with comparative objective disabilities.	page 32
2	Proportion of all patients awaiting either in-patient or out-patient treatment for neurasthenia in Ministry of Pensions' hospitals in the UK, 1921.	64
3	Percentage of awaiting neurasthenic pensioners in receipt of a treatment allowance.	75
4	Numbers of neurasthenic pensioners receiving in-patient and out-patient treatment in the UK, 1921–36.	108
5	Ministry of Pensions' hospitals operating in Ireland, 1929.	110
6	Cost of pensions per enlisted man, 1926–27.	124
7	Annual number of deaths in Irish asylums, 1913–19.	170
8	Percentage of diagnoses of dementia and melancholia in Service Patient populations.	189
9	The distribution of 375 Service Patients in Irish Free State mental hospitals, 31 December 1931.	198

List of figures

1	Leopardstown staff: the resident superintendent, matron and secretary surrounded by hospital nurses. Courtesy of the National Library of Ireland.	page 46
2	Leopardstown's 'croquet grounds' where patients participated in recreational games and activities. Courtesy of the National Library of Ireland.	47
3	Leopardstown's 'pleasure grounds' where patients were able to enjoy walks. Courtesy of the National Library of Ireland.	47
4	Leopardstown's recreation room. Courtesy of the National Library of Ireland.	48
5	Architectural drawing for Craigavon UVF Hospital. Figure taken from PRONI, LA/3/8/JA/12.	50
6	South Ireland and combined UK average figures of all patients awaiting either in-patient or out-patient treatment, 1921. Calculated from Bourke, 'Effeminacy, ethnicity and the end of trauma', 69.	64
7	Comparison between the UK and South Ireland for awaiting neurasthenic pensioners in receipt of a treatment allowance. Calculated from NA, PIN 15/56, Treatment of Neurasthenia, 1921–22.	76
8	The number of neurasthenic pensioners throughout the UK, 1921–38. Calculated from Ministry of Pensions Fourth Annual Report to Twenty-Second Annual Reports; Annual Reports covering the period 1 April 1920 to 31 March 1938.	107
9	A soldier-patient dressed in Hospital Blues. Taken from Manchester City Archive, GB124.DPA/690/19.	150
10	Belfast District Lunatic Asylum, c. 1890–1900. Taken from PRONI, T/418/1/86.	152
11	The age distribution of Irish lunatic patients, 1861–1911. Annual Report of the Inspectors of Lunatics, Ireland, 1913, xv.	166
12	Length of residence of male patients in Irish asylums who were discharged recovered and those who died in 1919. Annual Report of the Inspectors of Lunatics, Ireland, 1919, 9.	167

LIST OF FIGURES

13 Average annual number of deaths in Irish asylums over
    five-year periods, 1890–1919. Annual Report of the
    Inspectors of Lunatics, Ireland, 1919, xiv.   170
14 Number of Service Patients under treatment in
    Purdysburn Villa Colony, 1921–38. Calculated from
    Purdysburn Villa Colony Annual Reports, 1921–38; PRONI,
    HOS/28/1/5/9–12.   190
15 Number of Service Patient admissions and discharges in
    Purdysburn Villa Colony, 1921–38. Calculated from
    Purdysburn Villa Colony Annual Reports, 1921–38; PRONI,
    HOS/28/1/5/9–12.   191
16 Purdysburn House. Taken from PRONI, HOS/28/1/5.   193
17 Pleasure grounds at Purdysburn House. Taken from
    PRONI, HOS/28/1/5.   193
18 A regular villa. Taken from PRONI, HOS/28/1/5.   194
19 A villa dayroom. Taken from PRONI, HOS/28/1/5.   195
20 A villa dining hall. Taken from PRONI, HOS/28/1/5.   195

Series editors' foreword

You know a subject has achieved maturity when a book series is dedicated to it. In the case of disability, while it has co-existed with human beings for centuries the study of disability's history is still quite young.

In setting up this series, we chose to encourage multi-methodologic history rather than a purely traditional historical approach, as researchers in disability history come from a wide variety of disciplinary backgrounds. Equally 'disability' history is a diverse topic which benefits from a variety of approaches in order to appreciate its multi-dimensional characteristics.

A test for the team of authors and editors who bring you this series is typical of most series, but disability also brings other consequential challenges. At this time disability is highly contested as a social category in both developing and developed contexts. Inclusion, philosophy, money, education, visibility, sexuality, identity and exclusion are but a handful of the social categories in play. With this degree of politicisation, language is necessarily a cardinal focus.

In an effort to support the plurality of historical voices, the editors have elected to give fair rein to language. Language is historically contingent, and can appear offensive to our contemporary sensitivities. The authors and editors believe that the use of terminology that accurately reflects the historical period of any book in the series will assist readers in their understanding of the history of disability in time and place.

Finally, disability offers the cultural, social and intellectual historian a new 'take' on the world we know. We see disability history as one of a few nascent fields with the potential to reposition our understanding of the flow of cultures, society, institutions, ideas and lived experience. Conceptualisations of 'society' since the early modern period have heavily stressed principles of autonomy, rationality and the subjectivity of the individual agent. Consequently we are frequently oblivious to the historical contingency of the present with respect to those elements. Disability disturbs those foundational features of 'the modern.' Studying disability history helps us resituate our policies, our beliefs and our experiences.

Julie Anderson
Walton O. Schalick, III

Acknowledgements

I consider myself extremely fortunate to have had the opportunity to be part of the University of Liverpool's Institute of Irish Studies and to have enjoyed the considerable support and friendship of staff and colleagues throughout my academic career. In particular, I would like to thank Professor Diane Urquhart. Diane's patience, support and optimism have been fundamental in the completion of this work and in my personal and professional development. I do hope that this book pays sufficient tribute to her considerable contribution.

I am also indebted to Dr Julie Anderson, Professor Peter Barham, Professor Joanna Bourke, Dr Nick Bubak and Professor Brendan Kelly, who have all offered invaluable advice and timely guidance at various stages of my career and research. As a first-time author, I am very grateful for the patience and help which has been consistently on offer from the team at Manchester University Press. This project is only possible thanks to the invaluable archival work of various archivists who have preserved, restored and facilitated access to the records of both the Richmond War Hospital and various former Irish asylums. Thanks are also due to the Health Service Executive for providing privileged access to records that were otherwise closed to the public.

The Universities of Northumbria and Liverpool, the Irish Studies Doctoral Research Network, the British Association of Irish Studies and the Scouloudi Foundation generously provided funding to facilitate the research that underpins this book. Some material included in this book has also been accepted for publication in *War in History*. I am grateful to SAGE and the journal's editors for their permission to reuse material.

I would also like to thank all of my family and friends including the regulars of the Three Tuns Pub back home in Hetton-le-Hole. The existence of this book is a tribute to the unwavering and constant support of my late uncle Les and the friendship of my sister, Aimee. Finally, my thanks goes to my parents, Ken and Denise Robinson, for everything.

A note on language and anonymisation

The reader will be aware of instances where words and language are used which are insensitive by contemporary standards. They are employed throughout this book to remain historically true as they were widespread and often an acceptable ingredient of the official medical discourse. The inter-war period witnessed a shift in the medical nomenclature with lunatic asylums, for example, being redefined as mental hospitals. Thus, the names of facilities discussed in this study evolve with this development. Regarding the identification of mentally ill soldiers and veterans, this book adheres to the access conditions laid down by the archives in which they were initially identified. Thus, soldier-patients at the Richmond War Hospital and institutionalised Service Patients are anonymised to prevent their identification as I utilised records which were often otherwise closed to the general public. By contrast, the Ministry of Pensions' archive in London remains open to the public and, as such, disabled pensioners under discussion remain fully identifiable and are named.

List of abbreviations

CMS	Commissioner of Medical Services
DCMS	Deputy Commissioner of Medical Services
ESWS	Ex-Services Welfare Society
HC	House of Commons
HL	House of Lords
IRA	Irish Republican Army
NA	National Archives of England and Wales, London
NAI	National Archives of the Republic of Ireland, Dublin
PRONI	Public Record Office of Northern Ireland, Belfast
SILA	Southern Irish Loyalist Association

Introduction

In March 1921, 1,182,000 First World War veterans in Britain and Ireland were receiving a disability pension paid for by the Ministry of Pensions. Diagnostic categories, the severity of disablement and pension sum ranged on an individual basis, but each pensioner had a commonality: their disability was deemed attributable to or aggravated by their previous war service.[1] The hitherto unprecedented scale of pension infrastructure was the result of the intense and lethal reality of the First World War involving mass citizen armies experiencing static trench warfare, poisonous gasses, advanced heavy artillery and machine-gun fire. The innovative technological and industrial conduct of the Great War gave rise to physical injuries such as facial disfigurement, limb loss, paraplegia and blindness. Notable advances in military medical treatment, including developments in orthopaedics and the implementation of superior evacuation and medical systems at the Front, increased the likelihood of wounded servicemen surviving injury. Albeit their survival ensued with their bodies transformed: 'The science and technology of the First World War simultaneously destroyed and re-created the male body.'[2]

In addition to physical injuries, the British Army and the Ministry of Pensions also had to contend with a rise in psychoneurotic casualties. Observing the Russo-Japanese War, 1904–05, A. G. Kay, a Lieutenant-Colonel of the Royal Army Medical Corps, predicted an increase in the number of 'mental diseases' in any future conflict involving Britain, writing:

> The conditions of modern warfare calling large numbers of men into action, the tremendous endurance, physical and mental, required, and the widely destructive effect of modern artillery fire will undoubtedly make their influence felt in a future war, and we shall have to deal with a larger percentage of mental disease than hitherto.[3]

Kay's thesis disrupts previous arguments that military psychiatry was an unknown phenomenon before 1914.[4] Verifying Kay's prophecy, British Army personnel officially recognised over 80,000 cases of psychoneuroses during the First World War.[5] During the early stages of the conflict, an assortment of pre-existing diagnoses utilised in civilian medicine, including hysteria and neurasthenia, were applied by British Army medical officials. These established diagnoses described diverse and subjective neurological, physiological and psychological reactions to warfare.[6] Charles Myers formally recognised the description 'shell-shock' in a *Lancet* article in February 1915. Myers had been working with a medical unit of the British Army in France, and he admitted that he did not invent the term indicating it had already arisen in popular usage amongst frontline British soldiers.[7] Myers quickly realised the diagnosis was an 'ill-chosen' and 'harmful' description. A serviceman often suffered from mental symptoms due to the deleterious impact of warfare which wore down a man's nerves and resilience rather than being induced by the explosion or shock of a shell.[8] Active war service was not always necessary for breakdowns to occur, and there were numerous examples of psychoneurotic casualties who had never been exposed to frontline service. Subsequently, towards the end of 1915, the Army Council ordered medical staff to diagnose servicemen as 'Shell-Shock Wounded', where the ailment was a result of enemy action, or 'Shell-Shock Sick' where no such event like a shell explosion was traceable. After much contention and confusion, the label 'Not Yet Diagnosed Mental' became the primary diagnosis in mid-1917. Nevertheless, uncertainty remained. Military and medical officials, patients, politicians and the general public each had their own cognate definition of shell-shock. The term permeated but was never clearly defined nor understood as an exclusive medical, psychiatric or emotional disorder, a military administrative category or a cultural metaphor.[9] Four years after the Armistice, the War Office remained unable to define a clear and widely-held definition of shell-shock.[10] As a result, neurasthenia became the primary pensionable category. Like shell-shock, this diagnosis was incredibly broad including a variety of neuropsychiatric symptoms.[11]

Irishmen fought in the same uniform as their British comrades and experienced the same conditions and psychoneurotic afflictions both during the conflict as soldiers and in its aftermath as veterans. By 1921, an estimated 65,000 ex-servicemen were receiving a pension for the condition in the UK with around 12,420 pensioners residing in Ireland.[12] An additional category was the insane Great War veterans under treatment in the district asylum designated as 'Service Patients.' Like neurasthenic pensioners who returned to civil society, Great War veterans diagnosed with lunacy remained a charge on the Ministry of Pensions. In 1921, there were an estimated 6,300 institutionalised Service Patients in the UK with approximately 500 under treatment in Irish asylums.[13] With the formation of Northern Ireland and the Irish Free State in the early 1920s, mentally ill pensioners in Ireland continued to remain under the remit of the department charged with their after-care, namely the Ministry of Pensions. Their daily lives were shaped by distinct separate socio-economic and political conditions and by legislation enacted by the Parliament of Northern Ireland and the Dáil Eireann (Irish Parliament) respectively. Both Irish and British-based sources are required to reconstruct the lives of mentally ill Irish Great War veterans. Distinct socio-political and economic contrasts between Ireland and Britain are ever apparent in this study of post-war mentally ill communities in Ireland. Ireland's unique context impacted upon the functioning of the Ministry of Pensions, its rehabilitation of neurasthenic and insane Great War veterans permeating into the daily lives of individuals. There was never a singular experience of war-induced disability across the United Kingdom. British and Irish veterans were former comrades, received the same pensionable diagnoses and remained under the remit of the Ministry of Pensions; they were, however, subjected to varying levels of care and rehabilitative support on their return home.

Historiography

While this study addresses mentally ill ex-servicemen with a range of psychiatric or neurological diagnoses, it remains intimately associated with shell-shock. Shell-shock remains a culturally and historically evocative symbol of the First World War with afflicted serviceman a regular feature in memoirs, novels and poems. For example, Robert Graves' and Siegfried Sassoon's acclaimed post-war memoirs narrate their personal experiences of shell-shock.[14] Pat Barker's successful *Regeneration* trilogy further buttressed shell-shock as an essential British cultural reference point in its memory of the First World War.[15] Attention in these works, however, is exclusive to the officer class with the working-class private's torment comparatively concealed.[16] While veterans of conflicts have been described as 'neglected figures in histories of war and peace', the historical disregard of British Army veterans of the First World War has been manifested for those who had mental illnesses and who were members of the non-officer class.[17] Wendy Holden argues the post-Armistice treatment and experiences of traumatised Tommies are 'unquantifiable' and 'incalculable.'[18] Irish historians of the First World War accept a similarly overarching notion for its entire Great War veteran population. Tom Johnstone, for example, concludes 'most Irish ex-soldiers retired into historical oblivion' following their discharge.[19] This book disputes these narratives with an analysis of over ten thousand mentally ill servicemen who returned to Ireland.

An interest in combat syndromes during the First World War began in the 1970s with Paul Fussell's *The Great War and Modern Memory*, John Keegan's *The Face of Battle* and Eric Leed's *No Man's Land*.[20] These works analyse personal understandings of combat, with the Great War being a prevalent case study in their works. A small collection of publications also situates shell-shock within broader research into the medical history of combat neurosis.[21] Despite the significance of shell-shock as a cultural symbol of Britain's involvement in the First World War, Peter Leese offered the first in-depth and exclusive analysis of the British Tommy's experience of shell-shock in 2002 to reveal the traumatic struggles of shell-shocked Great War servicemen.[22] While the importance of Leese's work is undeniable, the underappreciation of the post-war lives of mentally ill veterans remains within the historiography.[23] Only a small number of academics have subsequently engaged with a post-war analysis.[24] Peter Barham's work largely focuses on the post-war experiences of institutionalised English Great War veterans.[25] Fiona Reid's broad study, *Broken Men: Shell-Shock, Treatment and Recovery in Britain, 1914–30*, examines shell-shock at the Front, shell-shocked veterans in post-war society, the treatment of institutionalised and insane Great War veterans, and leading veteran charity, Ex-Services Welfare Society (ESWS).[26]

Most recently, Tracey Loughran offered an academic study of the condition in *Shell-Shock and Medical Culture in First World War Britain*. Loughran assesses shell-shock's construction in the diagnostic nomenclature and within the medical culture in Britain. The book is thus unable to provide much information on the post-war experiences of mentally ill British Army veterans and omits engagement with Ireland.[27] The mentally ill Great War veteran in Ireland similarly remains absent in transnational studies of psychological trauma and combat neurosis in the aftermath of the First World War.[28] Barham is the only academic to explain his active omission of Ireland and Irish men by stating that the separate volumes of Irish archival material require a study of their own.[29] Joanna Bourke remains the sole historian to pay exclusive attention to the Irish Great War participants' experience of shell-shock.[30] The limited engagement with Ireland's experience of war-related mental disability echoes British-centric studies into physically disabled First World War veterans.[31]

In addition to perceived methodological shortcomings, the politicisation of the memory of the conflict in Ireland has influenced the absence of a post-war analysis of disabled Great War veterans. With the initial blessing of both the nationalist and unionist political mainstream, Irish servicemen were supported by the majority of the Irish public during the earlier stages of the conflict. The Easter Rising of 1916 shifted nationalist Ireland's backing of the war. After the execution of thirteen Easter rebels, widespread support arose for republicanism at the expense of Home Rule and the Irish Parliamentary Party.[32] The results of the 1918 General Election demonstrates the dramatic change in the political context. Despite not winning one seat during the 1910 General Election, Sinn Féin, espousing national self-determination for Ireland, won 73 out of 105 Westminster seats.[33] The following years saw the establishment of the First Dáil in 1919 and the Anglo-Irish War, 1919–21, resulting in the creation of the Irish Free State and Northern Ireland by 1922.

Following the formation of these respective states, two opposing national narratives emerged. Both emphasised identity and inclusion at the expense of the other. In the predominantly Protestant and unionist Northern Ireland, participation in the First World War was heralded as having helped to maintain the Union. The opposite was true among nationalists in the Irish Free State. As D. G. Boyce notes: 'The war was soon perceived as the wrong war, fought in the wrong place, and against the wrong foe – a view which became political orthodoxy.' Boyce thus described nationalists as having 'applied a sort of field dressing, in the shape of national amnesia, to the Great War experience.'[34] The Free State Government proved subsequently unwilling to patronise and observe Armistice Day ceremonies officially; its neutrality during the Second World War justified a scaling down of commemorative events. This detachment persisted after the cessation of the second global conflict.[35] While Northern Ireland did not have a national equivalent to the Cenotaph, sixty-two public war memorials were erected by 1939.[36] The Troubles in Northern Ireland further solidified the contestation of memory in Ireland. The Irish Republican Army (IRA) bombing of a Remembrance Day ceremony at Enniskillen Memorial, killing twelve people on 8 November 1987, highlights this intensification. As the peace process progressed, culminating in the signing of the Good Friday Agreement in 1998, the resulting quest for reconciliation between unionists and nationalists allowed the Great War to become a key point of reference to remember a period of shared experience.[37] The evolution of the memory of the First World War is essential when considering the silencing of the shell-shocked Irish veteran within the historiography. Traumatised populations are better able to have their experiences acknowledged publicly if their accounts are politically resonant and compatible with contemporary society.[38]

The subsequent increase in research regarding Ireland's involvement in the First World War has allowed notions of a 'historical revolution' to be declared.[39] It is, nevertheless, necessary to delve beyond actions in battle. There has been a surge in analyses of the relationship between medicine and the conflict in Ireland. This exploration has included research into Irish doctors, Irish nurses, maternal and infant health and medical networks during the First World War.[40] More extensive studies of Ireland during the revolutionary period reference British ex-servicemen. In particular, a debate rages as to whether republicans targeted ex-servicemen because of their prior service in the British Army.[41] Jane Leonard, for instance, contends that Irish Great War veterans became a marginalised and discriminated community who were spat on, physically intimidated, denied employment and targeted for reprisal by the IRA.[42] In 2015, Paul Taylor's *Heroes or Traitors? Experiences of Southern Irish Soldiers Returning from the Great War, 1919–39* finally considered Irish Great War veterans throughout the inter-war period. Taylor provides valuable insight into approximately 100,000 Great War veterans who returned to Southern Ireland later embodied as the Irish Free State.[43] This study adds to these works by offering an all-Ireland methodology and a case study of those who suffered from mental health problems following their service in the British Armed Forces. This book also regularly draws upon the vast English language literature of war trauma, mental illness, treatment and pensions across numerous combatant nations of the First World War. It also considers the treatment of disabled veterans of prior colonial conflicts such as the South-African War, 1899–1902, and the Irish revolutionary conflicts, 1919–23. This framework helps to foreground the simultaneous progressiveness and conservatism in the treatment of mentally ill Irish Great War veterans.

Methodology

As a disability history, *Shell-shocked British Army Veterans in Ireland, 1918–39* considers, contextualises and comprehends the lived experiences of disabled people in a past society. This approach poses a significant methodological challenge. Physically disabled Great War veterans left negligible personal records documenting their experiences.[44] This problem was manifested for those mentally ill as a result of war service. Mental breakdown carried an additional stigma in the legacy of Victorian masculinity, and the associated shame would have silenced some ashamed to articulate their suffering with others unable to due to illness. Periodic mental breakdowns frequently occurred during the inter-war years but went unrecorded.[45] One popular self-help book by a neurasthenic Great War pensioner published in 1933 stressed the importance for mentally-wounded servicemen to restrain from talking to anyone about their symptoms: 'To talk of troubles in a voluble, despairing way, merely piles on the agony and "plays-up" the emotions ... never display a wound, except to a physician.'[46]

The dearth of relevant historical source material further obscures Irish veterans. Their numbers were much smaller than their British counterparts. Approximately 4,280,000 enlisted in the British Army during the First World War in England, Wales and Scotland. This number equated to around 23 percent of the male population, while just 134,202 men from Ireland enlisted. This figure constitutes only over 6 percent of the male population.[47] These recruitments statistics impacted upon subsequent veteran communities including mentally and physically disabled communities. Second, Irish veterans in predominately nationalist areas may have been reluctant to exhibit their troubles due to the additional stigma often accompanying prior service in the British Army.[48] This case study of Ireland utilises a range of British and Irish sources to overcome these limitations. This monograph benefits from the Ministry of Pensions' archival collection currently held in the National Archives of England and Wales in London. The department established a system of national, regional and local administrative centres across the United Kingdom. In conjunction with private agencies, charities and employers, it administered pensions and provided medical care to the disabled pensioner. Ulster and South Ireland, with their headquarters situated in Belfast and Dublin respectively, constituted two of the eleven administrative regions defined by the Ministry of Pensions. Assisted by local committees, the Ministry's infrastructure continued to operate as an autonomous British governmental body in Ireland throughout the inter-war period. The Ministry of Pensions' archival records provides a wealth of qualitative and quantitative data dedicated to the disabled pensioner in Ireland including those in receipt of a disability pension for neurasthenia and lunacy.[49]

There has been opposition to using institutional sources as they have an inherent source-bias being written from the viewpoint of the non-disabled official interacting with the disabled person. As a result, they have been claimed to be 'inevitably one-sided in their account of the disabled people, presenting them as depersonalised objects of institutional care.'[50] While recognising the Ministry's files only reveal contact between Irish pensioners and the state, they still have immense historical value. The department's annual reports consistently portray an image of progress and professionalism to an external audience. The department's internal administrative material, by contrast, offers a more authentic insight into the treatment and experience of disabled pensioners residing in Ireland. Its archival records include financial data, minutes of conferences, information regarding in-patient and out-patient care, internal correspondence regarding bureaucracy, correspondence between local, regional and national staff and detailed observational reports produced by pensions staff working in Ireland.

The Ministry of Pensions' archive also contains pension files of individuals who were assisted by the department. Only a minority of these individual files dedicated to mentally ill veterans have survived.[51] This monograph benefits from the surviving medical and pension records of P. J. O'Ryan particularly. While his being a middle-class ex-officer and university educated adds to an over-reliance on the most affluent shell-shocked servicemen in existing works, O'Ryan lived in various areas of Ireland during the inter-war period and his files thus provide personal insight into the lived experience of mentally ill First World War veterans who returned to Ireland.[52] O'Ryan's pension records include a host of relevant information including regular medical reports provided by Ministry of Pensions officials, personal correspondence, transcribed attestations of O'Ryan's understanding and descriptions of his mental illness, and information on his employability, domestic arrangement and conduct in civilian society.[53] This life-course analysis echoes the work of Wendy Jane Gagen who has previously assessed the archive of an individual pensioner to provide a personal and intimate account of war-induced disablement.[54] Of course, each pensioner's life and understanding of mental illness would have been a subjective and individual experience. Individual case files, nevertheless, often verify the observations and descriptions in the Ministry of Pensions' administrative records. Collaborating the records of men like O'Ryan with those of the wider population of mentally disabled pensioners in Ireland helps to portray successful and unsuccessful attempts of rehabilitation, the propensity to relapse in times of financial and personal adversity, the importance of domestic caregiving, the stigma often associated with mental illness and the veteran's resulting exclusion from society. The unpublished memoirs of J. B. Arnold, a northern-Irish lawyer before the war, who enlisted in the Northumberland Fusiliers and served on the Western Front before being discharged from the army on account of a shrapnel wound to his thigh, further aids this study. In addition to detailing his experience of disability, Arnold became a Ministry of Pensions official in Ireland. As a Deputy Director in the Ministry's Dublin office and assisting on regional administrative issues, Arnold had a lofty position within the department supervising pension committees in Leinster, Munster and Connaught with numerous Ministry employees under his jurisdiction. Arnold's account thus provides unique information on the Ministry's establishment, remit and function during the initial post-war years in Ireland.[55]

The institutional records of Leopardstown Hospital in Dublin provide rare insight into the medical experience of mentally ill veterans who returned to civil society. This stately home, donated to the Ministry of Pensions by a wealthy philanthropist, acted as a treatment and rehabilitation centre for mentally ill pensioners throughout the inter-war period.[56] This study also utilises Parliamentary and Dáil debates alongside Irish national and regional newspaper accounts, as well as the *War Pensions Gazette*, a monthly journal for War Pensions Local Committees. These sources provide a contemporary discussion of the mentally ill pensioner, the disabled veteran and broader ex-service community in Ireland. *Shell-shocked British Army Veterans in Ireland, 1918–39* also coaxes out the mentally disabled pensioner's experience via an analysis of the records of the most prominent charitable bodies assisting British ex-servicemen, namely the British Legion, the Southern Irish Loyalist Association and the Ex-Services Welfare Society. This study integrates the records of the Ministry of Pensions, including its policymakers, welfare officials, medical practitioners and pensioners, alongside charity records and patient casebook records. In doing so, I seek to promote how assimilating social, political and policy histories can enrich our understanding of the past and, in this instance, the post-war lives of mentally ill Great War veterans in Ireland.[57]

This project does not restrict itself to neurasthenic pensioners. Previous estimates suggest that roughly 100,000 servicemen were demobilised back to

Ireland between the Armistice and May 1920.[58] By 1926, 34,500 disabled veterans in Ireland were in receipt of a pension from the Ministry of Pensions.[59] In addition to considering the broader population of 100,000 Great War veterans, it adheres to the methodology of Julie Anderson who argues that mentally and physically disabled ex-servicemen are better understood together rather than as separate entities.[60] Both Irish physically and mentally disabled veterans witnessed the bureaucracy of the Ministry of Pensions, widespread unemployment, a lack of treatment facilities, inflated waiting-list figures, poverty and stigma. A pensioner could also receive two separate pensions for a physical *and* a psychoneurotic condition. O'Ryan, for example, received a pension for both neurasthenia and a gunshot wound to his left leg. This study thus compares how both disabilities impacted on O'Ryan's civilian life and how the state attempted to rehabilitate and compensate him for *both* disabilities. In addition to mentally and physically disabled ex-servicemen in Ireland sharing experiences, a consideration of the entire ex-service population also helps to foreground differences in their rehabilitation depending on their disability. As will be demonstrated, veterans suffering from mental illness often faced additional barriers to rehabilitation, recovery and reintegration.

Shell-shocked British Army Veterans in Ireland, 1918–39 also assesses the treatment of mentally ill Irish Great War veterans who received institutional treatment. Following the precedent set by previous disability scholarship, this study uses the descriptions 'ex-serviceman' and 'veteran' from the moment it is clear a serviceman was not returning to active duty.[61] An analysis of the Richmond War Hospital (RWH) in Dublin falls within this definition. Although under the authority of the War Office, and with patients still officially remaining members of the British Army, the facility was, for all intents and purposes, a discharge centre. Once admitted, there was a negligible opportunity for patients to resume service. With these soldier-patients receiving 'observational' treatment for up to nine months, their residency offered medical staff the opportunity to assess whether the mentally ill patient was insane and suitable for admission into a district asylum. With their lunacy deemed attributable to their previous war service, they were labelled as 'Service Patients' and treated akin to private patients with the Ministry of Pensions paying associated expenses.

Research into soldier-patients receiving treatment in the Richmond War Hospital and Service Patients under care in a district asylum is possible by utilising institutional admission and discharge registers and patient casebook files. The casebook records of Belfast, Richmond and Cork asylums are assessed as these three institutions hosted the largest populations of Service Patients in Ireland. These medical sources are read 'from below' with the patient recognised alongside the doctor.[62] Admission and discharge registers allow for quantitative analysis of patient populations including diagnoses, length of residences and recovery rates. This study extrapolates a fuller picture of patient life via an analysis of psychiatric casebook records including information regarding a patient's war service, explanations for admission, regular updates on their state and conduct and, at times, transcriptions of the patient's testimony. This information helps to provide patient biographies and a voice to the previously marginalised.[63] This methodology is not without its challenges. Transcriptions were possibly paraphrased, and thus omit the patient's tone and fail to highlight the prompt that a patient was responding to. The process of transcribing clinical records rests on the doctor's perspective. David Armstrong acknowledges a patient's view was likely to be bypassed, and any historical analysis can only assess 'what is heard, not what is said.'[64] The larger Irish asylums, accommodating over 2,000 patients, would also have had difficulty in keeping accurate, in-depth and up-to-date records. Thus, descriptions such as 'No change' and 'Continues in the same mental and physical condition' to depict the state of long-term patients are commonplace. Ultimately, individual case notes only afford glimpses of a patient's experience of treatment.[65] Nevertheless, these institutional records still possess great historical value by providing insight unattainable in medical publications.

The annual reports of the Irish Lunacy/Mental Health Inspectorate further reveal the remit and functioning of the Service Patient scheme in Irish asylums. These records include vast quantitative and qualitative detail on the administration, patient and staff populations, and the state of mental institutions across Ireland during the inter-war period. Regional newspapers provide information regarding the meetings of various asylum committees which discussed the treatment and health of Service Patients. The Ministry of Pensions' archive holds detailed correspondence and reports regarding the Service Patient scheme and its remit and function in Ireland. Ministry inspection reports of the Belfast District Lunatic Asylum are also assessed. These detailed records include information regarding the accommodation delivered to Service Patients, their mental condition and conduct, their feedback regarding treatment, and how they spent their private allowances. These accounts do not feature in the annual reports of any other Irish asylum nor do they seemingly appear within the annual reports of British asylums. Their consideration in this study thus provides a unique insight into the Service Patient scheme and its impact on the everyday lives of insane Great War veterans.

This work also follows Jay Winter's recent advocation for the benefits of researching combat neurosis by incorporating the greater medical understanding of the subject in the aftermath of the Second World War and subsequent conflicts.[66] The official categorisation of PTSD in 1980 led to an upsurge in trauma within the clinical literature and medical humanities which, when applied retrospectively, can allow us to better understand the treatment and experiences of mentally ill Irish veterans of the First World War. Adopting this methodology to analyse mentally ill ex-servicemen in Ireland validates Barham's thesis that 'the historiography of the "silent working-class soldier" has obscured much of what were actually very noisy encounters.'[67] This revaluation applies equally to those who returned to civil society and those who received institutional treatment. This study does not profess to tell the *complete* story of these men's lives. In many ways, the everyday reality of mental impairment remains a hidden history with men and their families continuing to struggle in the private domestic sphere. This study instead demonstrates that it has been a mistake to assume the mentally ill Irish Great War veteran remains silent and untraceable.

Approach

Previous estimates suggest mental disorders equated to around 25,000 discharges of Irish troops during the First World War. Chapter 1 establishes Irishmen fighting in the same uniform as their British comrades also experienced psychoneurotic afflictions. How such instances amongst Irish troops were *perceived*, however, was unique. This chapter determines that the British Military establishment believed the Irish Tommy was susceptible to war neuroses. This observation was a continuation of long-held anti-Irish perceptions amongst Britons assuming the Irish were immature, emotionally volatile and susceptible to mental illness. The opening chapter explains how this prejudice was politically motivated, being induced by a 'pro-Union psychiatry' which helped to legitimise British rule in Ireland. This chapter sets the groundwork for the proceeding four chapters as this stereotype continued to permeate in the treatment of mentally ill ex-servicemen in Ireland throughout the inter-war period. Simultaneous to the continuation of such anti-Irish prejudices, this chapter also recognises the establishment of the Ministry of Pensions and its subsequent early rehabilitative attempts on behalf of neurasthenic pensioners in Britain and Ireland from 1917 until 1921. Exclusive in-patient and out-patient treatment was offered in Ministry hospitals throughout the United Kingdom. These facilities provided pensioners with psychological treatment. This infrastructure was far more progressive and innovative than is often assumed.

Chapter 2 demonstrates that infrastructure in South Ireland, the term applied by the Ministry of Pensions to the area of Ireland outside of the province of Ulster, however, was compromised. The region witnessed far higher waiting lists for neurasthenic pensioners awaiting in-patient and out-patient treatment in the United Kingdom. Ministry officials in London unfairly attributed the subsequent inflated waiting list figures to a longstanding racist assumption that the Irish were predisposed to mental illness. Any qualitative and quantitative evidence differentiating Ireland from the broader UK context must be contextualised within larger societal and administrative frameworks. Rather than an Irish biological disposition to mental illness, the ongoing Anglo-Irish War, 1919–21, better explains the high waiting list figures amongst neurasthenic pensioners in the region. The guerrilla conflict and republican political assistance caused much disruption in the rehabilitation of disabled Great War veterans. A study of the Ministry of Pensions' archival collection in London demonstrates pension officials operated in fear of IRA reprisals which had a detrimental impact on their functioning in Ireland. Correspondence from mentally ill pensioners also reveals that they too lived in fear of republican retribution during this hostile period. This unsuitable homecoming extended to Ulster where shell-shocked Catholic pensioners were subjected to sectarian and violent discrimination and abuse.

The second chapter examines the psychological impact this traumatising homecoming would have had on returning Great War veterans. The opportunity to work and provide for oneself was a fundamental component in the Ministry's rehabilitation of disabled pensioners. However, in addition to the stigma regarding mental illness, further discrimination attached itself to British ex-servicemen in increasingly nationalist areas where the British state was now viewed by many as an oppressive and occupying power. The lack of societal appreciation, training and treatment facilities increased the likelihood of unemployment amongst Irish Great War veterans. This reception, in turn, aggravated psychoneurotic symptoms and increased the likelihood of veterans turning to the Ministry for relief or applying to the department for medical treatment. Ultimately, the revolutionary period ensured that Ireland was the least suitable area in the United Kingdom for a mentally ill veteran to return.

Chapter 3 examines the subsequent experience of the mentally ill Great War veteran in the newly established Irish Free State and Northern Ireland between 1922 and 1939. The year of the outbreak of the Second World War, 1939, is an obvious cut-off point as the ensuing second global conflict lacked the shared involvement of its predecessor; southern Irish neutrality contrasted sharply with Northern Ireland enlistment. This section addresses an omission in the historiography with few shell-shock studies extending beyond the initial post-war years.[68] In addition to marking the significant diplomatic change in Anglo-Irish relations and political structure, 1922 also witnessed the publication of the War Office Report into Shell-Shock. Emphasising longstanding theories of predisposition and hereditary degeneration in the causation of shell-shock, the report helped to close the shell-shock debate throughout the UK. In the aftermath of this account, fewer researchers assessed war-induced neuroses or the plight of the mentally ill veteran in the UK. This restriction coincided with the infamous 'Geddes' Axe' enforcing a host of tax increases and economic cutbacks in the UK public sector. The austere management of public economies included the Ministry of Pensions' domestic policy; from 1922 onwards, there was a dramatic restriction in pension outlay and a reduction in exclusive Ministry-run medical facilities including the provision of progressive and innovative psychotherapeutic treatment. There was a resulting widespread assumption amongst medical and pensions officials that the neurasthenic pensioner was incurable. Mentally ill veterans were largely 'pensioned off' with little state intervention in their recovery. Crucially, unlike the revolutionary period, where the treatment of neurasthenic pensioners was much different in Ireland and Britain, their subsequent experience of Ministry policy and infrastructure was more of a shared one from 1922 onwards. Nonetheless, the broader Irish and British understanding of disability and rehabilitation were not identical.

As in Britain, the government of Northern Ireland provided employment and training assistance, and its society undertook philanthropic efforts to accommodate disabled ex-servicemen in both the public and the private sector. As the economy regressed from the 1920s onwards, opportunities for the disabled ex-serviceman decreased as the able-bodied and non-ex-service population competed for limited resources. In the Irish Free State, while hostility and discrimination was reduced, there remained an absence of societal and governmental concern for the Great War veteran. Returning veterans were unable to benefit from voluntary and governmental employment schemes enforced in Britain and Northern Ireland. Instead, preferential treatment was reserved for another ex-service population: veterans of the Free State National Army who helped defeat the anti-Treaty IRA in the Irish Civil War. Crucially, however, the Ministry of Pensions' financial outlay in the Free State to assist disabled ex-servicemen far exceeded relative ratios available in England, Wales, Scotland and Northern Ireland. These nuances and contradictions emphasise the multifaceted and complex treatment of disabled Irish Great War veterans.

The book's perspective then shifts to the treatment of institutionalised mentally ill ex-servicemen. Chapter 4 focuses on the Richmond War Hospital between 1918 and 1919. The hospital was a thirty-two-bed observational hospital in an adjunct building on the grounds of the Richmond District Lunatic Asylum. While officially remaining soldiers of the British Army during their residency, there was little expectation of redeployment. Instead, the military hospital primarily functioned as a discharge centre able to decipher whether a psychoneurotic serviceman was suitable for discharge into civil society or admission into a district asylum. The hospital was part of the British War Office's War

Hospital network established during the First World War throughout the UK. The facility was innovative in the context of contemporary mental health treatment. Patients remained under 'observation' for up to nine months in an exclusive military facility with a better standard of care than otherwise on offer in district asylums. War Hospitals were also established to cater for physical injuries, and all soldier-patients wore 'Hospital Blues' regardless of their ailment. For the first time in the history of the British Army, mental illness was deemed treatable in its early stages and on an equal footing to physical ailments. Despite the scope, complexity and novelty of the War Hospital scheme, the function of these facilities has escaped scholarly attention.[69] Utilising contemporary medical publications and War Office reports, this work situates the Richmond War Hospital alongside the other twenty-three war hospitals established on asylum grounds. Utilising the casebooks of soldier-patients, alongside the hospital's admission and discharge register, the daily running of the hospital mostly resembled the traditional Irish district lunatic asylum.[70] The soldier-patients' military status would, nevertheless, prove crucial. The years 1916 to 1918 were witness to a reduction in financial investment and staff as well as increased overcrowding resulting in a reduced standard of care and a subsequent increase in mortalities. Soldier-patients at the Richmond War Hospital were spared this fate due to their segregation from pauper lunatics and their amalgamation with physically wounded veterans.

Chapter 5 offers an all-Ireland analysis of the treatment of insane Great War veterans designated as 'Service Patients' in the public asylum. With their insanity deemed attributable to war service, Service Patients were identified as private patients with the added luxuries of private clothing, pocket money and segregated burial financed by the Ministry of Pensions to prevent their association with pauper lunacy. This chapter argues that being legally recognised as insane as a result of war service was mostly inconsequential. The contrasting conditions apparent in individual asylums were the most influential force in dictating a patient's daily life rather than their legal status. There were, nevertheless, notable differences in the remit and function of rehabilitative policy between Ireland and Britain. In 1923, the Ministry of Pensions extended attributability to all insane Great War veterans in Britain irrespective of whether the Great War veteran's insanity was caused by war service. While the extension of the scheme was a result of public and political pressure in Britain, the lack of similar outrage and lobbying on behalf of the British ex-serviceman in Ireland negated its implementation. A study of the Service Patient programme in Ireland provides crucial insight into how lobbying, public relations and financial concerns helped to shape the Ministry of Pensions' policy and the daily lives of disabled ex-servicemen.

Ultimately, there was not a collective understanding of disability amongst British Army veterans of the First World War. To better comprehend the post-war experiences of these forgotten men of Irish and British history, this study considers how mental illness and disability were culturally, politically and socially designed. It seeks to understand how Irish and British societies understood mental illness amongst their service populations, and how British medico-pensions officials comprehended and interacted with mentally disabled veterans in Ireland in comparison to the equivalent ex-service community in Britain. An objective bureaucracy did not always shape policy. Instead, shell-shock and post-war mental disability was a 'bio-psycho, social and cultural experience' which was 'significantly underpinned by the political concerns.'[71]

The stereotype that the Irish were predisposed to mental illness continued to permeate in the treatment of ex-servicemen in Ireland throughout the inter-war period. This narrative impacted upon the treatment of neurasthenic pensioners in civil society and the insane veteran in the post-war asylum. An analysis of this lingering narrative foregrounds the crucial variable of ethnicity and race which has remained overlooked in previous studies into shell-shock and post-war disability.[72] This consideration echoes a recent trend within the social history of psychiatry considering the relationship between psychiatric discourse and imperial governance.[73] While *Shell-shocked British Army Veterans in Ireland, 1918–39* contributes to a wealth of material attentive to the colonial asylum, the book's corresponding focus on neurasthenic pensioners in Irish society provides overdue attention to how colonial psychological narratives also featured amongst British officials in rehabilitative contexts and outside of asylum walls.

Connecting the histories of the Ministry of Pensions, charities, individual pensioners and mental health facilities, this study delivers a new perspective on disability history with an analysis of a previously unaccounted for community. This book reclaims the disabled Irish Great War veterans and gives them a voice often denied in their own lives. In addition to recovering these forgotten men of Irish and British history, this work situates itself within the broader historiographical debate centred on whether the First World War was a watershed moment in UK society.[74] Influential works by the likes of Paul Fussell have argued that the Great War ushered in modernity, presenting a clear break between the pre-and post-war eras.[75] Subsequent research has disputed this theory, emphasising the continuities evident before and after the war.[76] An Irish case study of post-war disability and mental illness contributes to this debate.

The truth was too complicated for either explanation. This Irish case study attests to the disparate treatment and reception of mentally ill veterans. For the first time, the state properly recognised mentally ill ex-servicemen alongside their physically disabled former comrades. Opportunities for medical treatment surpassed comparative treatment provided to mentally ill civilians, British Army veterans of prior conflicts and Irish veterans of the revolutionary conflicts. These progressive reforms co-existed with widespread stigma and prejudices and with longstanding assumptions of degeneration and, most relevant to this case study, the supposed Irish predisposition to mental instability. These assumptions continued to feature in societal, medical and rehabilitative discourse throughout the inter-war period. These inconsistencies are neither random nor unexplainable. Instead, one should interpret them as a concept. The First World War significantly altered British society but so too was there was a continuation of Victorian and Edwardian narratives which proved hard to alter. *Shell-shocked British Army Veterans in Ireland, 1918–39* emphasises evidence of simultaneous change and continuity in Irish and British society and rehabilitative culture in the aftermath of the First World War.[77]

Notes

1 Third Annual Report of the Ministry of Pensions, 1920–1921, 52.
2 Heather Perry, *Recycling the Disabled: Army, Medicine and Modernity in World War One Germany* (Manchester: Manchester University Press, 2014), 1.
3 A. G. Kay, 'Insanity in the army in peace and war and its treatment', *Journal of the Royal Army Medical Corps*, 18:2 (1912), 153.
4 John Hughes-Wilson and Cathryn Corns, *Blindfold and Alone: British Military Executions in the Great War* (London: Cassel & Co, 2001), 52; Edward Brown, 'Between cowardice and insanity: shell-shock and the legitimation of the neuroses in Great Britain', in E. Mendelsohn and P. Weingart (eds), *Science, Technology and the Military* (Dordrecht: Springer, 1988), 323–4.
5 Mark Harrison, *The Medical War: British Military Medicine in the First World War* (Oxford: Oxford University Press, 2010), 110.
6 Tracey Loughran, 'Shell-shock, trauma, and the First World War: the making of a diagnosis and its histories', *Journal of the History of Medicine and Allied Sciences*, 67:1 (2012), 101–2.
7 Charles Myers, *Shell Shock in France, 1914–1918: Based on a War Diary* (Cambridge: Cambridge University Press, 1940), 12; Fiona Reid, *Broken Men: Shell Shock, Treatment and Recovery in Britain, 1914–1930* (London: Continuum, 2010), 26.
8 Myers, *Shell-Shock in France*, 26; Stefanie Linden and Edgar Jones, '"Shell-shock" revisited: an examination of the case records of the National Hospital in London', *Medical History*, 58:4 (2014), 533–4.
9 Jay Winter, 'Shell-shock and the cultural history of the Great War', *Journal of Contemporary History*, 35:1 (2000), 7.
10 *Report of the War Office Committee of Enquiry into Shell-Shock* (London: HMJ, 1922) [hereafter The Southborough Report].
11 Myers, *Shell-Shock in France*, 27.

12 Edgar Jones, Ian Palmer and Simon Wessely, 'War pensions (1900–1945): changing models of psychological understanding', *British Journal of Psychiatry*, 180 (2002), 376; Irish approximations were calculated using Bourke's estimation that around 36 percent of ex-servicemen receiving disability pensions in the early 1930s were listed as suffering from a psychiatric ailment; Joanna Bourke, *Dismembering the Male: Men's Bodies, Britain and the Great War* (London: Reaktion, 1996), 109. In 1926, 34,500 disabled veterans in Ireland were in receipt of a pension from the Ministry of Pensions; NA, PIN 15/3640, Ministry of Pensions Minute Sheet, 26 February 1926.
13 Peter Barham, *Forgotten Lunatics of the Great War* (New Haven: Yale University Press, 2004), 375.
14 Robert Graves, *Goodbye To All That* (Harmondsworth: Penguin, 1929); Siegfried Sassoon, *Siegfried's Journey, 1916–1920* (London: White Lion, 1945).
15 Pat Barker, *The Regeneration Trilogy* (London: Penguin, 2014).
16 Arthur Kleinman, *Writing at the Margin: Discourse between Anthropology and Medicine* (California: University of California Press, 1997), 249.
17 David Gerber, 'Introduction', in David Gerber (ed.), *Disabled Veterans in History: From Ancient Greece to the conflict in Afghanistan* (Ann Arbor: University of Michigan Press, 2014), 1.
18 Wendy Holden, *Shell-Shock: The Psychological Impact of War* (London: Channel 4 Books, 2001), 7, 66.
19 Tom Johnstone, *Orange, Green and Khaki: The Story of the Irish Regiments in the Great War, 1914–18* (Dublin: Gill and Macmillan, 1992), 428.
20 Paul Fussell, *The Great War and Modern Memory* (Oxford: Oxford University Press, 1975); John Keegan, *The Face of Battle: A Study of Agincourt, Waterloo and the Somme* (London: Pimlico, 1975); Eric Leed, *No Man's Land: Combat and Identity in World War One* (Cambridge: Cambridge University Press, 1979).
21 Anthony Babington, *Shell-Shock: A History of the Changing Attitudes to War Neurosis* (London: Leo Cooper, 1997); Ben Shephard, *A War of Nerves* (London: Jonathan Cape, 2000); Edgar Jones and Simon Wessely, *Shell-Shock to PTSD: Military Psychiatry from 1900 to the Gulf War* (Hove: Psychology Press, 2005).
22 As Leese writes: 'I began my book to find out who the shell-shocked men were, to explore shell shock as they saw it'; Peter Leese, *Shell-Shock: Traumatic Neurosis and the British Soldiers of the First World War* (Basingstoke: Palgrave Macmillan, 2014), xii.
23 In a review of Leese's work, Roger Cooter prophesised: 'The final section of the sufferers' post-war experiences still retains a freshness, though an emergent literature on veterans and state pensions may soon overtake it'; Roger Cooter, 'Review', *Journal of Modern History*, 76 (2004), 955–6.
24 Reviewing the literature, Jason Crouthamel highlights the need for further analysis of war-induced mental illness writing: 'One of the areas that begs more research is the experience of traumatized men after 1918, in particular their struggle to restore themselves in work and family life'; Jason Crouthamel, 'Review of *Broken Men – Shell Shock, Treatment and Recovery in Britain, 1914–1930*', (review no. 997) www.history.ac.uk/reviews/review/997 [accessed 20 September 2014].

25 Peter Barham, *Forgotten Lunatics of the Great War* (New Haven: Yale University Press, 2004).
26 Fiona Reid, *Broken Men: Shell Shock, Treatment and Recovery in Britain, 1914–1930* (London: Continuum, 2010).
27 Tracey Loughran, *Shell-Shock and Medical Culture in First World War Britain* (Cambridge: Cambridge University Press, 2016).
28 Jason Crouthamel and Peter Leese (eds), *Psychological Trauma and the Legacies of the First World War* (Cham: Palgrave Macmillan, 2017).
29 Barham, *Forgotten Lunatics of the Great War*, 10.
30 Joanna Bourke, 'Shell-shock, psychiatry and the Irish Soldier during the First World War', in Adrian Gregory and Senia Paseta (eds), *Ireland and the Great War: 'A War To Unite Us All'?* (Manchester: Manchester University Press, 2002), 155–70.
31 This absence reflects broader historiographical trends. The literature regarding the history of disability in Ireland lags behind British scholarship; Ana Carden-Coyne and Julie Anderson, 'Enabling the past: new perspectives in the history of disability', *European Review of History*, 14:4 (2007), 455.
32 David Fitzpatrick, *Politics and Irish Life, 1913–1921: Provincial Experience of War and Revolution* (Cork: Gill and Macmillan, 1998), 109; Jason Myers, *The Great War and Memory in Irish Culture, 1918–2010* (California: Academica Press, 2013), 10.
33 John Coakley, 'The election that made the First Dáil', in Brian Farrell (ed.), *The Creation of the Dáil* (Dublin: Blackwater Press, 1994), 164.
34 D. G. Boyce, '"That party politics should divide our tents": Nationalism, Unionism and the First World War", in Adrian Gregory and Senia Paseta (eds), *Ireland and the Great War: 'A War To Unite Us All'?* (Manchester: Manchester University Press, 2002), 201.
35 Myers, *The Great War and Memory in Irish Culture*, 74, 206.
36 For an insightful study into these memorials, see Catherine Switzer, *Unionists and Great War Commemoration in the North of Ireland, 1914–1939* (Dublin: Irish Academic Press, 2007).
37 Adrian Gregory and Senia Paseta, 'Introduction', in Adrian Gregory and Senia Paseta (eds), *Ireland and the Great War: 'A War To Unite Us All'?* (Manchester: Manchester University Press, 2002), 6.
38 Joanna Bourke, "Remembering' War', *Journal of Contemporary History*, 39:4 (2004), 473.
39 Keith Jeffery, *Ireland and the Great War* (Oxford: Oxford University Press, 1998), 1.
40 David Durnin, *The Irish Medical Profession and the First World War* (Basingstoke: Palgrave Macmillan, 2019); Yvonne McEwen, *It's a Long Way to Tipperary: British and Irish Nurses in the Great War* (Dunfermline: Cualann Press, 2006); Patrick Casey, Kevin Cullen and Joe Duignan, *Irish Doctors in the First World War* (Dublin: Irish Academic Press, 2015); Fionnuala Walsh, '"Every human life is a national importance": the impact of the First World War on attitudes to maternal and infant health', 15–31; Patricia Marsh, 'The war and influenza: the impact of the First World

War on the 1918–19 influenza pandemic in Ulster', 31–45; Ronan Foley, 'From front to home and back again: geographical networks of auxiliary medical care in the First World War', in Ian Miller and David Durnin (eds), *Medicine, Health and Irish Experiences of Conflict, 1914–45* (Manchester: Manchester University Press, 2016), 125–39.

41 Peter Hart, *The IRA and its Enemies* (Oxford: Oxford University Press, 1998), 301–2, 312; *The IRA at War 1916–1923* (Oxford: Oxford University Press, 2003), 136.

42 Jane Leonard, 'Getting them at last: The IRA and ex-servicemen', in David Fitzpatrick (ed.), *Revolution? Ireland 1917–1923* (Dublin: Trinity History Workshop, 1990), 118–29; '"Facing the finger of scorn": veteran's memories of Ireland after the Great War', in Martin Evans and Ken Lunn (eds), *War and Memory in the Twentieth Century* (Oxford: Berg, 1997), 59–72; 'Survivors', in John Horne (ed.), *Our War: Ireland and the Great War*, (Dublin: Royal Irish Academy, 2008), 209–23.

43 Paul Taylor, *Heroes or Traitors?: Experiences of Southern Irish Soldiers Returning from the Great War, 1919–1939* (Liverpool: Liverpool University Press, 2015).

44 Meaghan Kowalsky, 'Enabling the Great War: Ex-servicemen, the Mixed Economy of Welfare and the Social Construction of Disability, 1899–1930' (PhD Thesis, University of Leeds, 2007), 48.

45 Reid, *Broken Men*, 5; Barham, *Forgotten Lunatics of the Great War*, 5–6; Eric Coplans, 'Some observations on neurasthenia and shell-shock', *The Lancet*, 31 October 1931, 960.

46 Scott Stossel, *My Age of Anxiety: Fear, Hope, Dread and the Search for Peace of Mind* (London: Random House, 2014), 24.

47 Gerard Oram, *Worthless Men: Race, Eugenics and the Death Penalty in the British Army during the First World War* (London: Francis Boutle, 1998), 5.

48 Neil Richardson, *A Coward If I Return, A Hero If I Fall: Stories of Irishmen in World War I* (Dublin: O'Brien Press, 2011), 212, 314.

49 In 1931, military researchers described the Ministry of Pensions' record collection as 'unique in character and pregnant with possibilities for research'; T. J. Mitchell and G. M. Smith, *Medical Services: Casualties and Medical Statistics of the Great War* (London: H.M. Stationary Office, 1931), 350.

50 Elizabeth Bredberg, 'Writing disability history: problems, perspectives and sources', *Disability and Society*, 14:2 (1999), 190–1.

51 The 'PIN 26' series is organised by pension type and then by alphabet. With every fiftieth file kept for archival purposes, 22,756 individual files regarding pension awards have survived which represents just 2 percent of the pensions awarded as a result of disablement. Extracting a relevant Irish case study was difficult and time-consuming. Over 60 percent of the surviving material relates to pensions awarded in the London region, and there is no search function to locate pensioners who returned to Ireland; Ian Beckett, *The First World War: The Essential Guide to Sources in the UK National Archives* (Surrey: Public Record Office, 2002), 159.

52 O'Ryan's census entries in 1911 note his previous residence in the affluent area of Castleknock, Dublin with surviving descendants of O'Ryan supporting notions of

his relative affluence; Interview with Ann O'Ryan and John O'Ryan, 23 February 2019.
53 As David Gerber has previously asserted: 'By shifting the perspective toward the experience of disability may we understand the nature of the veteran's own agency in attempting to shape his relations to the state around his own conception of his needs and aspirations'; David Gerber, 'Disabled veterans, the state, and the experience of disability in Western societies, 1914–1950', *Journal of Social History*, 36:4 (2003), 901.
54 Wendy Jane Gagen, 'Remastering the body, renegotiating gender: physical disability and masculinity during the First World War, the case of J. B. Middlebrook', *European Review of History*, 14:4 (2007), 525–41.
55 Brotherton Library, Leeds University, LIDDLE/WW1/GS/0047, J. B. Arnold's Typescript Recollections.
56 There has been a lack of research into these facilities. In 1917, Grafton Elliot Smith and Thomas Pear wrote that research into their operatives was 'urgently needed.' Its absence remains over a century later; Grafton Elliot Smith and Thomas Pear, *Shell-Shock and Its Lessons* (Manchester: Manchester University Press, 1917), 117.
57 Donald Critchlow, 'Integrating social history and the state: policy history through case studies', *The History Teacher*, 31:4 (1998), 460.
58 Taylor, *Heroes or Traitors?*, 11.
59 NA, PIN 15/3640, Ministry of Pensions Minute Sheet, 26 February 1926.
60 Julie Anderson, '"Jumpy stump": amputation and trauma in the First World War', *First World War Studies*, 6:1 (2015), 9–19.
61 Gerber, 'Introduction', 1.
62 Roy Porter, 'The patient's view: doing medical history from below', *Theory and Society*, 14:2 (1985), 175–6.
63 Jonathan Andrews, 'Case notes, case histories, and the patient's experience of insanity at Gartnavel Royal Asylum, Glasgow, in the nineteenth century', *Social History of Medicine*, 11:2 (1998), 279.
64 David Armstrong, 'The patient's view: doing medical history from below', *Social Science & Medicine*, 18:9 (1984), 737.
65 Daniel Rambaut, 'Case-taking in large asylums', *British Journal of Psychiatry*, 49 (1903), 45–6; Louise Hide, *Gender and Class in English Asylums, 1890–1940* (Basingstoke: Palgrave Macmillan, 2014), 2–3, 13.
66 Jay Winter, *War Beyond Words: Languages of Remembrance from the Great War to the Present* (Cambridge: Cambridge University, 2017), 181, 192.
67 Barham, *Forgotten Lunatics of the Great War*, 315.
68 For example, Marina Larsson, in her study of mentally ill Australian veterans, describes the 1930s as 'a postscript' in the historiography of shell-shock; Marina Larsson, *Shattered Anzacs: Living with the Scars of War* (Sydney: UNSW, 2009), 208.
69 As John Hopkins noted: 'Despite its scope and complexity, the Asylum War Hospitals Scheme as such, has almost entirely escaped scholarly attention'; John Hopkins, 'Problems, Politics and Personalities in the Treatment of Mental and Nervous

Casualties in the British Army, 1914–1918' (PhD Thesis, University of Leicester, 2003), 248.
70 Durnin, *The Irish Medical Profession and the First World War*, 94–5.
71 Ana Carden-Coyne, *The Politics of Wounds: Military Patients and Medical Power in the First World War* (Oxford: Oxford University Press, 2014), 5; this thesis is agreed upon in Tracey Loughran's assessment of shell-shock: 'Diagnostic categories were not only pragmatic modes of organizing knowledge, but also alive with social, political, and cultural dimensions relevant outside the medical world'; Loughran, *Shell-Shock and Medical Culture in First World War Britain*, 77.
72 This stands in contrast to studies of gender and class. For example, see Joan Busfield, 'Class and gender in twentieth-century British psychiatry: shell-shock and psychopathic disorder', in J. Andrews and A. Digby (eds), *Sex and Seclusion, Class and Custody: Perspectives on Gender and Class in the History of British and Irish Psychiatry* (Amsterdam: Rodopi, 2004), 295–322.
73 This historiography is extensive. For a generalist study, see S. Malone and M. Vaughan (eds), *Psychiatry and Empire* (Basingstoke: Palgrave Macmillan, 2007).
74 A succinct overview of this literature is provided in Alison Fell and Jessica Meyer, 'Introduction: untold legacies of the First World War in Britain', *War and Society*, 34:2 (2015), 85–6.
75 Paul Fussell, *The Great War and Modern Memory* (Oxford: Oxford University Press, 1975).
76 Adrian Gregory, *The Last Great War: British Society and the First World War* (Cambridge: Cambridge University Press, 2008); Dan Todman, *The Great War: Myth and Memory* (London: Continuum, 2005).
77 My case study of Ireland bolsters the so-called 'half-way house' theses offered by Mathew Thomson and Tracey Loughran in their studies of shell-shock and its impact on medical culture in Britain; Loughran, *Shell-Shock and Medical Culture in First World War Britain*, 214; Mathew Thomson, *Psychological Subjects: Identity, Culture and Health in Twentieth Century Britain* (Oxford: Oxford University Press, 2006), 185.

I

'A DEFINITIVE NEURASTHENIC TEMPERAMENT'? THE IRISH TOMMY AND VETERAN

Introduction

There was negligible medical provision for mental and nervous casualties before the First World War. The 955-bed Royal Victoria Military Hospital at Netley provided just 125 beds for such cases within its 'D Block.' The Lunacy Act of 1890 enabled discharge from the army, certification and a transferral to an asylum.[1] During the Second Anglo-Boer War, 1899–1902, severely mentally ill troops in both South Ireland and Ulster were discharged from the army and admitted into their local district asylum. Irish servicemen subsequently shared the ignominy and stigma associated with pauper lunacy.[2] The First World War would dramatically change the treatment of war-induced psychoneuroses. The War Office's official medical history of the conflict went so far as to write that shell-shock 'raised the psychoneuroses to the dignity of a new war disease before which doctors seemed well-nigh helpless.'[3]

An investigation of mentally disabled Great War veterans will begin where the majority of such illnesses manifested: the Western Front. Two-thirds of Irish battalions spent the entire duration of the war in this theatre which was responsible for almost 31,000 war-dead from Irish Regiments equating to 82 percent of fatalities.[4] The British military and medical authorities paid little heed to forewarnings that modern industrial warfare would contribute to a higher number of mental and nervous casualties. Mental and nervous casualties were treated on an ad-hoc basis during the early stages of the First World War. Casualties were cared for wherever they could be placed including military hospitals and wards in general hospitals.[5] A basic network of treatment facilities was established for psychoneurotic casualties by 1915. This infrastructure included a treatment facility set up at the No. 26 General Hospital near Etaples with 'insane' cases segregated and housed in a small hut. Additional 'mental blocks' were placed at other base hospitals throughout the war.⁶ In 1916, coinciding with the Somme Campaign where the British Army haemorrhaged manpower, an attempt to combat losses was made with the British Army introducing the concept of 'forward psychiatry'. This intervention established specialised treatment centres behind trench front lines. These units worked towards the 'PIE' system which focused on three core objectives: Proximity of treatment to the area of service; Immediacy of response to symptoms; Expectation of recovery. The most chronic and acute cases were referred to the United Kingdom for further treatment. The Royal Victoria Hospital in Netley, the No. 4 London General Hospital in Britain and the King George V Hospital in Dublin would often act as clearing stations in the UK. Following an initial assessment, servicemen were transferred to suitable hospitals for further treatment including, for example, the Red Cross Military Hospital in Maghull or the National Hospital for Paralysed and Epileptic, Queen Square, London.⁷ Psychoneurotic men were also sent to newly established War Hospitals established on district asylum grounds. Approximately 4,470 asylum beds were available for the treatment of servicemen's mental and nervous injuries.⁸ This number included a thirty-two-bed segregated Richmond War Hospital adjunct to the Richmond District Lunatic Asylum and the Belfast War Hospital which displaced the entire population and grounds of the Belfast District Lunatic Asylum.

Varying responses to shell-shock were apparent across these medical and military establishments as practitioners sought to balance caregiving without depleting manpower. Each medical centre's treatment philosophy largely echoed the professional backgrounds of its senior medical staff, although it was not uncommon for different medical judgements and approaches to be evident within the same institution. Some military and medical officials favoured a somatic explanation, believing shell-shock to be the result of physical shock or concussion. Failing these causative agents, a more disciplinary approach emphasising faulty hereditary explanations or moral degeneracy were to blame. This method was arguably most infamously personified by Dr L. R. Yealland's treatment of shell-shocked soldiers via faradism or electrical shock therapy. There was also a continuation of the long-established Weir–Mitchell treatment for neurasthenia which administered bromide medication, a milk diet, rest, recuperation, massage and drugs to assist in a soldier's recuperation. By contrast, psychotherapeutic treatment encouraged patients to adjust their thought processes when suffering from ailments such as anxiety and depression, rationalising negative thoughts and increasing the regularity and magnitude of positive ones.⁹ R. G. Rows preferred this ethos of abreaction for staff at Red Cross Military Hospital in Maghull, Liverpool, as did W. H. R. Rivers at his comparative hospital reserved for the officer class at Craiglockhart War Hospital in Edinburgh.[10] Edgar Jones assesses that the core change in ethos at Maghull was to reconvene diagnoses such as hysteria and neurasthenia not as 'functional nervous' disorders but as variants of 'psychoneurosis.' While some practitioners emphasised the pathological change in the nervous system of a soldier-patient, medical staff associated with Maghull disputed this claim underlining a mental or psychological reason. At its most basic level, these practitioners emphasised nurture over nature in explaining combat neurosis.[11] With this outlook and associated treatment, Leese argues that these hospitals were 'the most humane of the British centres' for neurasthenic servicemen.[12] The division between organic and psychological causation amongst the medical network was not total. Instead, individual facilities and staff often centred an emphasis on either outlook.[13] Thomas Webb writes that these differing treatment philosophies constituted a 'desperate and disparate set of responses to the problems posed by the reality of the shell-shock epidemic.'[14]

Irishmen experienced psychoneurotic afflictions alongside their British-born comrades during this evolution from a patchwork of military medical facilities to a more specialised treatment network. Sir John Collie, a leading authority of the Ministry of Pensions who helped organise payment of pensions and medical treatment of psychoneurotic veterans, supposed that around 200,000 soldiers were discharged from the British Army due to a mental breakdown, of which Irish troops constituted around 12.5 percent.[15] The war diary of the Medical Officer of the 1st Connaught Rangers contains rare medical references to mental and nervous casualties.[16] On 30 November 1914, one Captain was sent to a nearby military hospital after suffering from a 'nervous breakdown.' The most informed entry for a psychiatric-related transferral was provided on 17 November, noting: 'One mental sent to hospital ... the man had hallucinations of hearing and vision.' In a summary of diseases from 17 August to 31 December 1914, there was a total of twenty-eight diagnoses of 'nervous system' casualties, and 82 percent of these casualties were attributable to 'neuoritis' with the other 18 percent being made up of 'headaches', 'fits' and 'mental.'[1]

Private William Smith of the Irish Guards was knocked unconscious by a shell explosion. After regaining consciousness, Smith suffered from recurrent and extreme tremors and muscle spasms, depression and headaches. He was discharged from the army in September 1915 bringing an end to his twelve-year career in the British Army. Shrapnel badly injured Michael McGauly in 1915. Despite his twenty-five years of service in the British Army, and the healing of his physical wounds, the experience had a profound impact on his mental state: 'Ever since wounding has been nervous ... tremor of tongue and hands.' He was transferred to a convalescent home in Britain for treatment. Private John Morrison was relocated to a military hospital in Sheffield unable to keep his food down, suffering from persistent headaches and confessing to having nightmares and feeling frightened.[18] The Royal Enniskillen Fusiliers' Medical Officer described Irishman Patrick John O'Ryan, who had experienced active service on the Western Front for over three years, in 1917 as such:

> Very poorly suffering from nerve exhaustion and hard work. He has no organic disease and all he wants to make him quite fit for duty is a little absolute rest and quiet, for this reason, I must strongly recommend that he be granted an extension of leave, to return to duty now would mean a nervous breakdown from which it would take a considerable time to recover.[19]

This study foregrounds how the Medical Officer's fears of prolonged mental illness proved accurate.

F. Purser treated all nationalities in his role as a physician in a Military Hospital in Dublin and subsequently wrote: 'English, Scotch, or Irish seem all alike susceptible. Nationality makes no difference.'[20] How such instances amongst Irish troops were perceived, however, was unique. Irish nervous casualties experienced more dismissive and inferior treatment at the Casualty Clearing Hospitals owing to their nationality.[21] Non-white soldiers and labour corps under treatment at military hospitals could also be the subject of imperial prejudice and racial stereotyping. Ana Corden-Coyne writes that the British Army and the British Empire was 'one form of common discrimination' where white 'rank-and-file soldiers (including Irish, Welsh, and Scottish soldiers) were subject to ethnic and class scrutiny by their middle-class superiors.'[22] This book investigates this idea with a study of Ireland's experience of combat neurosis and mental health in the aftermath of the First World War. It echoes previous research into shell-shock which foregrounds the necessity to consider continuities with a pre-war discourse which survived beyond the First World War.[23] Synthesising a pre-war, war-time and post-war timeframe highlights the simultaneous progression and conservatism which attached itself to the Irish experience of shell-shock.

Perceptions of Irish mental instability before the Great War

Due to the notorious presence of Irish migrants in Britain from the mid-1830s onwards, perceptions of their supposedly innate dirtiness, criminality, violence and savagery arose amongst Britons. Contemporary research has countered that Irish migrant communities often settled in industrial areas which were already unhygienic, overcrowded and crime-stricken, an experience that was worsened by police discrimination, judicial bias and isolation from family networks. It was poverty, rather than biology, that explains why the Irish were especially prone to arrests due to drunkenness, theft, prostitution and fighting in Victorian Britain.[24] In the absence of this contemporary literature, the Irish Tommy during the First World War was perceived by the military establishment to be innately aggressive and an ideal shock troop, yet careless, ill-disciplined, prone to criminality and filthy. These stereotypes have again been refuted by modern-day historical research which demonstrates that the conduct of Irish soldiers within the British Army was not exceptional.[25] The Irish experience of shell-shock and trauma remains underexamined in comparison

The relationship between class and gender with shell-shock has been well covered by historians. Elaine Showalter offers an influential gendered reading of shell-shock arguing that the feminised condition constituted 'a crisis of masculinity.'[26] Loughran counters that military and medical officials were more likely to compare shell-shocked servicemen to children as they were to class, rank or gender.[27] Jessica Meyer's reading of shell-shock also cites that ideals of masculinity during the era were heavily associated with discourse relating to adult maturity over the immature child.[28] Grafton Elliot Smith and Thomas Pear, medical practitioners at the forefront of the shell-shock episode, similarly related war neuroses to maturity theorising that 'the neurotic's behaviour in the face of an insurmountable difficulty presents a considerable resemblance to that of a child.'[29] It is within this maturity discursive framework that the Irish experience of shell-shock is better understood.

Connotations denoting the childlike, volatile and emotionally unsuitable Irish soldier were longstanding in pre-war British thought. Widely read journal articles by racial determinists like Robert Knox promoted the childlike emotionality of the Irish who required paternalistic supervision by the British.[30] Such connotations would also appear in the medical literature. In an article for the *Journal of Mental Science*, published in 1894, Dr Thomas Draper, the Resident Medical Superintendent of Enniscorthy District Asylum, emphasised innate Irish mental instability:

> Temperament and racial characteristics have, no doubt, much to do with susceptibility to mental derangement, and here the Irish are at a disadvantage. An excitable brain is an easily disturbed brain; and the quick-witted, passionate, versatile and vivacious Celt has, for those qualities which made him so charming, too often to pay the price of instability.[31]

Like the supposed Irish predisposition to criminality, violence and drunkenness, there was empirical evidence to corroborate Irish mental instability. In 1851, Ireland's asylum population stood at 2,800 increasing to 24,815 by 1914.[32] Irish-born patients also constituted the most prominent ethnic identity after the native-born population in English asylums.[33] Occurring at the same time as widespread concern regarding high asylum numbers in Ireland, local British press and medical officials attributed their presence to a national predisposition for institutionalisation.[34] 'Bad Irish character' was referenced with nineteenth-century Irish asylum patients being portrayed as volatile, aggressive, criminal, ill-disciplined and in need of strict management from British asylum staff.[35] Academic research has since re-engaged with these stereotypes in an attempt to explain the augmentation in Irish lunacy figures. A range of more convincing explanations has been offered, including the psychological and demographic impact of the Irish Potato Famine, poverty, low marriage rates, the less stigmatised refuge of the asylum in comparison to the workhouse and the social isolation of Irish migrants in Britain.[36]

In the absence of alternative contemporary academic research, the British establishment corroborated Irish childishness and emotionality and its exceptionalism regarding mental ill-health within political frameworks. The existing political context would shape this corroboration. 'Revolutionary insanity' gained legitimacy in medical discourse from the French Revolution onwards.[37] In 1918, Grafton Elliot Smith similarly wrote: 'ever since the French Revolution every European War has stirred up discussion of the problems of nationality and the problems of nationalist and closely related questions of race and character ... The present war has been peculiarly fertile.'[38] In her research into madness and slavery in the USA, Diana Louis argues that 'pro-slavery psychiatry', the association between race and insanity in psychiatric thought and medical culture, persisted during slavery and continued after slavery had ended.[39] Psychological discourse foregrounding mental illness and psychotic outbursts were similarly used by the British establishment to dismiss nationalist movements in British East Africa in the early twentieth century.[40] These politically motivated diagnoses also became seamlessly interwoven into established derogatory views of the Irish.

A predisposition to less severe forms of mental illness was also assumed. Shortly before the commencement of the First World War, one article in *The Lancet* decreed that the nationality of a patient diagnosed with neurasthenia should be considered before recommendation for treatment.[41] Perceptions of functional nervous disorders were offered by high-profile British medical officers during the Victorian and Edwardian eras as particularly prevalent in counties which accommodated simpler and more impulsive populations.[42] These considerations also applied to descriptions of 'temperament' and those who were considered biologically culturally inferior and less civilised in pre-war British medical culture, including the Irish.[43] Perceptions of Irish immaturity, emotionality and mental instability undermined the Irishman's capability for self-government, buttressing English policy and control in Ireland.[44] The prejudice was politically motivated, legitimising a 'pro-Union psychiatry' which helped to support British imperialism in Ireland.[45]

One critic argued that the Irish were unsuitable to have their own government owing to their 'fierce passions' of which one unenviable trait was 'the unreasonableness of children.' In the aftermath of the United Irish rebellion in 1798, the *Morning Chronicle* wrote 'the minds of the insurgents are so diseased and so infatuated.' Those involved in the rebellion were depicted not as staunch rebels ideologically opposed to British rule but as momentarily mentally ill.[46] Fenian activities in the 1860s allowed the British press to repeat the supposed mental instability of the Irish agitators. The *Daily Telegraph* described 'a feeling that Ireland is inflicted with an incurable disease … we may use the strait-waistcoat for her mad fits.' The prognosis for recovery was also poor: 'we can have no certain hope of seeing her one day clothed and in her right mind.' Such associations were also evident in a cartoon published in the aftermath of the Fenian Clerkenwell Bombing in 1867 where the intervention of a paternal British physician, Dr John Bull, ensured Paddy was no longer a danger to himself or others by admitting him into an asylum.[47] The Land War of 1879–81 again prompted British press depictions of the mental and moral sickness of the Irish people.[48]

Reviewing the post-Easter Rising shift towards republicanism, British soldiers repeated the supposedly innate Irish tendency towards childishness and emotionality. S. J. Wallis wrote in October 1918: 'Ireland is the spoilt child of the family and kicks at England as a kid in a temper kicks his nurse.'[49] Even constitutional nationalists could equate more radical nationalists with the Irish propensity to mental illness. Denis Kilbride, an MP for the Irish Parliamentary Party, replied to Sinn Féin supporting agitators during a political address by stating: 'there were so many young men in the asylums in Ireland and so many damned lunatics outside.'[50] Such instances contradict assertions that views of the Irish being predisposed to mental illness did not influence Anglo-Irish political discourse.[51] Perceptions of the emotional Irish race being susceptible to mental instability were seemingly prevalent in Victorian and Edwardian England.[52] One way in which 'pro-slavery psychiatry' manifested itself was in the treatment of African-American soldiers, with racist aspersions that they were predisposed to break down which lingered throughout twentieth-century conflicts.[53] Permeations of pro-Union psychiatry similarly re-emerges in perceptions of the Irish Tommy during the First World War and in its aftermath.

The childlike and emotional Irish soldier

In his influential study, *Introduction to Social Psychology* (1908), William McDougall used scientific theory to argue that fighting characteristics were dependent on inherited national characteristics. Theories supporting an innate instinct in the Irish soldier were recurrent in public lectures, autobiographies, literature and publications such as the *Irish Ecclesiastical Record*.[54] Like Indian and Black African troops, descriptions of the Irish soldier were associated with the theory of 'martial races.' Irish soldiers were believed to be unruly, childlike and emotional.[55] Rudyard Kipling, the most famous war writer in Britain for the best part of three decades, embedded the foundations of this image.[56] Michael MacDonagh advanced this theory in his account of Irish troops at the Somme, summarising:

> It may well be that sometimes the English officers of Irish battalions are puzzled by the nature of their men – its impulsiveness, its glow, its wild imagery and over-brimming expression. It is easy to believe, too, that the changeful moods of the men, childlike and petulant, now jovial, now fierce, and occasionally unaccountable, may be a sure annoyance to officers who are formal and precise in matters of discipline.[57]

Other English commanding officers of Irish battalions repeated similar sentiments.[58] For example, Rowland Fielding, a battalion commander of the Connaught Rangers, wrote home to his wife stating: 'Ireland will always be Ireland. It is a land of children with the bodies of men.' Again like children, he confided to his wife that Irish troops were mentally fragile and 'easily made happy' but, also, 'easily depressed.'[59] Such perceptions were not limited to the Army. J. K. McLeod, a Lieutenant Commander in the British Navy, similarly attested to the ill-discipline and emotionality of Irish personnel under his command, writing: 'They are no good. They have no back bone. They weep occasionally. They disgust me.'[60]

Such a discourse appeared transnationally. French medical journals stated that immature and childlike soldiers in African and Muslims battalions were more likely to break down due to their innate emotionality and mental weakness.[61] In Austria, reputable medical practitioners held that negligible Germans and Austro-Hungarians suffered from combat neurosis, yet many troops from Czechoslovakia and Romania broke down. In a similar vein to British perceptions of shell-shock amongst Irish soldiers, breakdown was shaped by their disloyalty to the ruling monarchy.[62] In a summary of similar medical research, the *Journal of the American Medical Association* noted in 1917: 'From the literature the impression is gained that nationality and race play a considerable role in the biology of functional nervous disturbances.'[63] Mental illness attained racial and ethnic connotations before the outbreak of the First World. This relationship would continue in the experience of shell-shock during the conflict and the treatment of psychoneurotic veterans in its aftermath.[64]

As Mosse argues: 'shell-shock provides an excellent example of the fusion of medical diagnosis and social prejudice which had taken place during the previous century.'[65] This continuing prejudice would, however, co-exist with certain progressive efforts made in the state-funded after-care of disabled veterans.

The state and the disabled veteran, 1914–21

Disabled British Army veterans of previous conflicts relied heavily on voluntary philanthropic efforts for financial and societal assistance. Military pensions existed but were discretionary and without a statutory requirement. Only two exclusive facilities existed for the most infirm army veterans: the Chelsea Hospital in London and the Kilmainham Hospital in Dublin. This *laissez-faire* approach reflected the British Government's broader ethos of non-intervention in societal problems.[66] Reflecting the military's response to combat neuroses, the British state's treatment of returning veterans disabled as a result of war service also underwent a significant change as a result of the First World War.

Medico-pensions officials, ex-service journals and politicians all reference that the large-scale enlistment and conscription of a civilian army to participate in an industrial conflict roused an unprecedented public sense of solidarity and social justice to assist disabled veterans.[67] Following his discharge from the Northumberland Fusiliers, Arnold became an official for the Ministry of Pensions working in Ireland. He theorised that the establishment of the Ministry of Pensions across the UK was induced by the totality and brutality of the First World War wounding men on an unprecedented scale: 'Ministry of Pensions was the child of the war demanded by the appalling casualties of four years of hostilities ... It was the duty of the newly formed Ministry to award pensions to those disabled by the war, to look after their care and medical treatment, until such time if ever they were fit to return to civilian life.'[68] The public lobbying for political rights on behalf of veterans was influential. Ministry archival documents during its formation during the First World War repeatedly refer to 'popular sentiment' and the political necessity to increase generous provisions to returning ex-servicemen.[69] Conscription was never introduced in Ireland. Its absence was the result of the threat of its implementation solidifying all strands of nationalist opinion against the British Government culminating in a one-day national strike on 23 April 1918. The ratio of Irish enlistees thus lagged far behind comparative British figures. In comparison to almost one-quarter of England's male population enlisting in the British Armed forces, just 6 percent of the Irish male population enlisted.[70] Irish veterans disabled as a result of war service would still benefit from the government's increased involvement in the rehabilitation of veterans due to Ireland's political unity as part of the United Kingdom.

A moral claim to care for and compensate mentally ill veterans also arose.[71] A Medical Superintendent of a northern English district asylum cited an 'awakened consciousness' on behalf of a grateful public on behalf of the neurotic ex-serviceman's sacrifice of mental health.[72] One unnamed voluntary pensions worker similarly attested that the experience of shell-shock during the First World War had raised national awareness as to the need to assist mentally ill veterans on their return to society.[73] Arnold countered that the department's concessions were due to the Ministry's 'generous spirit' and not merely a by-product of political pandering.[74] While Arnold overplays his department's hand, he was correct in ascribing the causal agent in the establishment of the new department: 'Like many other things in the First World War this was a breaking of virgin soil.'[75]

The Ministry of Pensions was established in 1916. Initially administered by local and mostly volunteer local war pensions committees, arrangements were made to provide financial recompense and medical treatment to disabled veterans. Each committee consisted of around 25 primarily volunteer members with over 300 committees in operation in March 1918.[76] Unlike many physical disabilities, where pension payments generally followed much more objectively verifiable guidelines, pensions for mental illness were dependant on the adjudged severity of the ex-serviceman's condition (Table 1).

In response to continuing public and political lobbying on behalf of the disabled veteran, the War Pensions Acts of 1919 solidified the state's responsibility to disabled ex-servicemen. The legislation's most significant measures entrenched pensions as a statutory right, introduced independent appeal tribunals and secured an increase in the rate of pensions provided. In addition to providing a pension, the Ministry facility provided medical and rehabilitative treatment. The Ministry's treatment provisions initially revolved around utilising accommodation in civil hospitals and military hospitals as well as establishing its own specialist facilities.[77] Coinciding with the large-scale demobilisation of servicemen in 1919, the Ministry would go on to establish a more substantial network of exclusive rehabilitative facilities reserved for disabled veterans.[78] Medical and rehabilitative treatment were very much part of the Ministry's philosophy of 'reconstruction' which sought to facilitate the full-time employment of a disabled ex-serviceman. This rehabilitation aimed to save national welfare expenditure in the long term by diminishing the need for poverty-stricken ex-servicemen to claim for state-funded welfare. Ex-servicemen who required in-patient treatment

Table 1 Pension scale and payment in accordance with neurasthenic pensioners' condition with comparative objective disabilities.

Scale of pension and weekly payment	Neurasthenic condition	Other objective disabilities on identical rate
20%: 8s 6d	A constant threat of a relapse into a more serious mental condition. Nevertheless, with a supportive domestic set-up and suitable employment, a rehabilitation back into society was deemed possible	Loss of one finger on each hand
50%: 13s 9d	Able to re-enter civil society and enter employment but blighted by lethargy and a recurrence of neurasthenic symptoms	Leg amputated below the knee or arm below the elbow or had lost sight in one eye
80%: 22s	Unemployable and requiring constant admissions to receive medical treatment	Lost both feet, had a leg amputated at the hip, or arm at the shoulder joint, or total mutism
100%: 27s 6d	Seriously ill with no chance of recovery and needing constant supervision and care. Lunacy	Loss of two or more limbs, paraplegia, drastic facial injuries

Officers were paid on a higher scale for the same injuries and wounds than other ranks. Source: table formulated from Leese's analysis of individual pension files in the 'PIN 26' collection in the National Archives; Leese, *Shell-Shock*, 147–54.

were provided with a maximum pension entitled a 'treatment allowance', regardless of the grading and severity of their disability, to entice them to undergo rehabilitative care.[79]

The new department struggled to accommodate disabled ex-servicemen, particularly in the initial post-war period as millions of men were demobilised out of the British Armed Forces. The bureaucracy of the national Ministry set up in Britain in the immediate post-war years was 'a shambles.' Staff regularly proved unable to cope with the vast swathes of demobilised men with as many as 30,000 demobilisations occurring daily in 1919. It could often take over twelve months for ex-servicemen to receive a reply regarding a disability query. During this early phase, the jurisdiction for assessing pensioners rested on the largely autonomous local war pensions committees. This provincial system also proved imperfect with varying standards and policies enforced on a regional basis. Accusations of regional differences in the interpretation of Ministry guidelines, bias and even collusion with pensioners were commonplace amongst high-ranking Ministry officials.[80] A subsequent desire to streamline workloads and Ministry control of expenditure blunted the department's most overburdened and benevolent elements with a policy of decentralisation and the establishment of eleven regional centres across the UK: Scotland, Northern, North-Western, Yorkshire, Wales, West Midlands, East Midlands, South Western, London, Ulster and South Ireland.[81]

Arnold became a Ministry inspector observing Irish administration in 1919. Arnold oversaw the transferral of authority from the local war pensions committees to regional headquarters in Belfast and Dublin for Ulster and South Ireland respectively. Arnold held that Ireland desperately required the decentralisation of authority. During his supervision of war pension committees in Munster, for example, he noted that members of local war pensions committees were, for example, overcharging the Ministry for remuneration for loss of time to participate in meetings. The financial pull of sitting on committees also led to councils gerrymandering appointments ensuring that preferred candidates were on the Ministry payroll. Arnold wrote 'the ramifications of appointments made by local authorities in Southern Ireland is one about which a whole book might be written.' Arnold again foregrounded supposed regional characteristics in South Ireland asserting that 'like the peoples of the east the inhabitants of Southern Ireland thrive in brokerage.'[82] One Ministry of Pensions' memo on South Ireland similarly complained: 'The ministry must assume a more direct and effective control over the expenditure of Local Committees if a serious waste of money is to be avoided.'[83]

In what would become a constant ethos underlying most Ministry ventures, an austere policy shift was deemed necessary throughout the UK: 'In a department which requires the taxpayer to provide an annual sum of over 100 million, financial control is obviously of first class importance.'[84] Local powers were subsequently reduced from 1920 onwards. The Ministry transferred significant jurisdiction regarding policy and expenditure, including the certification and arrangement of treatment, to the eleven regional officers headquartering the eleven areas of the United Kingdom.[85] Under the jurisdiction of a regional headquarters' Director-General, much of the medical-related work was now placed under the authority of a Commissioner of Medical Services (CMS) and Deputy Commissioner of Medical Services (DCMS). The CMS and DCMS oversaw the function of medical pensions, treatment and the general bureaucracy of all medical related matters.[86] Two regional headquarters in Belfast and Dublin assumed policy for Ulster and South Ireland respectively. As one Ministry report explains:

> The great distinction to be drawn between the Ministry of Pensions, London, and its twelve Regional Directors (with their Staffs) on the one hand, and Local Committees on the other hand, is that the former are purely official whereas the latter are representative bodies constantly in touch with the community as a whole. Thus the main duty of a War Pensions Committee is to discuss the Ex-Serviceman's affairs with him in person, or the affairs of his family, and generally to put forward his point of view as against the official point of view.[87]

Regional Directors stationed at regional headquarters were granted authority over local authorities, and it was their job to oversee Ministry guidance to foster a universal policy for local authorities.[88]

Ireland had forty-one local Ministry of Pensions' committees and seven district committees, alongside its two regional headquarters in Dublin and Belfast. Medical and pension examinations were administered via private practitioners, whose fees were paid by the Ministry of Pensions, at out-patient clinics, or via special medical boards consisting of Ministry-appointed specialists. It was, however, only under a region's CMS that treatment could be finalised. As South Ireland's CMS, Harold Sugars was responsible for the administration of assessment boards, arranging treatment and general administration of medical infrastructure in the region. Sugars was ideally placed for this role. He had joined the Royal Army Medical Corps in 1915 following seven years in the Colonial Medical Service. His attachment to the Yorkshire Light Infantry led to both awards for bravery and permanent disability due to his shattered leg received as he cared for a soldier suffering from a severed artery while under heavy fire. As will be demonstrated, Sugars' doughty defence of wounded servicemen would continue in his role for the Ministry of Pensions until his untimely death in 1929.[89]

While the Ministry of Pensions initially held the responsibility to allocate employment, this task shifted to the Ministry of Labour in June 1919 in a further attempt to streamline Ministry policy and reduce the department's hectic workload.[90] On assuming responsibility for the employment of disabled ex-servicemen in Ireland, the Ministry of Labour described the existing infrastructure as 'hopelessly chaotic', 'past belief' and a 'public scandal.' The medical commissioners in Belfast and Cork were found to be living permanently in Dublin. One medical commissioner for the Dublin region was contended to be too old and of little use, and the Dublin office was without the use of a working telephone. The Ministry of Labour criticised the 'casual way in which these matters are generally conducted in Ireland' describing 'the ultra-casual way' in which the

Ministry of Pensions operated, believing it to be 'good reasons for anxiety.' In the Cork Branch, 2,000 unopened or only partially dealt with employment files were on open display. Even the Ministry of Pensions in Dublin was unable to deny that their infrastructure was in 'a very unsatisfactory state.' The Irish Federation of Discharged and Demobilised Soldiers, one of the ex-service charities which would amalgamate to formulate the British Legion in 1921, similarly referenced 'the deplorable conditions' of the Ministry of Pension offices in Dublin, complaining that ex-servicemen and their families were in a 'stifling and unsanitary atmosphere for four, five and a many as seven hours a day.' They lamented 'the moral effect of this treatment on broken heroes.'[91]

In addition to state assistance in the form of the Treasury-funded Ministries of Labour and Pensions, voluntarism and the incorporation of societal schemes to reintegrate the disabled Great War veteran remained central to Britain's rehabilitation philosophy. In 1919, E. T. Devine, an American academic, described the UK system as being a 'mosaic of two elements' shaped by 'the constant interplay of state activity and private effort.'[92] The King's National Roll scheme exemplifies this mosaic. The King's National Roll was a British state programme which encouraged employers to ensure at least 5 percent of their workforce were ex-servicemen in receipt of a disability pension. Launched in Britain in 1919, employers who participated were included on a national 'Roll of Honour' with the privilege of using the King's Seal in correspondence.[93] Such an effort helped to create a sense of duty and appreciation for the disabled ex-service population. Previous research into the scheme has highlighted its worthiness as almost 24,000 employers participated in helping 259,000 disabled ex-servicemen attain employment in 1921.[94]

The input of ex-service charities was also hugely significant. The British Legion, a philanthropic organisation born via the amalgamation of several ex-service charities in 1921, was a mixed and composite body assisting ablebodied and disabled veterans alike. The charity assisted pensioners and claimants with training opportunities, providing personal advice on disabilities and rehabilitative care, distributing financial donations in particularly desperate times, offering personal representation in ex-servicemen's' dealings with the Ministry and lobbying politicians.[95] The ESWS also helped over 25,000 mentally ill veterans during the inter-war period. Many veterans were assessed by the organisation's medical officers before their claims were forwarded on to the Ministry, as well as helping to provide additional medical care, accommodation, allowances, relief and even tobacco and confectionary to insane veterans. While operating on a much-reduced scale in comparison to the British Legion, the ESWS praised itself for being as 'a potent representative of the mentally disabled ex-serviceman.'[96] This engrossment of philanthropic and societal ventures helped to shield the British state from the political and economic consequences of veteran and public ire.[97]

Neurasthenia as a pensionable diagnostic category comprised of all functional disorders of the nervous system, ensuring that its remit remained incredibly far-reaching and ill-defined.[98] An analysis of 200 randomly selected pension files reveals a broad and varied array of symptoms including exhaustion, heart palpitations, sleep problems, muscle tremors, recurring headaches and joint and muscle pain.[99] The seemingly minimal measure of officially diagnosing mentally ill veterans was significant. Modern research into trauma argues that sharing a common diagnosis with a community is the first step to allowing a person to understand their own condition better and appreciating that they are not alone and that others are similarly suffering.[100]

The Ministry faced a huge challenge in assessing neurasthenic veterans. In 1921, Sir Arthur Lisle Webb, the Ministry's Director General for Medical Services, pronounced the neurasthenic pensioner to be 'one of the most difficult' aspects within the department's remit. Webb supposed that complications were unavoidable due to the military and medical establishment's inexperience with psychoneurosis.[101] The standing start of military psychiatry at the outbreak of the First World War ensured an absence of medico-pensions and assessment officials with expertise and knowledge of psychoneurotic conditions. Even authors who published on war-induced neuroses had little experience of the subject due to the shortage of specialists.[102] In comparison, the Ministry's assessment of physical disabilities often included a range of medico-pensions officials, private practitioners and civilian doctors who assessed claimants and pensioners by payment per report. Due to the intricacies and lack of experience with psychoneurotic ailments, the Ministry required assessment boards comprising of specialists and chaired by specifically selected medical men.[103] In Ireland, W. R. Dawson, an Inspector of Lunacy in Ireland before the First World War, and subsequently enlisted by the War Office during the conflict to help manage the treatment of mentally ill soldier-patients, became the president of the Special Medical Boards assessing neurasthenic men in Dublin and Belfast.[104] Approval for pensions and treatment relied solely on the judgement of a region's Commissioner of Medical Services and the Special Medical Boards who examined mentally ill ex-servicemen.[105]

The legitimacy and causation of a neurasthenic pensioner's disability claim, which had dogged the shell-shock debate during military service, persevered. One official report recognised the dangers of subjective diagnosis:

> It is unwise to place too much reliance upon a nervous manner, coarse tremor or marked stammering alone, for these are often induced, or unconsciously exaggerated at the time of examination. The prognosis of Functional Nervous

Disease is always difficult, and the difficulty is much enhanced when it depends upon accurately gauging the alleged subjective symptoms that a patient alleges he feels is always very real to him, but unhesitatingly to accept statements and award gratuities or pensions at these examinations in the absence of physical corroboration would in many cases be to an injustice to the State and harm to the individual.[106]

Unlike physical disabilities, where pension payments followed more objectively verifiable guidelines, pensions for neurasthenia were dependant on the severity of the condition. This facet was also recognised by the ESWS who argued that the war's responsibility for mental illness was doubted in a way that a missing limb or a gunshot wound was not. While the latter remained comparatively stationary in its severity and condition, psychoneuroses could vary widely daily. The charity's Chairman suggested that the lack of objective visibility of the disability, in opposition to missing limbs or blindness, reduced societal and governmental sympathy bestowed on mentally ill veterans.[107]

Difficulties in assessment manifested over time and with fresh claims for war-induced mental illness arising after demobilisation. Navy veteran and Belfast-born Peter Fitzpatrick was awarded a 40 percent pension in 1920. Fitzpatrick suffered from headaches, drowsiness, sleeplessness, hurried conduct, tremulous hands and worry attributable to the intense and traumatic impact of working landing strips under fire near German East Africa. Fitzpatrick's pension was reduced from 40 to 20 percent in 1921 with Ministry board officials deeming his mental state to have improved.[108] O'Ryan experienced numerous pension boards during the inter-war period. His pension scale fluctuated between 80 and 100 percent. Due to his physical wounds attained on the Western Front, O'Ryan was unable to walk more than five miles without experiencing pain.[109] One Ministry of Pensions' official who assessed O'Ryan commented that the assessment of neurasthenia was 'so largely a matter of personal opinion.' While it was noted by assessment officials that his mental 'condition appears to vary from time to time', his medical reports describe a nervous and reclusive man who avoided large crowds and suffered from 'battle dreams' with accompanying somatic 'nervous signs' such as tremulous limbs, a chronic spasm in his neck and a rapid pulse.[110] In addition to providing a pension to First World War veterans like O'Ryan and Fitzpatrick, the option for Ministry-funded treatment was available.

Institutional treatment for mentally ill veterans

Civil hospitals and the existing public health infrastructure were regularly used to treat physically disabled veterans with the Ministry financing treatment via capitation grants.[111] The organisation to cater for Great War veterans suffering from Pulmonary Tuberculosis was, for example, already established owing to the illness's frequency in pre-war British society. The Ministry of Pensions, the Ministry of Health and local authorities collaborated to enable tubercular ex-servicemen to be treated in existent civil sanatoriums.[112] Treatment of insane Great War veterans adopted a similar infrastructure. By May 1916, 3,000 servicemen were estimated to have been discharged as pauper lunatics in the UK since the outbreak of the war.[113] In August 1917, Pensions Minister Sir Frederick Milner noted: 'There is nothing which the public regard with greater or more natural dread than the possibility of being shut up in an asylum.'[114] The lack of treatment available in the district asylum was recognised by the Ministry of Pensions, which regarded these facilities as a 'cemetery of hopeless cases.'[115] The Ministry established the Service Patient scheme to counter this failing. Categorised alongside private patients, with their maintenance paid for by the Ministry of Pensions, Service Patients would benefit from a weekly allowance of 2/6d for 'additional comforts' while under treatment. Should they pass away while under treatment, they were spared burial within the asylum cemetery in a pauper's grave with financial assistance provided to family and friends for a private burial. They were also permitted to wear distinct civilian clothing to differentiate them from the regular asylum population to spare them from the stigma of pauperism.[116]

Ireland particularly needed the Service Patient scheme. Owing to a misprint in the Lunacy (Ireland) Act 1901, the word 'prisoner' instead of the word 'person' ensured that any serviceman admitted into an Irish asylum was legally classified as a 'Criminal Lunatic.' The cost of running an asylum was shared by local councils who provided a suitable charge on the poor rate, and this was assisted by a capital grant raised by local taxation.[117] The maintenance of these 'Criminal Lunatics' was, therefore, paid by the Imperial Exchequer. While there were accusations that the War Office discontinued a man's pension to make up for the additional cost of maintenance, this practice appears to have stopped with amendments to the 1909 Army Act.[118] Pension authorities, government bodies and the Irish Lunacy Inspectorate were all at pains to stress that this amendment ensured ex-servicemen were 'Criminal Lunatics' in name only, and there was no difference with regards to their treatment.[119] Regardless, the situation ensured that Irish soldiers were legally designated as criminally insane alongside those guilty of heinous crimes.[120] Under such conditions, even the Belfast War Pensions Committee, who were previously sceptical as to the usefulness of the Service Patient scheme, recognised the situation required redress.[121] The Ministry of Pensions also recognised the injustice meted out to institutionalised ex-servicemen in Ireland: 'the present state of the law cannot be defended and immediate steps should be taken to amend the act.'[122]

Instructions related to the classification and treatment of servicemen as Service Patients in Irish asylums were distributed on 28 August 1919, which was over two years after the scheme's introduction in Britain.[123] 'Criminal Lunatics' were believed to require more supervision, so the cost of their maintenance was higher than for the regular asylum population.[124] There were financially-motivated complaints regarding the extension of the Service Patient scheme in Ireland. The Superintendent of the Waterford Asylum wrote to the Ministry of Pensions office in Dublin on 22 October 1919: 'These men are criminal lunatics by Act of Parliament and the Committee of this Asylum will not accept any other classification which means a loss in the cost of maintenance.'[125] The Ministry of Pensions' agreement to pay a uniform sum of 3s 9d per week, in addition to the cost of maintenance and providing extra distinctive clothing for each Service Patient admitted, ensured the new scheme operated without a loss to the asylum or local authorities. The introduction of the Service Patient scheme also relieved the asylum and local authorities from the future cost of maintenance. With these conditions made clear, the lunacy authorities subsequently endorsed the implementation of the scheme.[126]

While tubercular and insane veterans would share asylums with consumptive and insane populations from civil society, the Ministry also established its own exclusive facilities for the treatment of disabled veteran communities. The department was again aided by previous medical experience in pre-war public health, ensuring that the Ministry often had a body of pre-1914 medical practice to draw upon. The Ministry's orthopaedic facilities hugely benefitted from its staffs' prior experience and knowledge of caring for disabled children and those disabled in industrial accidents.[127] This experience would seemingly advance the treatment of this disabled veteran population. The artificial leg distributed to a disabled pensioner would evolve into a metallic limb. The British Legion, medico-military staff and contemporary historians have assessed that the British metal leg limb was world-leading with regard to durability and flexibility.[128] In Ireland, this experience benefitted limbless veterans undergoing rehabilitative treatment at Blackrock Hospital, a former Industrial School in Meath, purchased by the War Office. Catering for 500 soldier-patients, the facility dedicated itself to orthopaedics and artificial limb manufacture and replacement.[129] Two years after the war's conclusion, the facility was transferred to the Ministry of Pensions who continued to operate the facility to benefit limbless veterans. Surviving footage of the hospital from 1921 advertises one armless in-patient's ability to use an artificial limb for productive labour work.[130] Ulsterman Arnold was discharged from the British Army in 1917 owing to German artillery shrapnel penetrating his thigh and restricting his manoeuvrability. He was grateful that the Ministry's specialist orthopaedic practitioners helped to rehabilitate him back into civilian life:

> I cannot give too much praise to the way in which the surgeons dealt with my limb, and beyond very slight pain when the wind blows it has never given me any trouble. A surgical boot with a one inch elevation had corrected my lameness and I owe an everlasting debt of gratitude to the Ministry of Pensions for their kindness and efficiency in effecting the necessary renewals.[131]

Having been unable to walk long distances due to the stiffness of his thigh, Arnold credited the intervention of Ministry treatment in allowing him to pursue his passion for mountaineering that would continue into later life.[132]

No such foundational blocks or established medical culture existed for psychoneurotic veterans. As early as 1915, an official government committee reported that transferring a mentally ill veteran who was not a danger to himself or others to a lunatic asylum was not the most suitable aid to a man's recovery.[133] A prominent Treasury official similarly wrote in 1921:

> The matter is, as you know well, far from being a simple one, and the present circumstances of the country do not make it any easier. We have been in touch with the best and most eminent opinion of the civil medical profession on the subject for the last four years, and are constantly taking the best specialist's advice. One difficulty is that the profession itself has come to no final or static view on the subject, and I believe I am right in saying that in comparatively recent times, very various opinions have held the field in turn.[134]

As was the case with assessing neurasthenic veterans, the Ministry had to found a suitable medical infrastructure itself. Interpreting subjective psychiatric symptoms and deciding the best course of treatment proved difficult. As one British military doctor assessed: 'The symptoms themselves are hardly ever the same twice over.'[135] The official history of the British Army's Medical Services summarised the complexity facing the Ministry of Pensions in their diagnosis of neurasthenic pensioners:

> The diagnosis and treatment of cases of neurosis and psychosis needed much more time, skill and patience. In their more acute forms these conditions presented many novel features, and amidst the various theories and therapeutic suggestions it was difficult at the outset to decide on the most effective form of treatment.[136]

The Ministry initially pursued the Maghull model of psychotherapy. The Commanding Officer of Maghull, Rows, was a former district asylum advisor during peacetime who was interested in psychoanalysis. Rows affirmed that Maghull was the first military institution to provide 'definitive teaching in mental illnesses and [where] psycho-therapy was given.'[137] He expanded on the treatment offered:

> The work of this hospital, therefore had been directed to: – (1) Explaining to the patient the mechanism concerned in mental processes. (2) Discovering the incident or series of incidents on which the disturbance depends. (3) Educating the patient so that he may see the relation of cause and effect between the incident and the associated emotional state in his own case – may be enabled to regard it from a fresh and broader point of view, and so be led to face his problem to solve it.[138]

This method of narrative-focused treatment was a precursor to treatment that would today be labelled Cognitive Behavioural Therapy (CBT). Both Rows and modern-day CBT practitioners engage with their anxious and depressed patients by attempting to adjust their thought processes in the hope of rationalising negative thoughts and increasing the consistency and extent of positive ones. Treatment thus constituted a 'top down' method allowing sufferers to connect with others and better understand their symptoms while processing the memories of the causal trauma.[139] Smith and Pear observed transnational research to argue that the opportunity for such personal and concentrated care could assist in preventing a serviceman's symptoms from deteriorating.[140] They held that the treatment was 'a great experiment in preventative medicine', signifying 'conclusively that the exercise of scientific care during the early phases of mental disorder would save many from such a complete breakdown as would necessitate certification and removal to an asylum.'[141] One patient's reflection on his experience of this treatment affirmed its merits: 'I understand now; it is not my muscles which require treatment so much as the mind.'[142] Abreaction therapy and hypnosis improved the hysterical paralysis of one Irish soldier-patient who was experiencing a loss of mobility due to his hand's persistent motioning as if grasping an imaginary rifle. It was during psychotherapeutic treatment with a military specialist that the Irish soldier's experience of having suffered from multiple bayonet wounds was unearthed. Memories of the traumatic event were discussed and relived during treatment, and a relationship to the man's current symptoms and defensive paralysis was drawn and understood to the betterment of the Irishman's symptoms and mental state.[143]

The Maghull's Hospital's Committee described the wartime treatment offered to soldier-patients as having 'produced an enormous improvement … the patients now highly appreciate the value of the attention paid to them.'[144] Rows attested that it 'demonstrates the value of explaining the origin of the disability to the patient. Many have said that they have been able to overcome slight returns of the disability by remembering the explanations that had been given to them.'[145] Ex-service newspapers also describe the general steady improvement amongst soldier-patients receiving such treatment at facilities like Maghull.[146] Maghull treated 3,638 soldier-patients between its opening in 1914 until its transferral to the Ministry of Pensions in mid-1919.[147] This number included Irishmen and men serving in Irish units, including Private John Cox from the 3rd Royal Irish Regiment who had served over three decades in the British Army. Transferred from a Military General Hospital on the Western Front on 27 February 1915, Cox told medical staff 'that he went out to France at the end of January has been in the trenches and states that he became broken up by the strain.' His case notes describe a listless man with wandering attention, albeit without suffering from temper outbursts, hallucinations or delusions. Rows also noted that on describing his service at the Front, Cox 'became very emotional and had crying attacks when questioned.' Cox was seemingly able to make a substantial improvement in his mood within a month of undergoing treatment at Maghull.[148] Soldier-patients of the officer class at Craiglockhart went so far as to portray their Commanding Officer, Rivers, as a wizard, such was his apparent ability to attain remarkable results in their mental state. Prejudices did not cease, however. Rivers, for example, was frustrated in his dealings with working-class patients in Maghull due to their supposed inability to articulate fully during sessions and their simple dreams.[149] Nevertheless, assessing Maghull and Craiglockhart, Barham wrote that 'the circumstances of the war provided the conditions for more relaxed and egalitarian treatment regimes that were not entirely subjugated by traditional military values.'[150] In the closing stages of the First World War, asylum staff working in nearby regional district facilities even arranged for observations of the psychoanalytic treatment of soldier-patients at Maghull Hospital to learn more about the nature and extent of the treatment provided.[151] In becoming 'the first school of clinical psychopathology in Britain', Shephard went even further describing Maghull as a 'landmark in psychiatric history.'[152]

The Ministry's treatment of mentally disabled veterans initially pursued Maghull's ethos of abreaction. The unpreparedness of the Ministry to accommodate mentally ill veterans, and its lack of qualified medical staff to provide psychotherapy, quickly became evident.[153] Maghull thus became crucial in the redress of this imbalance with a teaching facility headed by Rows. As RAMC practitioners received teaching in Maghull for the treatment of soldier-patients, Ministry medical officers also underwent training in residence including for those who were to sit on tribunals to assess claimants and pensioners. They were educated on dream analysis, 'talking therapy' including word association, and hypnosis for work in the Ministry's in-patient and out-patient facilities.[154] The Ministry was proactive in training new medical staff, even including advertisements in medical journals requesting that GPs transfer any psycho-neurotic veteran in their surgeries to them for treatment by their practitioners in training.[155] Maghull's educational ethos subsequently incorporated tens of thousands of British soldier-patients and neurasthenic pensioners. This broad remit led Holden to describe the facility as 'a seedbed of British psychology.'[156]

The *War Pensions Gazette* best summarised the function of the Ministry's resulting in-patient network which utilised these newly trained practitioners: 'the Home is a hospital, yet it is not a bit like a hospital. It much more resembles a very comfortable country house.'[157] The Ministry's 'Country House Scheme', established from 1917, involved private residences donated to the Ministry of Pensions to provide pensioners with up to three months of recuperation.[158] In-patient treatment provided for 'chronic cases' offered a dual form of therapy. Psychotherapy aimed to advance a neurasthenic pensioner's mental condition while occupational therapy was intended to facilitate their employment in civil society after their discharge.[159] Ministry in-patient and out-patient facilities were reserved for 'nerve shattered soldiers.' This discourse and appropriate facility stood in stark contrast to the lunatic population institutionalised in an asylum deemed a 'burden on the nation.' There remained an emphasis on 'immediate action being taken by which these poor men may be treated, and be re-equipped for a fresh start in life.'[160] In contrast to the asylum, patients were unable to be admitted or detained against their will, and were not legally certified as insane.[161] Ministry in-patient and out-patient facilities sought to treat neurasthenic pensioners 'at the earliest opportunity.'[162] Believing that the continuation of the immediate treatment afforded to soldier-patients would also help veterans to recover, Ministry facilities offered a rare opportunity for the early treatment of mental symptoms. As Smith and Pear observed: 'In our own country, mental disorder is seldom treated in its early stages. Nearly all our elaborate public machinery for dealing with this distressing form of illness is devised, and in practice is available, only for the advanced cases.'[163] Out-patient evening clinics were established to make attendance more convenient for neurasthenic pensioners in full-time employment.[164] Out-patient treatment was considered beneficial within a sixteen-week timeframe and focused primarily on psychotherapy.[165] One Regional Director of a Ministry of Pensions' out-patient clinic in Oxford stressed the role of psychopathology and the work of Sigmund Freud and Carl Jung as heavily influencing the mode of treatment at these facilities.[166] Out-patient facilities treating neurasthenic pensioners who had a 'promising prognosis' were considered beneficial within a sixteen-week timeframe.[167]

Previous internal memos and correspondence by Ministry officials advanced that the most appropriate treatment for neurasthenia was the transfer of a neurotic ex-serviceman from his home to a suitable Ministry of Pensions' institution to receive treatment. Transferral was explicitly reserved for unemployed men.[168] John Harry Hebb, the Ministry's Director General of Medical Services for much of the 1920s and 1930s, disclosed that employed neurasthenics should be 'disturbed as little as possible' by transferrals for in or out-patient treatment.[169] Out-patient facilities catered for neurasthenic pensioners in possession of employment so as not to disturb their income.[170] The emphasis on employment within both in-patient and out-patient facilities again reflected the Ministry of Pensions' broader philosophy of 'reconstruction' aiming to facilitate the full-time employment of a disabled ex-serviceman in the aftermath of treatment.[171] The emphasis on vocational and physical therapy continued a nineteenth-century tradition of 'moral therapy' aligning mental illness with physical causes and remedies.[172] While the ethos of wartime psychotherapeutic treatment was to return men to duty, its post-war function was to restore mentally disabled men as employable, able to attain a full-time wage and thus save the British Treasury money in the long term.[173]

By 1921, the Ministry had established twenty-three exclusive in-patient facilities and forty-eight out-patient clinics for neurasthenic pensioners: approximately 3,283 neurasthenic pensioners were receiving in-patient treatment in a Ministry facility, and 8,698 were receiving out-patient care throughout the United Kingdom.[174] Two Ministry in-patient services were available to neurasthenic ex-servicemen in Ireland: a Ministry of Pensions facility in Leopardstown, Dublin and Craigavon UVF Hospital outside of Belfast. Ireland had additional out-patient facilities regularly accommodating a handful of pensioners per session. A clinic was held at Ministry of Pensions' Ulster headquarters in Belfast five evenings per week. Similar arrangements were in place at Dublin Headquarters and then in the Ministry's central office in Cork.[175]

In the absence of surviving institutional records, it remains challenging to verify how individual pensioners responded to in-patient and out-patient treatment.[176] Nevertheless, like the soldier-patient who received treatment in Maghull, it appears that neurasthenic pensioners often initially benefitted from the treatment provided. One neurological expert working for the Ministry of Pensions believed a 'distinct and definitive reduction' of a pensioner's neurasthenic condition was possible.[177] Another Ministry memo in March 1918 praised 'the results obtained [which] have proved to be extremely satisfactory'.[178] One practitioner who worked at the Ministry's Lancaster Clinic similarly attested to the beneficial treatment provided to neurasthenic pensioners via in-patient and out-patient psychotherapy, including for those who had previously repressed their thoughts, feelings and experiences of trauma, and those whose recovery had stagnated through relying on conservative remedies such as tonics, drugs and bromides.[179] At their most basic level, sharing in-patient facilities and out-patient sessions with fellow neurasthenic pensioners would offer therapeutic value via what was later termed as 'Rap Sessions' for American veterans of the Vietnam War. This terminology denotes formal sittings of veterans diagnosed with PTSD discussing their symptoms and hearing other ex-servicemen's' stories of their wartime experiences and resulting trauma which could initiate a better understanding of their symptoms and suffering.[180] One fundamental failure of the Ministry, however, was the dearth of the facilities. A Ministry inquiry in 1921 would lament the lack of in-patient facilities. Waiting lists of neurasthenic pensioners awaiting out-patient treatment far outweighed the equivalent data for other war-related ailments.[181]

The progress of the Ministry's infrastructure is significant despite this shortage. Ministry facilities operated at a time when the treatment of mental illness outside of the asylum was very much in its infancy in inter-war Britain.[182] As Bedford Pierce, an asylum superintendent and future Lunacy Commissioner to the Board of Control, wrote in 1917: 'At present, broadly speaking, no person unable to pay its cost can receive adequate treatment until he is certified as of unsound mind.'[183] The prominence of psychoanalysts operating in Britain before the First World War has been equated to a 'toehold.' The majority of the medical establishment, including asylum superintendents, largely dismissed psychotherapy and psychoanalysis.[184] Such was psychoanalysis' infancy and the controversy that accompanied it that Smith and Pear did not cite the term until more than halfway through *Shell-Shock and its Lessons* in fear of provoking 'unnecessary and acrimonious discussion on any particular doctrinal aspect of the question which this term may be taken to imply.'[185]

The Ministry's psychotherapeutic approach was also criticised by non-medical professionals. One British MP described the treatment as 'torture' which was unfairly 'experimenting with shattered lives.'[186] The First World War would even cause dispute amongst the small body of committed psychoanalysts.[187] The opportunity for a working-class former 'Tommy' to experience expensive, intensive and controversial psychotherapeutic treatment was thus confined to Ministry facilities.[188]

Leopardstown and Craigavon hospitals

By October 1917, the necessity to treat neurasthenic southern Irish ex-servicemen as in-patients was 'urgent.'[189] The benevolence of Gertrude Dunning partially addressed this shortage when she leased her estate and mansion of Leopardstown Park in Dublin rent-free to the Ministry of Pensions (Figure 1).[190] The home was initially not ready for such a role. The purchase of furniture, medical

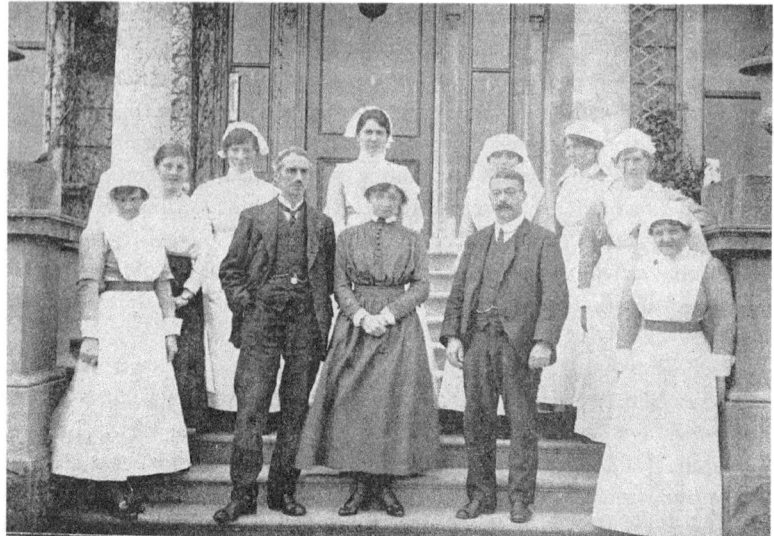

Figure 1 Leopardstown staff: the resident superintendent, matron and secretary surrounded by hospital nurses.

equipment and general supplies was required alongside the renovation of most rooms.[191] The finances were mainly raised through grants from the Ministry of Pensions and by fundraising £5,000 in the USA with a noted dearth of voluntary philanthropic contributions in Ireland.[192] The committee of management for the facility included a range of men and women with an assortment of experience in the military, public and medical affairs and staff including a resident medical officer, a matron, a secretary, a nursing sister, nurses, a cook/housekeeper and three servants.[193]

The Leopardstown Hospital had 100 acres of arable and picturesque land and was self-sufficient in its production of food (Figures 2, 3 and 4). Such facilities were very much part of the Ministry of Pensions' philosophy of 'reconstruction' which sought to facilitate the full-time employment of a disabled ex-serviceman. The facility provided curative therapy with workshops providing treatment in joinery, carpentry, leathery and gardening.[194] One member of the hospital's management committee protested against the employment of a gardener stating that 'the work which the patients would do in the garden would be an integral part of the cure.'[195] Sugars wrote that few facilities existed in Ireland which emphasised vocational therapy but which remained 'absolutely necessary.'[196]

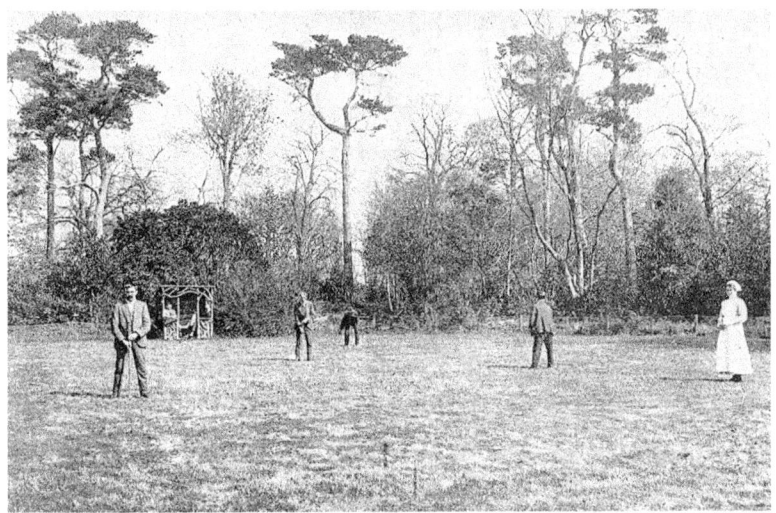

Figure 2 Leopardstown's 'croquet grounds' where patients participated in recreational games and activities.

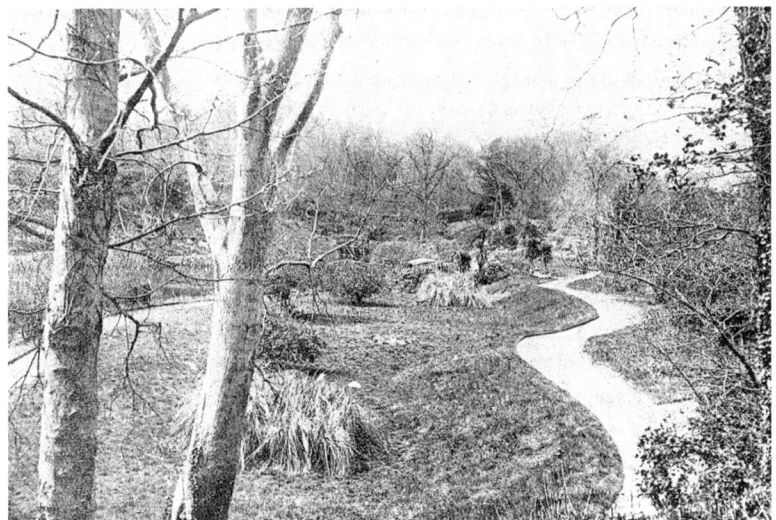

Figure 3 Leopardstown's 'pleasure grounds' where patients were able to enjoy walks.

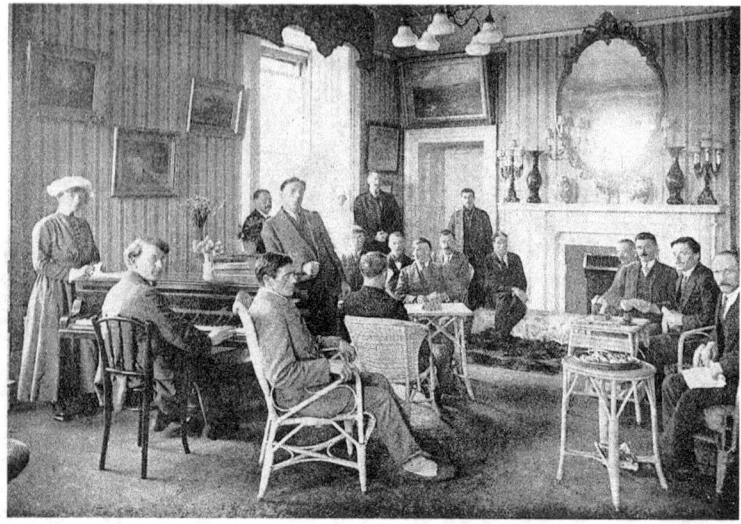

Figure 4 Leopardstown's recreation room.

As regards size, Leopardstown resembled the private asylum much more than the more immense district asylum. The average population size in the twelve private asylums in the Irish Free State was seventy patients.[197] In contrast, larger district asylums in Ireland could exceed 1,000 patients. Ministry institutions ensured that soldier-patients could receive attentive individual care not afforded to civilian patients.[198] Unlike the asylum, where individuals could be admitted and detained against a patient's will, Leopardstown required a voluntary decision to receive treatment with no obligation to be held against an ex-serviceman's will. This voluntarism in public health facilities would not be established in Northern Ireland until 1930 and the Free State until 1945.[199] In Strandtown, Belfast, the UVF Craigavon Hospital was also converted from a country mansion donated by James Craig MP, a prominent leader of the Ulster Unionist Party and future Prime Minister of Northern Ireland. Like Leopardstown, its establishment was overdue. Craigavon already had a backlog of a 'considerable number of cases' awaiting treatment before the hospital's opening.[200] The hospital could accommodate seventy-five patients and provided idyllic amenities as patients were provided with massages, baths, a healthy diet, quietness and solitude.[201] Situated three miles outside of Belfast in what the *Irish Times* described as 'picturesque surroundings', the rehabilitation of shell-shocked men again emphasised the necessity of allowing in-patients to become employable and self-sufficient on their discharge.[202] At the official unveiling of the hospital, the Minister of Pensions, G. N. Barnes MP, repeated the Ministry's core ethos of ensuring the employability of pensioners, warning society that it 'must not be content with giving a man a pension; it must build him up and return him a self-supporting and self-respecting unit to the community.'[203]

Patients were taught skills such as gardening, pottery, motoring, metalwork, basket weaving, poultry, farming, rabbit breeding, brush making and tailoring. The Ministry of Pensions provided £322, with a £300 annual subsidy, to establish a vegetable patch within the grounds of the hospital to sustain healthy eating within the institution, as well as produce items for sale for the local population.[204] In the absence of any surviving photographs, the architectural drawing (Figure 5) for the facility provides some indication of its infrastructure.

The Ministry of Pensions and British Treasury were financially liable for the running and financial maintenance of these two facilities donated by wealthy philanthropists.[205]

Conclusion

The First World War induced a fundamental change in the state's treatment of disabled ex-servicemen. The newly created Ministry of Pensions established legal pension rights and acknowledged accountability for the medical treatment and rehabilitation of disabled veterans. Nowhere is this development better exemplified than in the treatment of psychoneurotic ex-service personnel. Neurasthenic pensioners were in a much more favourable position than mentally ill British Army veterans of the preceding South African War who were, by comparison, regularly denied financial recompense and treated within the highly stigmatised and conservative public asylum. Diseases only joined wounds as eligible for disability pensions in 1901, and it was not until the First World War that the extent to which war service could affect the nervous and mental system of a soldier was adequately recognised.[206] The Ministry would establish financial recompense and progressive psychotherapy for returning veterans with shattered nerves despite the relative infancy of the treatment of psychoneurosis in UK society and the lack of modern developments crucial to a contemporary understanding of anxiety and mental health disorders.

The remit and function of the Ministry of Pensions were not, however, absolute nor without significant drawbacks. Inherent problems permeated the medical treatment of neurasthenic pensioners. A myriad of intensely personal reasons and even non-war related factors dictated progress or regression during treatment. As specialists concluded at a conference of regional DCMS in 1921:

> A general discussion ensued on this point and it was agreed that no definitive medical standard could be laid down as to requirements of treatment. Some DCsMS had attempted to work on such a basis but had found it impracticable for it was quite possible that a man with 80% disability was incapable of receiving

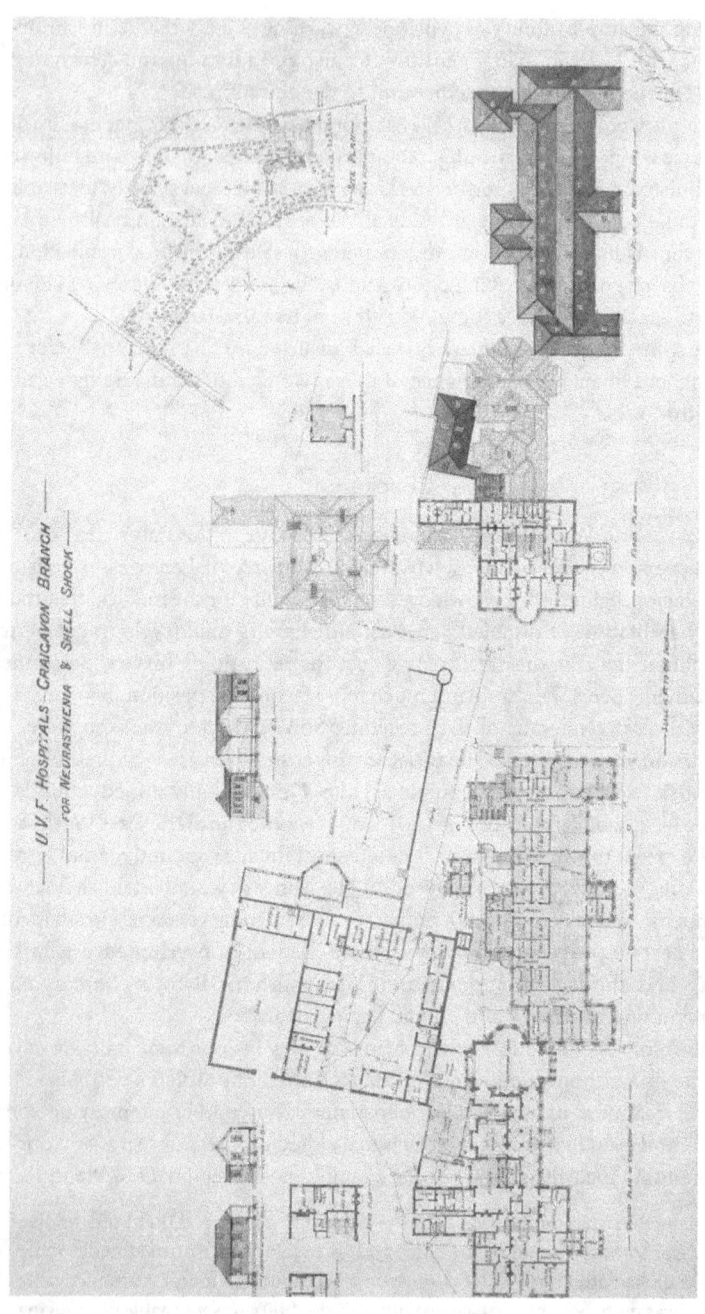

Figure 5 Architectural drawing for Craigavon UVF Hospital.

any further improvement by treatment. While a man with 5% or 10% might be completely cured by appropriate treatment, it was therefore necessary to deal with each case on its merits.[207]

The British Army's official medical history of the war cites similar problems.[208]

Despite the increased state intervention in the wellbeing of returning disabled veterans, voluntarism, philanthropy and employment remained central to the Ministry's rehabilitative strategy. This societal involvement would fatally compromise the Ministry's attempts to rehabilitate mentally ill veterans. While recognising the financial assistance and opportunity for medical treatment offered by the Ministry, the unpredictable nature and pervasive stigma attached to mental illness often prevented many neurasthenic pensioners attaining employment. A case study of Ireland during its revolutionary period centres the Ministry's failure to establish a seamless 'mosaic' of state and societal infrastructure to rehabilitate the mentally ill veteran. The Ministry's policy and infrastructure were severely undermined in Ireland with waiting list figures for neurasthenic in-patient and out-patient treatment far outweighing comparative figures in Britain. To help explain these numbers, long-held and widely established prejudices that Irishmen were biologically predisposed to mental illness returned. Worse still, they were articulated by the very government department officials charged with the care and wellbeing of disabled Irish Great War veterans.

Notes

1. Leese, *Shell-Shock*, 68; Shephard, *A War of Nerves*, 6.
2. PRONI, HOS/28/1/3/3/1, Belfast District Lunatic Asylum, General Register of Patients, 1846–1932; HOS/28/1/3/3/2, Belfast District Lunatic Asylum, General Register of Patients, 1882–1955; Luke Diver, 'Ireland and the South African War, 1899–1902' (PhD Thesis, Maynooth University, 2014), 189–94.
3. William Macpherson, *Medical Services: Diseases of the War, vol. 2*, (London: HMSO, 1923), 9.
4. Nicholas Perry, 'Nationality in the Irish Regiments in the First World War', *War and Society*, 12:1 (1994), 66.
5. Leese, *Shell-Shock*, 68; Barham, *Forgotten Lunatics of the Great War*, 384; Reid, *Broken Men*, 29; William Macpherson, *Medical Services: General History, Volume 1* (HMSO: London, 1921), 71.
6. Harrison, *The Medical War*, 113.
7. Jones and Wessely, *Shell-Shock to PTSD*, 17–8.
8. This figure equated to around 14 percent of the accommodation that was provided on asylum property; Charles Read, *Military Psychiatry in Peace and War* (London: H. K. Lewis & Co, 1920), 42; Barham, *Forgotten Lunatics of the Great War*, 45.

9   The historiography on the wartime medical debate and response to shell shock is extensive. A suitable introduction is provided in Peter Leese, '"Why are they not cured"?: British shell-shock treatment during the Great War', in Mark Micale and Paul Lerner (eds), *Traumatic Pasts: History, Psychiatry, and Trauma in the Modern Age, 1870–1930* (Cambridge: Cambridge University Press, 2001), 205–21.

10 The wide-ranging psychodynamic programme adhered to at Maghull during the war is discussed in Edgar Jones, 'Shell shock at Maghull and the Maudsley: models of psychological medicine in the UK', *Journal of the History of Medicine and Allied Sciences*, 65:3 (2010), 368–95; W. H. R. Rivers, *Instinct and the Unconscious: A Contribution to a Biological Theory of the Psycho-neuroses* (Cambridge: Cambridge University Press, 1920), 185–204.

11 Jones, 'Shell shock at Maghull and the Maudsley', 382–3.

12 Leese, *Shell-Shock*, 89.

13 Jones, 'Shell shock at Maghull and the Maudsley', 394.

14 Thomas Webb, 'Dottyville: Craiglockhart War Hospital and shell-shock treatment in the First World War', *Journal of the Royal Society of Medicine*, 99:7 (2006), 346.

15 Norman Fenton, *Shell-Shock and its Aftermath* (St Louis: The CV Mosby Company, 1926), 166; Peter Reid, 'The Institutional Management of Soldiers with Shell Shock in Ireland, 1916–19', (MA Thesis, University College, Dublin, 2014), 19; Bourke, 'Shell-shock, psychiatry and the Irish Soldier', 156–7.

16 A Medical Officer played a fundamental role in the frontline management of health care, often acting as the first point of contact with a sick or wounded serviceman. Thus, their interpretation and medical judgement of a physical or mental wound often proved decisive in dictating whether a soldier was transferred for treatment and, if so, if they were redirected to an Advanced Dressing Station, a Base Hospital or evacuated to Britain; Leese, *Shell-Shock*, 33–4.

17 NA, WO 95/3923/2, 1st Battalion Connaught Rangers, Medical Officer.

18 NA, MH 106/2101, Medical Sheets, 1914–1915.

19 NA, PIN 26/22244, Patrick John O'Ryan, Pension File, The Royal Inniskilling Fusiliers, 1918–1979.

20 F. C. Purser, 'Transactions of the Academy of Medicine in Ireland', *Dublin Journal of Medical Science*, 35 (1917), 228.

21 Joanna Bourke, 'Effeminacy, ethnicity and the end of trauma: the sufferings of "shell-shocked" men in Great Britain and Ireland, 1914–39', *Journal of Contemporary History*, 35:1 (2000), 62.

22 Barham, *Forgotten Lunatics of the Great War*, 82, 221; Carden-Coyne, *The Politics of Wounds*, 198.

23 Brown, 'Between cowardice and insanity', 123.

24 Don MacRaild, *Irish Migrants in Britain, 1750–1922* (Basingstoke: Palgrave Macmillan, 1999), 164; Liz Curtis, *Nothing But The Same old Story: The Roots of Anti-Irish Racism* (Belfast: Sasta, 1984), 10; John Harrington, *The English Traveller in Ireland: Accounts of Ireland and the Irish through Five Centuries* (Dublin: Wolfhound Press, 1991), 65, 88–9; Andrew Hadfield and John McVeagh, *Strangers to that Land: British Perceptions of Ireland from the Reformation to the Famine* (Gerrards Cross:

Colin Smythe, 1994), 46; Roger Swift, 'Crime and the Irish in nineteenth century Britain, 1871–1921', in Roger Swift and Sheridan Gilley (eds), *The Irish in Britain, 1815–1939* (London: Pinter 1989), 165–78; Alan O'Day, 'Varieties of anti-Irish behaviour, 1846–1922', in Panikos Panayi (ed.), *Racial Violence in Britain in the Nineteenth and Twentieth Centuries* (Leicester: Leicester University Press, 1996), 30–1; F. Finnegan, *Poverty And Prejudice: A Study of Irish Immigrants in York, 1840–75* (Cork: Cork University Press, 1982), 153; Jacqueline Turton, 'Mayhew's Irish: the Irish poor in mid nineteenth-century London', in Roger Swift and Sheridan Gilley (eds), *The Irish in Victorian Britain: The Local Dimension* (Dublin: Four Courts Press, 1999), 146; Walter Ralls, 'The Papal aggression of 1850: A study in Victorian Anti-Catholicism', *Church History*, 43:2 (1974), 244.

25 Joanna Bourke, '"Irish Tommies": The construction of a martial manhood 1914–1918', *Bullan*, 6 (1998), 13–30; Nicholas Perry, 'Maintaining regimental identity in the Great War: the case of the Irish infantry regiments', *Stand To: The Journal of the Western Front Association*, 52 (1998), 5–11; Terence Denman, 'The Catholic Irish soldier in the First World War: the "racial environment"', *Irish Historical Studies*, 27:108 (1991), 352–65.

26 Elaine Showalter, *The Female Malady: Women, Madness, and English Culture, 1830–1980* (London: Virago, 1987), 167–95.

27 Loughran, *Shell-Shock and Medical Culture in First World War Britain*, 144.

28 Jessica Meyer, 'Separating the men from the boys: masculinity and maturity in understandings of shell shock in Britain', *Twentieth Century British History*, 20:1 (2009), 4–5.

29 Smith and Pear, *Shell-Shock and its Lessons*, 71; again, foregrounding the confused and contradictory nature of discourse regarding combat neurosis, Peter Barham describes Smith and Pear as 'progressive thinkers and practitioners' in the field of psychoneurosis. Jay Winter, however, also notes that the former was partial to repeating prejudicial tropes regarding the mentally weak shell-shocked soldier; Barham, *Forgotten Lunatics of the Great War*, 151; Winter, *War Without Words*, 186.

30 Arnold also prominently voiced the view that the Irish were incapable of self-governance in *On the Study of Celtic Literature* (London: David Nutt, 1910); L. Curtis, *Apes and Angels: The Irish in Victorian Caricature* (Newton Abbott: David and Charles, 1971), 18, 44; Harrington, *The English Traveller in Ireland*, 265; L. Curtis, *Anglo Saxons and Celts: A Study of anti-Irish Prejudice in Victorian England* (New York: New York University Press, 1968), 53–5; Edward Lengel, *The Irish Through British Eyes: Perceptions of Ireland in the Famine Era* (London: Praeger, 2002), 131.

31 An edited copy of 'On the Alleged Increase of Insanity in Ireland', by Dr Thomas Draper, Resident Medical Superintendent, Enniscorthy District Asylum, XL (1894), 518–47; 'Voices of doctors and officials', in Pauline Prior (ed.), *Asylums, Mental Health Care and the Irish: Historical Studies 1800–2010* (Dublin: Irish Academic Press, 2012), 282.

32 Pauline Prior, 'Overseeing the Irish Asylums: the Inspectorate in Lunacy, 1845–1921', in Pauline Prior (ed.), *Asylums, Mental Health Care and the Irish 1800–2010* (Dublin: Irish Academic Press, 2012), 227.

33 Catherine Cox, Hilary Marland and Sarah York, 'Itineraries and experiences of insanity: Irish migration and the management of mental illness in nineteenth-century Lancashire', in Catherine Cox, Hilary Marland and Sarah York (eds), *Migration, Health and Ethnicity in the Modern World* (Basingstoke: Palgrave Macmillan, 2013), 36; Elizabeth Malcolm, '"A most miserable looking object" – The Irish in English Asylums, 1851–1901: Migration, poverty and prejudice', in John Belchem and Klaus Tenfelde (eds), *Irish and Polish Migration in Comparative Perspective* (Essen: Klartext Verlag, 2003), 121; Prior, 'Overseeing the Irish Asylums', 227.

34 Cox, Marland and York, 'Itineraries and experiences of insanity', 47, 55.

35 Catherine Cox, Hilary Marland and Sarah York, 'Emaciated, exhausted and excited: the bodies and minds of the Irish in nineteenth-century Lancashire asylums', *Journal of Social History*, 46:2 (2012), 512–17.

36 Bourke, 'Effeminacy, ethnicity and the end of trauma', 61; Damien Brennan, 'A theoretical exploration of institution-based mental health care in Ireland', in Pauline Prior (ed.), *Asylums, Mental Health Care and the Irish: Historical studies 1800–2010* (Dublin: Irish Academic Press, 2012), 289–92; Mark Finnane, *Insanity and the Insane in Post-Famine Ireland* (London: Croon Helm, 1981), 143; Elizabeth Malcolm, '"Ireland's crowded madhouses": the institutional confinement of the insane in nineteenth- and twentieth-century Ireland', in Roy Porter and David Wright (eds), *The Confinement of the Insane: International Perspectives, 1800–1965* (Cambridge: Cambridge University Press, 2003), 323; Damien Brennan, *Irish Insanity, 1800–2000* (New York: Routledge, 2014), 81; Elizabeth Malcolm, '"The house of strident shadows": the asylum, the family, and emigration in post-famine rural Ireland', in Greta Jones and Elizabeth Malcolm (eds), *Medicine, Disease and the State in Ireland, 1650–1940* (Cork: Cork University Press, 1999), 186; Malcolm, 'A most miserable looking object', 131; Cox, Marland and York, 'Itineraries and experiences of insanity', 55; Dermot Walsh, 'Did the Great Irish Potato Famine increase schizophrenia?', *Irish Journal of Psychological Medicine*, 29:1 (2012), 7–15.

37 Martin Miller, 'The concept of revolutionary insanity in Russian history', in Angela Brintlinger and Ilya Vinitsky (eds), *Madness and the Mad in Russian Culture* (Toronto: University of Toronto Press, 2007), 105–6.

38 John Rylands Library, University of Manchester, GES/2, 'Race, Nationality and Character' (1918) by Grafton Elliot Smith.

39 Diana Louis, 'Peculiar Institutions: Representations of Nineteenth-Century Black Women's Madness and Confinement in Slavery and Asylums' (PhD Thesis, Emory University, 2014), 77–117.

40 Sloan Mahone, 'The psychology of rebellion: colonial medical responses to dissent in British East Africa', *The Journal of African History*, 47:2 (2006), 241–58.

41 J. S. R. Russell, 'Treatment of neurasthenia', *The Lancet*, 22 November 1913, 1453–6.

42 Andrew Scull, *Madness: A Very Short Introduction* (Oxford: Oxford University Press, 2011), 61–2.

43 Tracey Loughran, 'Hysteria and neurasthenia in pre-1914 British medical discourse and in histories of shell-shock', *History of Psychiatry*, 19:1 (2008), 37–41; Tracey

Loughran, 'Shell-shock in First World War Britain: An Intellectual and Medical History, c. 1860–c.1920' (PhD Thesis, Queen Mary, University of London, 2006), 61; Tracey Loughran, *Shell-Shock and Medical Culture in First World War Britain*, 72–7; Bourke, 'Effeminacy, ethnicity and the end of trauma', 61.

44 Curtis, *Anglo-Saxons and Celts*, 54–5.
45 I expand upon this thesis in 'Perceptions of the mentally ill Irish population during the nineteenth and early twentieth centuries', *Études Irlandaises*, 42:2 (2017), 59–71.
46 Michael Di Nie, *The Eternal Paddy: Irish Identity and the British Press, 1798–1882* (Wisconsin: University of Wisconsin Press, 2004), 59.
47 Ibid., 165.
48 Ibid., 215.
49 Brotherton Library, Leeds University, INDEX/LIDDLE/GA/2020, S. J. Wallis Correspondence, 8 October 1918.
50 Paul Redmond, 'Denis Kilbride M. P. 1848–1924' (MA Thesis, University of Maynooth, 2003), 318.
51 Loughran, *Shell-Shock and Medical Culture in First World War Britain*, 76–7.
52 Curtis, *Anglo Saxons and Celts*, 53–5.
53 Margaret Humphreys, *Intensely Human: The Health of the Black Soldier in the American Civil War* (Baltimore: Johns Hopkins University Press, 2008), 9, 55–6; R. F. Jefferson, '"Enabled courage": Race, disability, and black World War II veterans in postwar America', *The Historian*, 65:5 (2003), 1104; E. Dwyer, 'Psychiatry and race during World War II', *Journal of the History of Medicine and Allied Sciences*, 61:2 (2006), 143.
54 Bourke, 'Irish Tommies', 18.
55 Thomas Bartlett and Keith Jeffery, 'An Irish military tradition?', in Thomas Bartlett and Keith Jeffery (eds), *A Military History of Ireland* (Cambridge: Cambridge University Press, 1996), 18.
56 Curtis, *Anglo Saxons and Celts*, 55.
57 Bourke, 'Irish Tommies', 20.
58 Timothy Bowman, *Irish Regiments in the Great War: Discipline and Morale* (Manchester: Manchester University Press, 2003), 19.
59 Bourke, 'Irish Tommies', 20.
60 Brotherton Library, Leeds University, INDEX/LIDDLE/GA/2018, Lieutenant Commander J. K. McLeod, Royal Navy, correspondence.
61 Frankwood Williams, *Neuropsychiatry and the War* (New York: War Work Committee, 1918), 117; Didier Fassin and Richard Rechtman, *The Empire of Trauma: An Inquiry into the Condition of Victimhood* (Oxford: Princeton University Press, 2009), 53, 56.
62 Henri Ellenberger, *Discovery of the Unconscious: The History and Evolution of Dynamic Psychiatry* (New York: Basic Books, 1970), 826.
63 A closer analysis of breakdowns in German medical publications disproved these theories with breakdown rates broadly similar for all nations represented in the

German and Austro-Hungarian Armies; Williams, *Neuropsychiatry and the War*, 264–5.
64 George Mosse, 'Shell-shock as a social disease', *Journal of Contemporary History*, 35:1 (2000), 103; Bourke, 'Effeminacy, ethnicity and the end of trauma', 60; Fiona Reid, *Medicine in the First World War: Soldiers, Medics, Pacifists* (London: Bloomsbury, 2017), 83–4.
65 Mosse, 'Shell-shock as a social disease', 101.
66 Deborah Cohen, *The War Come Home: Disabled Veterans in Britain and Germany, 1914–1939* (Berkeley: University of California Press, 2001), 5.
67 J. L. Llewllyn and Arthur Jones, *Pensions and the Principles of their Evaluation* (London: William Heinemann, 1919), 22–3; *Reveille*, 1 (August, 1918), 55–6; *Reveille*, 3 (February 1919), 390–2; Mitchell and Smith, *Medical Services*, 311; Bettinson, 'Lost Souls in the House of Restoration', 19–25.
68 Arnold's Typescript Recollections, 126.
69 Cohen, *The War Come Home*, 24.
70 This percentage was also considerably smaller than Wales, Scotland Canada, Australia, New Zealand and South Africa; Oram, *Worthless Men*, 5.
71 Harrison, *The Medical War*, 110.
72 Combat Stress Archive, Surrey, Annual Report for 1933, 10.
73 A Voluntary Pensions Worker, *Pensioners of the Great War* (London: Robert Scott, 1922), 31.
74 Arnold's Typescript Recollections, 126.
75 Ibid.
76 Bettinson, 'Lost Souls in the House of Restoration', 159.
77 Mitchell and Smith, *Medical Services*, 308–9.
78 Ibid. More information on these facilities can be found in the Ministry of Pensions' annual reports.
79 Anon, 'Treatment of disabled soldiers: work of the Ministry of Pensions', *The Lancet*, 16 April 1921, 827; Llewllyn and Jones, *Pensions and the Principles of their Evaluation*, 47–8; James Hogge and T. H. Garside, *War Pensions and Allowances* (London: Hodder and Stoughton, 1918), 301.
80 Bettinson, 'Lost Souls in the House of Restoration', 178–9, 267.
81 Mitchell and Smith, *Medical Services*, 309.
82 Arnold's Typescript Recollections, 127.
83 NA, PIN 15/789, Ministry of Pensions Undated Minute Sheet.
84 Departmental Committee of Inquiry into the Machinery of Administration of the Ministry of Pensions Report to Ian Macpherson, MP, Minister of Pensions, 1921, 6.
85 For more information on complicated process of decentralisation see Nineteenth Annual Report of the Ministry of Pensions, 1935–1936, Part 2, 3–4.
86 Bettinson, 'Lost Souls in the House of Restoration', 210.
87 NAI, FIN/1/216, Proposal for establishment of Ministry of Pensions in Ireland. The reference to 12 Regional Directors here would seem to be an error.

88 Bettinson, 'Lost Souls in the House of Restoration', 210.
89 Anonymous, 'Dr. Harold Saunderson Sugars Obituary', *British Medical Journal*, 3567 (1929), 935.
90 Kowalsky, 'Enabling the Great War', 98–9.
91 NA, LAB 2/855/ED5412/13/1921, Ministry of Labour, to Ministry of Pensions, 13 March 1921, Irish Federation of Discharged and Demobilised Soldiers, February 1920; LAB 2/522/TDS1636/1919, Training Department: General Correspondence regarding the establishment of training schemes in Ireland, Memorandum, 18 November 1919, 2; LAB 2/855/ED5412/7/1921; Ministry of Pensions, note, 12 March 1920; LAB/2/522/TDS3949/2/1919, Ministry of Labour, Dublin, to Ministry of Labour, London, 30 May 1919; LAB 2/528/TDS1181/1921, Application of Training, Attached Minute, 11 July 1922.
92 E. T. Devine, *Disabled Soldiers and Sailors, Pensions and Training* (Oxford: Oxford University Press, 1919), 94.
93 Taylor, *Heroes or Traitors?*, 92.
94 For more information on the scheme see Meaghan Kowalsky, '"This honourable obligation": the King's National Roll Scheme for disabled ex-servicemen 1915–1944', *European Review of History*, 14:4 (2007), 567–84.
95 For more information on the British Legion's remit and function during the inter-war period, see Niall Barr, *The Lion and the Poppy: British Veterans, Politics, and Society, 1921–1939* (Westport: Praeger, 2005), 62.
96 Combat Stress Archive, Surrey, ESWS Chairman's Report for 1926, 10.
97 Bettinson, 'Lost Souls in the House of Restoration', 38.
98 Mitchell and Smith, *Medical Services*, 318.
99 Edgar Jones and Simon Wessely, 'Battle for the mind: World War 1 and the birth of military psychiatry', *The Lancet*, 384:9955 (2014), 1708.
100 Judith Herman, *Trauma and Recovery: The Aftermath of Violence from Domestic Abuse to Political Terror* (New York: Basic Books, 2015), 158.
101 NA, PIN 15/56, Ministry of Pensions, London, to Ministry of Pensions, Dublin, 21 December 1921.
102 Loughran, 'Shell-shock in First World War Britain', 32–3.
103 A Voluntary Pensions Worker, *Pensioners of the Great War*, 31; Mitchell and Smith, *Medical Services*, 310.
104 Eoin Kinsella, *Leopardstown Park Hospital, 1917–2017: A Home For Wounded Soldiers* (Dublin: Heritage, 2017), 39.
105 NA, PIN 15/56, Director General of Medical Services to Reginal Directors (All Regions), 23 June 1921.
106 NA, PIN 15/54, Ministry of Pensions, Instructions for 'Special Medical Board', 2.
107 Combat Stress Archive, Surrey, ESWS Annual Report for 1934, 17; ESWS Chairman's Report for 1927, 9; ESWS Appeal 1938.
108 NA, PIN 26/16836, Leading Seaman Peter Fitzpatrick Pension File.
109 NA, PIN 26/22244, O'Ryan Pension File.

110 Ibid.
111 For example, the Ministry financed the treatment of disabled ex-servicemen in the private Shankiel Hospital in Cork, Ireland; Bettinson, 'Lost Souls in the House of Restoration', 38; Durnin, *The Irish Medical Profession and the First World War*, 183.
112 Fifth Annual Report of the Ministry of Pensions, 1921–1922, 13; NA, T 136/2, Treasury to the Ministry of Pensions, 8 October 1918; Mitchell and Smith, *Medical Services*, 340.
113 Barham, *Forgotten Lunatics of the Great War*, 104.
114 Ibid., 293.
115 Ibid., 327.
116 Barham describes segregation of soldiers and pauper lunatics at burial as 'perhaps the most affecting symbol' of the entire Service Patient scheme; Ibid., 57; NA, PIN 15/896, Instruction Relating to the Classification and Treatment of Soldiers and Sailors as Service Patients.
117 Reid, 'The Institutional Management of Soldiers with Shell Shock in Ireland, 1916–19', 9.
118 Bourke, 'Shell-shock, psychiatry and the Irish soldier', 165–6; NA, PIN 15/896, Ministry of Pensions, note, 13 August 1917.
119 NA, PIN 15/897, Ministry of Pensions, note, 11 December 1918; Westminster House to County Down War Pensions Local Committee, 2 November 1918; War Office Note, 2 October 1918; PIN 15/898, I. O. Regent's Park, 8 August 1919.
120 Pauline Prior, *Mental Health and Politics in Northern Ireland* (Aldershot: Avebury, 1993), 23.
121 NA, PIN 15/897, Chief Inspector's Note, 27 August 1918.
122 NA, PIN 15/896, Ministry of Pensions, note, 15 January 1917.
123 NA, PIN 15/899, Instructions relating to the classification and treatment of soldiers and sailors as Service Patients, Office of Lunatic Asylums, Dublin Castle, 28 August 1919.
124 Ibid., Office of Lunatics asylums, Dublin Castle, to Ministry of Pensions, London, 12 March 1920.
125 Ibid., Asylum Superintendent of Waterford Asylum to Ministry of Pensions, Dublin, 22 October 1919.
126 Ibid., Office of Lunatics asylums, Dublin Castle, to Ministry of Pensions, London, 12 March 1920.
127 Jeffrey Reznick, *Healing the Nation: Soldiers and the Culture of Caregiving in Britain during the Great War* (Manchester: Manchester University Press, 2004), 118.
128 *British Legion Journal*, 3 (August, 1923), 43; Mitchell and Smith, *Medical Services*, 339; for more information on the superior design of the British metallic limb, see Mary Guyatt, 'Better legs: artificial limbs for British veterans of the First World War', *Journal of Design History*, 14:4 (2001), 307–25.
129 Kinsella, *Leopardstown Park Hospital*, 94.

130 British Pathé Archive, Online, 'Demonstration of Artificial Arms at Blackrock Special Hospital', 27 June 1921.
131 Arnold's Typescript Recollections, 123.
132 Ibid.
133 Report of the Committee Appointed by the President of the Local Government Board upon the Provision of Employment for Sailors and Soldiers Disabled in the War (1915), 134.
134 NA, PIN 15/55, George Chrystal note, 31 May 1921.
135 Mark Humphries and Kellen Kurchinski, 'Rest, relax and get well: a re-conceptualisation of Great War shell shock treatment', *War and Society*, 27:2 (2008), 92.
136 Mitchell and Smith, *Medical Services*, 341.
137 War Office, *History of the Asylum War Hospitals in England and Wales* (London: War Office, 1920), 69; Holden, *Shell-Shock*, 53–4.
138 War Office, *History of the Asylum War Hospitals in England and Wales*, 71.
139 Bessel Van Der Kolk, *The Body Keeps the Score: Mind, Brain and Body in the Transformation of Trauma* (London: Penguin, 2015), 3; Christopher Frith and Eve Johnstone, *Schizophrenia: A Very Short Introduction* (Oxford: Oxford University Press, 2003), 143.
140 Smith and Pear, *Shell-Shock and its Lessons*, 82–4.
141 Ibid., 108–9.
142 War Office, *History of the War Hospitals in England and Wales*, 70.
143 Bourke, 'Shell-shock, psychiatry and the Irish soldier', 161–2.
144 The surviving medical sheets of soldier-patients admitted into the facility indicate a general improvement in their psychoneurotic condition; Liverpool Record Office, M614 MAG/1/3, 'Medical Case Sheets'; M614 MAG/1/1, Committee Minute Book, Maghull Military Hospital, 7 October 1915;
145 War Office, *History of the War Hospitals in England and Wales*, 70.
146 *War Pensions Gazette*, 8 (December, 1917), 103.
147 Jones, 'Shell shock at Maghull and the Maudsley', 375.
148 Liverpool Record Office, M614 MAG/1/3, Medical Case Sheet – Private John Cox.
149 Holden, *Shell-Shock*, 60–2.
150 Barham, *Forgotten Lunatics of the Great War*, 284.
151 Liverpool Record Office, M614 Mag/1/3, Letter from T. Stewart Adair, Resident Medical Superintendent Asylum, Kirkburton Asylum, to Colonel Rows, Maghull Military Hospital, 1 May 1918.
152 Ben Shephard, '"The early treatment of mental disorders": R. G. Rows and Maghull 1914–1918', in Hugh Freeman and G. E. Berrios (eds), *150 Years of British Psychiatry, Volume 2, The Aftermath* (London: Athlone Press, 1996), 450.
153 Anon., 'Mental disease in ex-servicemen: work of the Ministry of Pensions', *The Lancet*, 31 December 1921, 1388.

154 Liverpool Record Office, M614 MAG/1/3, Letter from Mary Dendy to Dr Robertson 24 August 1918; Rivers, *Instinct and the Unconscious*, 5; Leese, *Shell-Shock*, 87; Jones and Wessely, *Shell-Shock to PTSD*, 132; Frederick Mott, *War Neuroses and Shell-Shock* (London: Hodder & Stoughton, 1919), 155–6; Millais Culpin, *Recent Advances in the Study of the Psychoneurosis* (London: Churchill, 1931), 20.

155 Martin Stone, 'The Military and Industrial Roots of Clinical Psychology in Britain, 1900–1945' (PhD Thesis, London School of Economics, 1985), 185.

156 Holden, *Shell-Shock*, 53.

157 *War Pensions Gazette*, 8 (December, 1917), 104.

158 Leese, *Shell-Shock*, 62.

159 NA, PIN 15/56, Memorandum on Conference of Neurological D.Cs.M.S. held at Headquarters, 17 June 1921; To Commissioners of Medical Services. All Regions: Treatment of Neurasthenia, 15 October 1921.

160 NA, PIN 15/53, Recuperative Hospitals, 3 January 1917.

161 HC Debates, 18 August, vol. 119, cols 1929-30W1929W.

162 NA, PIN 15/56, Ministry of Pensions, London, to Regional Directors, Treatment of Neurasthenia, 15 October 1921.

163 Smith and Pear, *Shell-Shock and its Lessons*, 24.

164 NA, PIN 15/56, Ministry of Pensions, note, 15 November 1921.

165 NA, PIN 15/2946, Neurological Cases – Out-patient treatment with or without allowances, and Home Treatment with allowances; Jones and Wessely, *Shell-Shock to PTSD*, 132.

166 A. Ninian Bruce, 'The out-patient treatment of early mental disorder: the neurological clinic, and some of its functions', *British Journal of Psychiatry*, 68 (1922), 385.

167 NA, PIN 15/2946, Neurological cases: Out-patient treatment with or without allowances, and Home Treatment with allowances; Jones and Wessely, *Shell-Shock to PTSD*, 132.

168 NA, PIN 15/54, Special Medical Board, 6.

169 Barham, *Forgotten Lunatics of the Great War*, 275.

170 Mitchell and Smith, *Medical Services*, 342.

171 Anon., 'Treatment of disabled soldiers: work of the Ministry of Pensions', *The Lancet*, 16 April 1921, 82; Llewllyn and Jones, *Pensions and the Principles of their Evaluation*, 57.

172 Brendan Kelly, *Hearing Voices: The History of Psychiatry in Ireland* (Kildare: Irish Academic Press, 2016), 178–9.

173 Llewllyn and Jones, *Pensions and the Principles of their Evaluation*, 56; NA, PIN 15/130, Ministry Clinics – Proposals to Establish Use of Military Orthopaedic Centres, 1917–1918 for discharged disabled men, Memorandum, 4 April 1917; Leese, *Shell-Shock*, 83.

174 Fourth Annual Report of the Ministry of Pensions, 1920–1921, 9, 32–4; NA, PIN 15/56, Provision of Treatment for Neurasthenia, 25 November 1921; Ministry of Pensions, Dublin, to Ministry of Pensions, London, 24 November 1921.

175 NA, PIN 15/56, Ministry of Pensions, note, 26 May 1921; Ministry of Pensions, London, to Ministry of Pensions, Dublin, 24 November 1921; PIN 15/2946, Out-Patient Neurological Returns for February and March.
176 There has been a lack of research into these facilities. In 1917, Smith and Pear wrote that research into their operatives was 'urgently needed.' This request remains unheeded over a century later; Smith and Pear, *Shell-Shock and its Lessons*, 117.
177 NA, PIN 15/56, Ministry of Pensions, Dublin, to the Ministry of Pensions, London, 13 December 1921.
178 NA, PIN 15/132, Circular on Psychotherapeutic Clinics, March 1918.
179 One prominent example of this pertained to a traumatised ex-serviceman who wished to be admitted into an asylum. Following prolonged and intensive therapeutic treatment, the soldier was able to recover a repressed memory of seeing a little girl killed in Belgium; *War Pensions Gazette*, 28 (August, 1919), 353.
180 Jeffrey A. Lieberman, *Shrinks: The Untold Story of Psychiatry* (London: Weidenfeld & Nicolson, 2015), 260.
181 Out-patient facilities did not cater for demand regardless of their innovative nature. It had, for example, almost 27 percent of pensioners deemed requiring treatment awaiting it in 1921. This compared to less than 2 percent for general medical and surgical out-patient care, and just one-tenth of a percentage for tubercular treatment; Departmental Committee of Inquiry into the Machinery of Administration of the Ministry of Pensions Report to Ian Macpherson, MP, Minister of Pensions, 1921, 98.
182 Of course, we know far more about how to treat mental illness today than during the period discussed in this study. For example, the use of anti-psychotic drugs is a relatively modern phenomenon; Frith and Johnstone, *Schizophrenia*, 145.
183 Smith and Pear, *Shell-Shock and its Lessons*, 79.
184 Martin Stone, 'Shellshock and the psychologists', in W. F. Bynum, Roy Porter and Michael Sheperd (eds), *The Anatomy of Madness: Essays in the History of Psychiatry. Volume 1: People and Ideas* (London: Tavistock, 1985), 242–3.
185 Smith and Pear, *Shell-Shock and its Lessons*, 74; the continued resistance and scepticism towards psychoanalysis is also cited in Jones and Wessely, *Shell-Shock to PTSD*, 49.
186 NA, PIN 15/56, Copy of House of Commons Question and Answers Session from 7 July 1921; Leese, *Shell-Shock*, 124.
187 British practitioners generally cited the shell-shock experience to dismiss Freudian theses regarding sexual motivations in causing neuroses. Dreams were also revised so as not to represent wish-fulfilments but, instead, provide an unconscious symbolic message to be interpreted; Stone, 'The Military and Industrial Roots of Clinical Psychology in Britain', 200–1.
188 Lease, *Shell-Shock*, 89; Shephard, *A War of Nerves*, 164.
189 NA, T 1/12508/12092, Ministry of Pensions, Leopardstown Park, 11 October 1917.
190 Ibid., Office of Public Works, Dublin, to the Treasury, London, 22 November 1919.

191 Ibid.
192 Ibid., Ministry of Pensions, London, to Treasury, London, 10 February 1920; Ministry of Pensions, Leopardstown Park, 11 October 1917; 'Leopardstown Park', *Irish Life*, 10 May 1918, 102.
193 Ibid., Ministry of Pensions, Leopardstown Park, 11 October 1917.
194 'Victims of the War: Treatment for Shell-Shock', *Irish Times*, 10 June 1924, 7; Anon, 'Treatment of disabled soldiers: work of the Ministry of Pensions', *The Lancet*, 16 April 1921, 827.
195 NA, T 1/12508/12092, Leopardstown, Management of the Committee memo, 23 October 1917.
196 NA, PIN 15/56, Facilities for Treatment of Neurasthenia in Ireland – South Region.
197 Annual Report of Irish Free State Mental Hospitals, 1929, 50.
198 Jones, 'Shell-Shock at Maghull', 368.
199 Brendan Kelly, 'The Mental Treatment Act 1945 in Ireland: an historical enquiry', *History of Psychiatry*, 19:1 (2008), 47–67.
200 The rush in converting the private residence into a hospital led to the accidental sale of Lady Cecil Craig's grand piano; PRONI, DI4151/B/38, diary of Lady Cecil Craig; NA, PIN 15/54, unknown author to the Earl of Derby, War Office, 29 May 1917.
201 W. Arthur Eakins, *The Somme: What Happened to the Casualties?* (Belfast: Eakins, 2008), 36–7.
202 'Sir Edward Carson in Belfast: Hospital for Neurasthenia and Shell-Shock Opening Ceremony', *Irish Times*, 23 July 1917, 6.
203 Bourke, 'Effeminacy, ethnicity and the end of trauma', 66.
204 Eakins, *The Somme*, 36–7.
205 NA, PIN MH 120/48, Schedule C.
206 Kowalsky, 'Enabling the Great War', 34; Jones and Wessely, *From Shell-Shock to PTSD*, 17; Barham, *Forgotten Lunatics of the Great War*, 120.
207 NA, PIN 15/56, Memorandum on Conference of Neurological D.Cs.M.S. held at Headquarters, 17 June 1921.
208 Mitchell and Smith, *Medical Services*, 341.

2

NEURASTHENIC PENSIONERS IN REVOLUTIONARY IRELAND

Introduction: 1921 DCMS conference

As part of the Ministry's attempt to better understand its remit, function and expenditure, Ministry headquarters in London contacted the eleven regional authorities throughout the United Kingdom requesting neurasthenic numbers, waiting lists and treatment allowances. This communication sought to establish a more objective and consistent policy framework regarding transferrals for treatment and the distribution of treatment allowances.[1] By November 1921, with Leopardstown operating at full capacity, 510 men were awaiting care. An additional 273 men were receiving treatment at an out-patient clinic with a further 254 on the waiting list.[2] The opening of an out-patient clinic in Cork subsequently reduced waiting list figures by another 101 men three weeks later. Inflated waiting lists in South Ireland persisted despite these increases.[3] This continuation would cause significant debate at the conference of Deputy Commissioners of Medical Services held at Ministry headquarters in London on 17 June 1921. One in five neurasthenic pensioners were receiving or awaiting treatment. In comparison, this ratio amounted to every two out of three men in South Ireland.[4] Waiting list figures in South Ireland substantially outweighed the Ministry's other ten designated regions (Table 2). The Ministry held that 'there ought not to be any Region [with] a variation of more than 5% from the average for the United Kingdom.'[5] Figures in South Ireland exceeded this limit, as shown in Figure 6.

At the 1921 conference, Dr A. Baldie attributed this difference to two explanations: 'a definitive neurasthenic temperament that was prevalent amongst the South Irish' and the 'special political conditions ruling in Ireland.'[6] Ulstermen were thus detached from the former assumption.[7] Grafton Elliot Smith

Table 2 Proportion of all patients awaiting either in-patient or out-patient treatment for neurasthenia in Ministry of Pensions' hospitals in the UK, 1921.

Area	Percentage awaiting in- and out-patient treatment	Percentage awaiting in-patient treatment	Percentage awaiting out-patient treatment
Scotland	2.5	21.0	0
North	7.5	0	13.5
North West	37.1	22.5	56.3
Yorkshire	20.9	7.3	24.5
Wales	4.5	5.3	7.6
North Midlands	49.9	22.2	53.1
Midlands	58.6	39.2	64.8
South West	7.6	8.7	7.3
London	7.2	32.8	5.9
Ulster	22.2	42.1	4.3
South Ireland	69.0	87.9	48.2

Source: Bourke, 'Effeminacy, ethnicity and the end of trauma', 69.

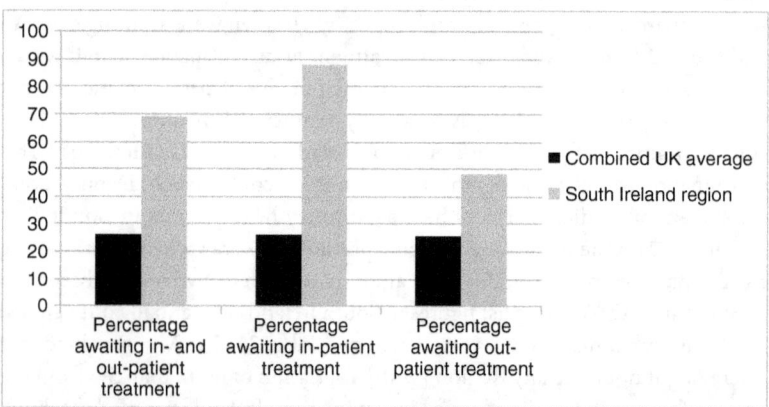

Figure 6 South Ireland and combined UK average figures of all patients awaiting either in-patient or out-patient treatment, 1921. Calculated from Bourke, 'Effeminacy, ethnicity and the end of trauma', 69.

better explained the exemption of the predominantly unionist and protestant Ulster:

> Community of race and speech, though important bonds of union, doesn't constitute nationality. By a nation we mean, broadly speaking, a population united by common interests, common institutions, common sympathies and a common history, and a consciousness of unity which leads it to desire a common government. Geographical circumstances do not determine nationality.

With this criterion in mind, Smith avowed that 'Ulster is not a part of the Irish nation.'[8] Dr Wallace held that it was 'indisputable' that those who were unfit recruits were more likely to enlist in South Ireland which 'included a large proportion of mentally defective and those subject to nervous disorders.' Wallace emphasised that assessments and waiting lists were inflated for all disabilities in the region, reinforcing his thesis: 'The case of South Ireland was admittedly out of the ordinary, and their assessments for treatment were persistently high not only for Neurasthenia but for all disabilities.'[9] The contents of the DCMS meeting, lasting from 11.30 to 5 pm, were not transcribed verbatim. The nine-page report on the conference only included the essential issues and conclusions further demonstrating the currency of such views. The fact that Wallace's and Baldie's testimonies were reproduced, seemingly without any disagreement or challenge from the other seventeen Ministry of Pension officials present, is telling of their perceived authenticity.[10] The memorandum was also sent out to Regional Directors of the Ministry of Pensions ensuring that these opinions were widely circulated.[11]

There is little evidence to suggest physically inferior or mentally unstable recruits were more likely in Ireland than in Britain.[12] Do not view Baldie and Wallace's quotes in isolation. The inaugural Minister of Pensions, George Barnes, MP, for example, claimed in Parliament in 1917 that some disabled pensioners did not receive a full pension as they were 'veritable weeds.' Barnes further explained this in his memoirs six years later: 'Many were freaks, some were lunatics who had joined up in a lucid moment.'[13] One contemporary commentator noted in 1918 that the Pensions establishment was plagued by 'countless prejudices.'[14] These partialities included anti-Irishness.

The medical establishment in Ireland was not immune to such theories. Charles Burtchaell had such cases in mind when he told the Royal Academy of Medicine in Ireland in 1920 that some mental casualties were 'only to be expected [seeing that] a large number of men who joined the Army were temperamentally unfitted for a soldier's life. Such men got into a nervous state before they came under fire.'[15] Contemporary researchers re-evaluated the inflated Irish representation in pre-1914 asylum data by analysing broader the social and cultural forces which could shape diagnosis and perceptions of mental ill-health. This methodology similarly contextualises the 1921 waiting list figures, helping to dismiss the prejudicial theses of Wallace and Baldie.

Unemployment and stunted recovery

There was still a shortcoming of 787 beds for neurasthenics in 1921 despite the Ministry of Pensions allocating 2,670 beds across the UK.[16] One Ministry official described this as 'deplorably inadequate in most regions and is causing grave harm.'[17] The lack of facilities also impacted upon standards with hasty and short-term treatment being carried out to accommodate more pensioners.[18] Integrating the research methods of disability historians proves beneficial here as they regularly foreground how disability is socially structured alongside being medically and administratively defined. In other words, broader public perceptions and cultural values shape the treatment and experiences of disabled people in past societies.[19] A crucial factor in explaining the shortage of beds for neurasthenics, a deficiency magnified in South Ireland, was the socio-economic reception of neurasthenic pensioners *outside* institutional facilities. Existing socio-cultural values compromised the effectiveness of the British Government's mixed economy of combining state pensions, treatment and training with public voluntarism.

Military and medical research, politicians, senior civil servants and Ministry of Pensions' medical staff endorsed the therapeutic importance of employment during the conflict and in its immediate aftermath.[20] Even Charles Myers, the first British medical official to pen the term 'shell-shock', held that the lack of post-treatment employment in civil life largely negated any progress made during abreaction therapy.[21] Hebb wrote in December 1921 that 'more and more we have become convinced that the work factor is the all-important one with the Neurasthenic.'[22] The Ministry of Pensions' subsequent annual report repeated the correlation between recovery and employment: 'The most successful and permanent results have been obtained by means of occupational treatment during a stay in hospital, especially if it is followed by the immediate return to employment on discharge.'[23] A popular self-help publication for mentally ill ex-servicemen published during the war stressed the benefits of work and employment in providing focus and distraction.[24] Empirical evidence exists to highlight this relationship. Northern England and Wales had the lowest waiting list figures for in-patient and out-patient neurasthenic treatment across the Ministry's eleven district regions. Ministry officials subsequently countered that many ex-servicemen worked in the mining industry and were thus better able to attain employment.[25] Indeed, previous research into disabled veterans who returned to South Wales and the North-East, regions whose economies largely depended on the coal industry, highlights how many were able to resume their old mining jobs or attain 'light work' at a colliery.[26] The connection between employability and neurasthenia was repeated internationally by former allies and enemies alike.[27] The correlation between welfare and unemployment is similarly evident amongst non-veteran populations. Research into inter-war National Health Insurance documents foregrounds how unemployment and mental illness were intrinsically linked in British society.[28] Research into US Army veterans of recent campaigns in Iraq and Afghanistan concludes that unemployed veterans may be disposed to incorrectly attributing their depression, anxiety and helplessness to Post-Traumatic Stress Disorder (PTSD).[29] Allan Young has compared this phenomenon to 'method acting' with veterans experiencing authentic psychological symptoms but not solely induced by war service.[30] While understanding that PTSD is not an ahistorical diagnosis, a captivating relationship between unemployment and neurasthenia cited by Pensions' staff during the inter-war period is apparent.[31]

Unemployment did not just stunt recovery amongst neurasthenic pensioners but induced claims for recompense from the Ministry of Pensions. One Ministry official noted the 'vicious circle' a neurasthenic pensioner often found himself during 'economic stress' which had a detrimental impact on a veteran's symptoms.[32] The Ministry of Pensions' neurological expert, Dr E. L. Forward, provides a clear explanation of this socio-psychological reaction:

> They are of the opinion that the bulk of the cases now being treated are of genuine War Neurosis, but that economic conditions such as unemployment etc., have enhanced the strain under which these men are living and probably rendering these patients worse than they otherwise might have been. It is difficult, if not impossible, to say where the one cause ends and the other begins.[33]

A report into neurasthenic pensioners in Scotland also stated that widespread unemployment in Glasgow ensured that a 'secondary economic neurasthenia' arose as a result of unemployment and the accompanying financial stress.[34] A small number of chronic neurasthenic pensioners were assessed to have deteriorated due to unemployment and their symptoms worsening on their return home and to their domestic unit.[35] Notions of hereditary deficiencies and degeneration remained prevalent in British society during this period.[36] A recognition of the broader context further magnifies the insurmountable challenge facing the Ministry of Pensions in rehabilitating the neurasthenic pensioner during the inter-war period. Contemporary prejudices of the mentally ill would contradict the Ministry's emphasis on the rehabilitative centrality of employment.

Unlike missing limbs and gunshot wounds, which were more objectively verifiable disabilities induced by war service, psychologically damaged veterans were hampered by the doubtful causation of their disability. A post-war transnational study produced by the Red Cross disregarded medical treatment, pension payments and employment, countering that 'a necessary feature of any program for restoring the disabled soldier to self-respect and self-support is a campaign of public education to convert the general attitude towards the crippled and handicapped.' There was a supposed 'signal failure to appreciate the value of public education' in Britain to change perceptions of those disabled as a result of war service.[37] This feature increased for those suffering from a psychiatric illness. In *The Future of the Disabled Soldier* (1917), specific physical disabilities were matched with particular occupations. Blind pensioners were apparently suitable basket makers; deaf veterans could become tailors; tubercular ex-servicemen should become golf caddies. No career, however, was seemingly appropriate for the veteran suffering from mental illness.[38] The Regional Director for the West Midlands region recognised these societal prejudices regarding the employment of neurasthenic pensioners. He wrote that occupational treatment was pointless as 'difficulty is experienced with the employers, who are often unwilling to accept men after they had heard details of their disability.'[39] Such fears had a foundation. Peter Fitzpatrick lost over a month in working days in just over a year working as a trainee in the boot and shoe trade in Belfast owing to his neurasthenic symptoms. Unsurprisingly, Fitzpatrick's tenure in this post did not last and he became unemployable on account of his unpredictability and costliness in the economic market.[40]

Writing in a publication aimed at veterans of the British Armed Forces, an American specialist of post-war disability emphasised that any scheme to rehabilitate disabled men would fail without an adjoining public consciousness to properly understand and fully support the reintegration of pensioners into civil society and employment.[41] Despite the advances made in the state's treatment of psychoneurotic veterans, the societal stigma surrounding mental ill-health fatally undermined the Ministry's attempts to rehabilitate the neurasthenic pensioner. The Ministry's policy of voluntarism and incorporation of civil society in the reintegration of disabled veterans proved particularly detrimental to neurasthenic ex-servicemen. A case study of the treatment and experience of neurasthenic pensioners in Ireland both exemplifies this failing and explains the inflated waiting list figures in the south.

The Anglo-Irish War

The ongoing Anglo-Irish War, 1919–21, fought between the British state and the IRA, compromised the rehabilitation of disabled veterans in post-war Ireland. Violence between the two sides would escalate during the conflict, encompassing assassinations of British agents including administrative staff and intelligence officers, the British utilisation of the irregular 'Black and Tan' forces to escalate engagement with the militant republicans, and the formation of IRA 'flying columns' employing guerrilla tactics. Simultaneous to the armed conflict, a political dispute ensued with the newly elected majority of Sinn Féin candidates declaring Ireland to be a republic and establishing a separatist government to delegitimise British administration in Ireland centred at Dublin Castle.[42] Significant civil disobedience also aimed to undermine British rule in Ireland, including a boycott by rail workers to transport British troops or British military supplies. Recent research by Steven O'Connor demonstrates that British ex-servicemen played an active role in this conflict by enlisting in both the opposing IRA and the Royal Irish Constabulary.[43] The conflict had a detrimental impact on the Ministry of Pensions' function and interaction with the disabled British ex-service community. Officials in Dublin noted significant delays in responding to requests from colleagues in London regarding neurasthenics owing to the difficulty in attaining information on the subject.[44] Arnold cited the boycott of Irish railway workers as further problematising his duties in Ireland: 'the break down of transport added enormously to the difficulties of our job.'[45] The curtailment of rail services also affected disabled veterans in Ulster with isolated communities having to be transported for treatment across Ireland via Ministry-funded car journeys, increasing departmental costs.[46]

Paramilitary activity and the guerrilla nature of the conflict even led to Ministry staff fearing for their wellbeing: 'It is of course, necessary to collect satisfactory information locally, but I do not in the least like suggestions that anyone should go to Ireland to collect it because one knows that the officer deputed would necessarily go at some personal risk.'[47] Sugars stated home-visits to meet and assess disabled Great War veterans were 'absolutely dangerous.'[48] It was even suggested that staff should not undertake such duties: 'The daily position at present does not justify an officer risking his life in doing out-door work, or work where he is not known, in Ireland, as in all cases, strangers are regarded with suspicion, and may be shot on sight, through no fault of their own.'[49] Sugars' fears appear justified. Ministry officials had come under fire when visiting areas outside of Dublin.[50] One clerk employed by the County Cork Local Committee was kidnapped and killed in May 1921.[51] Travel to and from Dublin also proved hazardous. The Inspector of Artificial Limbs in Belfast wrote: 'Every time I go to Dublin I am in or near ambushes or shootings of kinds which of course mean considerable personal risk.'[52] Research into Irish medical personnel who had previously served in the Royal Army Medical Corps similarly attest to their fear of being targeted for violent reprisal or being caught up in the crossfire during a guerrilla skirmish.[53]

Disabled Great War pensioners receiving in-patient treatment became unfortunate fatalities of the conflict. William McGrath, who lost an arm fighting for the Leinster Regiment during the First World War, was one accidental victim hit by a stray bullet fired by British forces in Cork, providing a tragic metaphor for the circumstances in which disabled British ex-servicemen now found themselves.[54] There were eleven separate incidents of damage to Ministry property or staff across Ireland during the revolutionary period.[55] Those perceived to be agents of an illegitimate British state in Ireland became targets of republican reprisal. For example, on 24 November 1920, the Cork City Pensions Office was raided by armed IRA men, during a well-organised heist, who stole £819.[56] Such robberies extended beyond facilities aiding the disabled ex-serviceman. Shops, banks and post offices were regularly targeted by IRA forces during the period.[57] By the start of 1920, policemen and British soldiers were beleaguered by IRA reprisals.[58] The Ministry also became a legitimate or accidental target of republican violence, with damage caused to Ministry property reflecting wider acts of damage done to government, including RIC barracks, Customs and Excise Offices, Inland Revenue Offices and even Coast Guard stations.[59] High-ranking officials at Dublin Castle involved in political administration were provided with armed police protection or even moved to permanently reside in the castle along with their families. Constituting the largest employer within the civil service in Ireland, postmen also became victims of the IRA on account of the important information they could carry.[60]

Arnold provides a commentary on his observations of RIC members being targeted and assassinated by militant republicans, and similarly notes the precautions necessary as a Ministry official working in Ireland: 'Such a soil was not very propitious to the betterment of the returned British soldier and even in the lowly province of a government inspector, the situation called for a good deal of careful handling.'[61] Arnold, nevertheless, downplayed the threats posed to Ministry officials in comparison to high-ranking civil servants or members of the RIC. Citing the department's 'somewhat privileged position amid this welfare of blood and confusion ... we of the Ministry of Pensions continued to go on with our work during the troubles and with some trifling exceptions were not molested.' To explain the comparatively fortunate position of Ministry officials, Arnold held that Sinn Féin and militant republicans did not oppose its remit to medically treat and provide pensions to veterans as it helped to extract money from the British Treasury.[62] Reflecting on this anti-British climate, the Ministry's Regional Director for South Ireland doubted the 'impartiality' of inspecting Medical Officers to assess a veteran's eligibility for treatment allowances: 'If the travelling D.C.M.S. cuts off a man's treatment allowances, it is notorious that he becomes unpopular, and it is dangerous for him to visit the same district again.'[63]

The preceding complaints from Ministry of Labour officials that the Ministry of Pensions was 'very chaotic', and inspection officers of pensioners and treatment and training facilities had no definite relationship with regional war pensions committees, appear harsh in this political context.[64] The chaotic administration, lack of intelligence and threat to the personal safety of pensions' officials appear to have had a crippling effect on the department's functioning throughout the region. Ministry staff in Ireland deserve credit for continuing to operate under such appalling conditions. Indeed, the impact of the conflict was not solely dependent upon the Ministry of Pensions; workhouses also struggled to manage the poor law in hostile areas such as Cork.[65] Writing to the Treasury in the summer of 1920, the loyalty and dedication of Ministry staff working in South Ireland was noted by its Regional Director, C. A. Sim, despite 'the extraordinary conditions under which we have to work [and] the risks and anxieties caused by reasons with which you are only too familiar.'[66] Arnold repeated this praise of his colleagues writing 'considering the difficulties it was wonderful how much was done.'[67] The significant shortage of treatment facilities in the region further highlights the commitment of Ministry staff working in South Ireland.

Lack of facilities

The conviction that Irishmen were more liable to suffer from war neurosis did not ensure more substantial facilities to counter this supposed national failing. Irish provisions were wholly insufficient.[68] In a damning indictment of the available facilities, following an inspection of ex-servicemen in Ireland in March 1921, Forward wrote: 'the present hospital accommodation, the number of clinics, and the supply of trained medical officers needed to deal with neurasthenic patients are much below the actual requirements.'[69] The lack of facilities in Ireland also impacted upon standards with treatment being carried out on a much-reduced scale to accommodate more pensioners.[70]

Sugars requested assistance and alleviation from the Ministry of Pensions in London to increase facilities at the Leopardstown Park Hospital: 'I think that unless the neurasthenic institutions in England are able to help us, there is little prospect of the waiting list being reduced in less than eighteen months to two years, and then only allowing for a short course of treatment for each case.'[71] A list of one hundred men was submitted for transferral to the Ministry of Pensions in charge of the London region for treatment in Ashurst War Hospital in Oxfordshire and Ewell War Hospital in Surrey to combat the dearth in treatment facilities.[72] One month later, however, the Ministry alerted all Regional Directors that all neurological hospitals in the London region were unable to admit any further cases to their waiting lists.[73] With regards to out-patient care, only one facility was in operation at Dublin headquarters until the end of 1921. This setup was 'very inadequate for Dublin City cases let alone being sufficient for the whole region.' The necessity of establishing a similar clinic at Cork was stressed. Travelling clinics, allowing neurological pension officials to treat men at local Ministry of Pension branches, were also needed where 'a sufficient number of pensioners were available in any district.' Their establishment would benefit men in Limerick, Waterford, Athlone, Mullingar and Sligo. Sugars wrote that it had 'frequently been found difficult' for pensioners to receive the attention of a medical or pension official.[74]

The revolutionary period also impacted upon neurasthenic treatment in Ulster by preventing the establishment of a centre for the treatment of the 438 neurological cases who resided in Londonderry. Any progression was postponed until 'as soon as the state of the country allows.'[75] Under financial strain, Craigavon was almost transferred into a sanatorium for consumptives just three years after its opening.[76] With the proposed allocation of an extra fifty beds for the fifty-three men awaiting treatment in Craigavon Hospital, the provision for in-patient treatment was, nevertheless, described as 'fair' with the prospects of managing the six men awaiting treatment in an out-patient clinic catering for 134 men in the region remaining 'excellent.' To put the chaotic situation in South Ireland into context, numerous regions in the United Kingdom were seemingly content with the availability of Ministry treatment facilities. Regional Ministry of Pension reports attest that waiting lists were 'negligible' in the West Midlands region, 'comparatively small and can be dealt with by the present accommodation' in the Yorkshire Region, while numbers awaiting in-patient treatment in Northern England amounted to 'nil.' In Newcastle, there were even fifty-six unoccupied beds at Shotley Bridge Hospital.[77] Forward recognised that neurasthenic treatment was confined to specialist centres in Dublin, Cork and Belfast. Thus, the expansion of existing facilities, a policy favoured by Sugars, would have provided little incentive to men in rural parts of Ireland unable or unwilling to receive treatment so far away from home. A clinic was only set up in Ulster in the comparatively sanguine year of 1917, as having to travel to Dublin from Belfast 'was rather a serious matter for men shaken by shell-shock.'[78] The travel of pensions' officials was dangerous during the revolutionary period, and it is possible that mentally ill British ex-servicemen may have been similarly reluctant to travel to receive treatment, further increasing waiting list figures.

Arnold described the breakdown of traditional legislative and administrative procedure during his employment as a Ministry inspector in revolutionary

Ireland. Not only had the RIC been heavily compromised due to assassinations, but the court systems stopped functioning effectively with the alternative government established by Sinn Féin often carrying out a de-facto judicial system.[79] Additional problems arose in the treatment of insane British ex-servicemen in Ireland due to the Anglo-Irish War. It was only after the admission to an asylum that a Great War veteran was classified as a Service Patient.[80] The 1838 Dangerous Lunacy Act (amended in 1867) enabled a family member to alert the police to a person's 'derangement of mind.' Certification was undertaken with the signature of two magistrates and a medical officer.[81] This process broke down in revolutionary Ireland where, except in Dublin, the police were severely compromised during the revolutionary period. As Ministry of Pensions officials in South Ireland noted: 'Under present conditions in Ireland, the arresting of lunatics is in abeyance, owing to other difficulties.'[82] High-profile republicans urged people to ignore and bypass the official court system before the Dáil announced the establishment of national arbitration courts in the summer of 1919. By June 1920, owing to the intimidation of witnesses and jurors in the British courts, the Royal Irish Constabulary noted that the popular 'Sinn Féin Courts' had superseded the conventional legal system.[83] Lunatics in numerous unspecified areas of Ireland were admitted via the partisan police force of the Irish Republic rather than the official Royal Irish Constabulary.[84] The Ministry of Pensions recognised their assistance would be unwelcome and extremely problematic with regards to insane British ex-servicemen. The Regional Director of the Ministry of Pensions in South Ireland noted the unsuitability and indignity of bringing ex-servicemen before legitimate police courts, describing it as 'a very undesirable method' due to the fact any dangerous lunatic often had to endure a night in a police cell before appearing before a magistrate the following morning.[85]

Despite the eventual introduction of the Service Patient scheme following a two-year delay, the Ministry in South Ireland accepted 'difficulties still arise owing to the present condition of asylums in Ireland.'[86] Grants from the government heavily subsidised Irish district asylums. Many local authorities in Ireland refused to recognise the government so did not submit their accounts for audit. Government grants were subsequently withdrawn, as were government subsidies on commodities such as flour, coal and sugar.[87] Asylums were forced to operate 'in a very reduced manner, and not admitting any patients if it is possible to avoid doing so.'[88] The Ministry of Pensions in Dublin recognised that 'owing to the local political difficulties there is not much tendency to assist the [insane] ex-soldier.'[89] The Ministry also wrote that the political situation was 'so acute that it is extremely difficult to get the superintendent of the asylum to take patients who have to be so transferred.'[90] Writing of the reluctance of admitting servicemen under treatment at Dublin military facilities into the Richmond Asylum in Dublin, the Ministry of Pensions clarified these difficulties:

> It is not the desire of the committee of this asylum at present instituted to have anything to do with service patients, and however the Ministry may meet them on this occasion, until there is some resettlement of a lasting nature of the present position in Ireland, there will be perpetual friction with this committee.[91]

In addition to public asylums, numerous Boards of Guardians similarly refused to admit British veterans into workhouse hospitals.[92]

Sugars noted relatives 'in a great number of cases refuse' to process the admission of an insane relative. The regulations of the Service Patient scheme stipulated that a doctor's fees for certification were only reimbursed by the Ministry of Pensions following classification as a Service Patient. Some relatives were unwilling to assume initial payment for certification.[93] The Ministry recognised that if a family member was unable to persuade an ex-serviceman to go to the asylum, then admission would also prove difficult.[94] This issue was also a problem in Britain.[95] On 15 March 1921, a special neurological board for the Ministry of Pensions in Dublin identified a combination of these issues which was problematising the certification of insane ex-servicemen in Ireland.[96] Ministry officials in London thus observed: 'It seems to be nobody's business to see these cases go to asylums.'[97] An unspecified number of mentally ill Irish Great War veterans were denied institutionalisation and may have instead sought Ministry treatment, further increasing its waiting lists.

Treatment allowances

In March 1921, 1,320 neurasthenic pensioners were awaiting out-patient or in-patient treatment in South Ireland for neurasthenia. This cost the Ministry £2,000 a week and £104,000 a year in the form of treatment allowances which provided maximum pensions to those awaiting treatment.[98] Neurasthenic pensioners were assumed by Ministry officials in London to prolong or exaggerate their symptoms to receive a bigger pension.[99] As one Ministry official in the West Midlands wrote: '[there is] a tendency to prolong these periods of out-patient treatment the patients not being ill, but being retained on the list for the sake of allowances.'[100] This scepticism was repeated in South Ireland with Forward reporting: 'In many instances I am convinced that men are kept on treatment allowances and in hospital solely on humanitarian grounds, and because they have no prospect of employment.' Forward reasoned that such 'action seems to be almost justifiable when all conditions are taken into considera-tion, and it is regarded that the only alternative is to stop allowances and allow the men to drift or starve.'[101] He further complained that 'a large sum is being annually expended on pensions and allowances', but 'no appreciable progress is being made.' [102] Dr Kaye, the Director of Medical Services for the Ministry of Pensions, observed that a liberal interpretation by Ministry officials in South Ireland in the transferral of pensioners for treatment helped to explain the bloated waiting list figures in the region by Ministry officials in South Ireland.[103]

A tightening in the distribution of treatment allowances by 1922 irked the British Legion. While accepting that the allocation of treatment allowances had been initially too liberal, the Legion held that they had now become too restricted.[104] The potential financially lucrative appeal of a provision of maximum treatment allowances does not fully explain high waiting list figures in South Ireland (Table 3 and Figure 7).

The 1921 War Pensions Act was introduced in the summer of 1921. The legislation initiated time limits on claims and final awards for disabilities that were judged to have reached permanency. As will be demonstrated in the proceeding chapter, these implementations would have huge implications on both the Ministry of Pensions and First World War veterans throughout the 1920s and 1930s. The 1921 War Pensions Act's ethos was to reduce the power of local pensions committees and to bring greater control and efficiency to

Table 3 Percentage of awaiting neurasthenic pensioners in receipt of a treatment allowance.

Region	Percentage of awaiting in-patients receiving treatment allowance	Percentage of pensioners receiving out-patient treatment receiving treatment allowance
Scotland	100	33
North	N/A	35
North Western	96	46
Yorkshire	100	35
Wales	100	43
North Midlands	30	0.5
Midlands	72	62
South West	42	4
London	69	26
Ulster	13	2
South Ireland	33	30

Percentages calculated from information provided in NA, PIN 15/56, Treatment of Neurasthenia, 1921–1922.

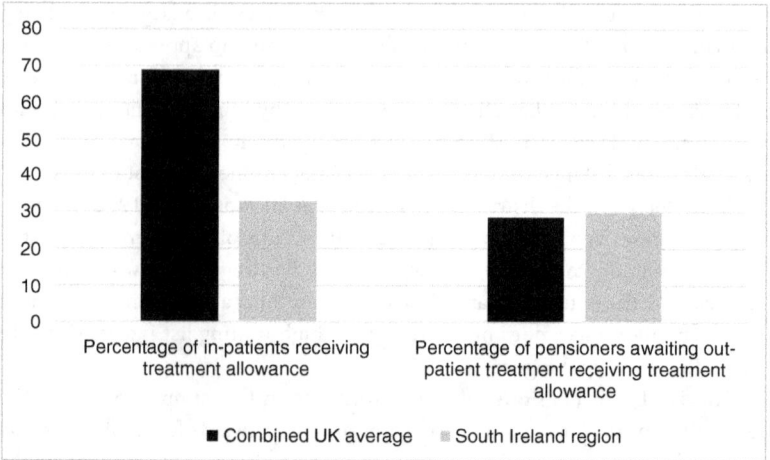

Figure 7 Comparison between the UK and South Ireland for awaiting neurasthenic pensioners in receipt of a treatment allowance. Percentages calculated from information provided in NA, PIN 15/56, Treatment of Neurasthenia, 1921–22.

permanent Ministry officials and to its central headquarters in London.[105] An analysis of correspondence discussing transferals for treatment amongst neurasthenic pensioners in South Ireland between regional Ministry officials in Dublin and those at London headquarters during the winter of 1921 illustrates the administrative clashes during this transitional period.

Despite a streamlining in waiting list figures and treatment allowances distributed in South Ireland, officials in London remained unsatisfied with the state of conditions in the region.[106] With the majority of neurasthenic pensioners in South Ireland not receiving treatment allowances, Ministry officials in London assumed that these men were 'capable of working and supporting their families.' Hebb wrote to Sugars asking 'are you convinced that those cases who are not in receipt of treatment allowances while waiting, do, in fact, require treatment at all.'[107] Sugars baulked at the query: 'The number of men on treatment allowances has been considerably reduced. This, apparently, does not satisfy you, but it would seem you want us to go further and say that these pensioners do not need treatment.' He further argued that the 229 cases 'fit for work' but still deemed as requiring treatment were 'very carefully investigated ... the opinion was definitely expressed by the specialist making the examination that the cases required neurological treatment.' Sugars assumed this as the correct procedure owing to the Ministry's repeated stress on employment in civil society on account of its therapeutic benefits: 'Your remarks suggest that in cases where, though recommended for treatment, a neurasthenic pensioner is, in the meantime, considered fit for work, it may not be necessary to consider the provision of such treatment. This is not what we have understood in this region.' Sugars described Hebb's position as 'very disconcerting' and 'points to a complete reversal of what was the policy of the Ministry.' He further queried: 'Is it to be understood that treatment should only be recommended for men in receipt of treatment allowances, or that the Ministry are of opinion that a pensioner not on treatment allowances is, ipso facto, not in need of treatment?'[108] In an attempt to defuse the situation, Hebb responded: 'I do not think you have been quite fair to my minute which was one rather asking a question than laying down a definitive law.' He assured Sugars that he and his staff should 'weigh the evidence in each case and act accordingly' before describing the comparative figures as both 'satisfactory' and 'remarkable.' Hebb went on to describe the neurasthenic pensioner as 'one of the most difficult' aspects within the department's entire jurisdiction. He reassured Sugars' confusion was expected as it was a process of 'getting experience.'[109]

Hebb's retreat was unsurprising due to the remit and function of the Ministry's regional setup. He had previously recognised the regional autonomy officials like Sugars possessed: 'the regions have it in their power to control the treatment of nervous disorders' and that it was 'impossible' to 'over-ride' their jurisdiction.[110] There was a discussion to provide more objective and uniform guidelines to ensure a level of conformity throughout the UK, but this was deemed impossible to achieve on account of the subjective nature of mental illness. Officials inspecting and dealing with neurasthenic pensioners could only assess 'each case on its merits.'[111] Hebb nonetheless still encouraged Sugars to make further enquiries as to investigate the accuracy of diagnoses. Repeating his opinion on the importance of employment, Hebb wrote:

> More and more we have become convinced that the work factor is the all-important one with the Neurasthenic, and that so long as a man is able to earn his livelihood the best remedy for his disease is to leave him at that occupation, unless it is entirely unsuitable, rather than to take him off and provide him with treatment in an institution where he will again on discharge have to find his place in the world, the result so frequently being that before he has obtained work his condition had become, through anxiety, worse than it was before the treatment commenced.[112]

Sugars initially followed Ministry policy by reducing the number of men awaiting treatment and those receiving treatment allowances. Despite pressure to make additional cuts to the waiting list figures, however, Sugars resisted further reductions.

Despite efforts to streamline waiting lists and reduce the number of those receiving treatment allowances, medico-pension officials like Sugars and Dawson who oversaw the assessment and treatment of neurasthenic pensioners in South Ireland may have been keener than their colleagues in Britain to recommend patients for treatment. In the absence of any records, it is possible that staff were aware of the dire outlook facing the neurasthenic pensioner. In July 1921, the Ministry in Ulster wrote that 'in a very large proportion of cases of the examination is valueless' owing to the leniency shown by medical referees associated with the Ministry.[113] Sugars could have challenged Dawson's recommendation as president of medical boards assessing neurasthenic claims and pensioners in Ireland. Yet, he seemingly backed Dawson's medical judgement and ignored urges from London to implement further reductions. While staff throughout South Ireland appear more inclined to recommend pensioners for treatment than their colleagues in Ulster or across the Irish Sea, available facilities did not match this preference.

Following his inspection in March 1921, Forward wrote of the inevitable 'congestion and stagnation' regarding Irish neurasthenic pensioners awaiting treatment owing to the lack of treatment facilities available.[114] He restrained on advocating for a vast increase in facilities assessing that 'no amount of psychotherapy' could alleviate the 'super-imposed anxiety' of unemployment and hostile reception a neurasthenic pensioner was likely to experience owing to the existing conditions in the region.[115] This observation is critical. While the lack of treatment facilities was unfortunate, Forward felt that the crucial problem was the experience of neurasthenic pensioners *outside* pension facilities and their treatment by contemporaries in civil society. In addition to policy disagreements and infrastructure and administrative problems persisting in revolutionary Ireland, it is necessary to look *beyond* the remit and function of the Ministry. This comprehensive contextual engagement centres the unfavourable societal reception and economic context which shaped mental ill-health and stunted veterans' recovery, contributing to the inflated waiting lists for associated treatment.

Social and political unrest

The Irish Federation of Discharged and Demobilised Sailors and Soldiers in Ireland wrote to the British Government in 1921 stressing 'that thousands of unemployed ex-servicemen in Ireland, particularly in the City of Dublin, are forced to line up in queues and accept charity.'[116] One report produced by the Southern Irish Loyalists Association (SILA), described the change in socio-political circumstances between 1914 and 1918: 'When the war was over these men returned to their own country to find it in the throes of a political upheaval which culminated in the Rebellion against the rule of the British government for whom they had been fighting in every part of the world.'[117] South Ireland would provide the neurasthenic pensioner with the least favourable homecoming conditions in the UK.

Following his review of Ireland in 1921, Forward wrote to colleagues in London that it is impossible to 'meet and overcome the existing difficulties occasioned by social and political unrest ... it cannot be expected that any reduction will take place in the numbers of men listed for treatment for neurasthenia.'[118] The ineffectiveness of increasing treatment capacity in the existing political climate was further explained: 'Regarding the stress to which men are now subjected owing to internal troubles, I am inclined to anticipate that the numbers are more likely to increase than decrease.' Forward reasoned that the Ministry of Pensions would achieve little to justify either its current or additional financial expense in the region.[119] Forward acknowledged the increased difficulties for veterans in South Ireland:

> These patients, in addition to their nervous disabilities resulting from the stress of War, all have the super-added anxiety states occasioned by the hopeless outlook for the future in respect of their obtaining employment, and in earning the means wherewith to maintain themselves and their dependants.[120]

Unemployment was a common experience for neurasthenic veterans due to the societal stigma which attached itself to their diagnosis. This problem was especially acute in South Ireland.

Bleak employment opportunities were evident in Ireland. Except for Belfast, the economic, labour and industrial context in Ireland was recognised by the Ministry of Labour as being 'fundamentally different' to Britain.[121] Ireland between 1920 and 1921 constituted a period of economic austerity followed by a deep depression.[122] While emigration had allowed an estimated 30,000 Irish men and women to emigrate annually before 1914, it was banned during the conflict, further inflating the labour market.[123] Great War veterans were also likelier to be amongst the unskilled and illiterate section of the labour force, further compromising their employability.[124] The estimated unemployment rate amongst the ex-service community across Ireland amounted to 46 percent in comparison to just 10 percent in Britain.[125] Even preceding the escalation of violence in Ireland, the Ministry of Transport estimated that there were 40,000 unemployed ex-servicemen in Ireland.[126] In addition to the unfavourable economic conditions prevalent for citizens throughout the UK, there is evidence to suggest that British ex-servicemen were actively discriminated against. Arnold remained a Ministry official in South Ireland following the decentralisation of

Ministry authority to regional headquarters. Arnold summed up the dramatic shift in the socio-political context ensuring the country Irishmen left in the early years of the war was fundamentally changed by the time of their return:

> The political strife which had at first boiled up in Southern Ireland at the Rebellion of Easter 1916 was seeming more and more menacing. At the elections in the autumn of 1918 the Sinn Fein party had swept the board in Ireland. Almost every constituency outside Ulster returned Sinn Féin candidates who pledged to secure the independence of Ireland: there was only seven of the old nationalist party left. Ever since 1916 the war had been unpopular in southern Ireland ... the whole tenor of the country was one of opposition of British rule.[127]

Arnold's identification of a change in public sentiment and growing anti-Britishness is verified by Wilfred Rhodes on active service in Athlone with the Royal Field Artillery. In 1917, Rhodes described the town as 'a seething bed of Sinn Féinism.'[128] As early as January 1918, the Ministry of Pensions was able to pick up on 'apathy' and 'anti-British feelings' amongst the southern Irish population. Local populaces often did little to engage with local war pension committees, with local councils even refusing to cooperate with or contribute financially to their operations.[129] Arnold's role as a Ministry official required him to travel across the region, and he noticed the detrimental impact that the Anglo-Irish War was having on departments like his own, writing: 'The sands of British administration in Southern Ireland now "the Republic" were running low and we saw them disappear in blood and misrule.'[130] This opposition to British rule would shape the reception of returning British ex-servicemen, including those disabled by war service.

The mentally and physically disabled would often share homecoming conditions. Forward concluded his report on Ireland with the thesis: 'I may add that my personal concern is with those men who are suffering from Neurasthenia but the same conditions, and suggestions put forward, are equally applicable to those suffering from other disabilities.'[131] A Ministry of Labour report into the position of British ex-servicemen in Ireland in March 1921, similarly recognised that the wider socio-economic and political conditions prevalent in South Ireland had a detrimental impact on all disabled Great War pensioners regardless of their ailment.[132] Henry Dale, a former professional soldier and veteran of the Royal Irish Rifles in receipt of a 40 percent pension for a gunshot wound of the left leg, pleaded with Ministry officials in South Ireland to increase his pension. Alluding to the existing 'state of things of Ireland' in 1920, Dale wrote: 'I cannot get work. I am at present living in the height of poverty ... I never knew that by serving my king and country little did I think when I was pouring my blood out on the fields of Belgium and France that I would be placed in such poverty and starvation afterwards.'[133] Writing to the office of David Lloyd George in February 1920, the National Federation of Discharged and Demobilised Sailors and Soldiers in Dublin commented on the plight of ex-servicemen like Dale:

> There is, as you know, an enormous amount of unrest in the country at the present moment and the many injustices under which the ex-servicemen are labouring are calculated to do anything but alleviate their unrest. The plight to the ex-servicemen in Ireland is getting more and more serious as the time goes on. As you know, as far as employment is concerned they are totally and absolutely boycotted and I think their case calls for special attention.[134]

The Ministry of Labour similarly conveyed that unemployment was by 'far the most important factor' for the ex-serviceman community, becoming an 'urgent problem' that required intervention. The department accredited the lack of employment squarely on an 'upheaval' in the 'political atmosphere' which occurred in the region in the aftermath of the Easter Rising: 'Since the signing of the Armistice the discharged and demobilised Irish solder has been returning to Ireland, only to find that his own people have nothing but contempt to offer him for his patriotism and sacrifice, and he is denied the right to work or live in the country in which he fought.'[135] Under such circumstances, disabled ex-servicemen were 'seething with discontent at nothing having been done for them and were mocked at for having served in the British Army.'[136]

Forward reasoned that employers were reluctant to employ Great War veterans due to intimidation from republicans or in fear of upsetting republicans already on the payroll. The 'crime' of serving in the British Army was 'regarded as sufficient grounds to merit such hostile treatment.'[137] The Irish Federation of Discharged and Demobilised Sailors and Soldiers in Ireland agreed: 'The majority of their employers have had no military or naval service and are members of political organisations which have openly expressed their hostility to the ex-servicemen.'[138] Service in the British Armed Forces marked some ex-servicemen as outsiders. On becoming a postman in Cork, for example, one British Army veteran received a threatening letter emphasising that 'no ex-soldiers are wanted' and demanding that he relinquished his post.[139] Several unemployed Great War veterans believed that their previous service was a detriment to their employability prospects.[140] The Ministry of Labour failed to provide universal employment and felt impotent operating in Ireland during the period: 'It is not within the power of the Ministry of Labour however effectively staffed to provide any radical solution to the problem of the disabled soldier.'[141] Another report explained this bleak prognosis: 'So long as the present political attitude is maintained, it is almost hopeless to expect to find after employment for the disabled ex-service man.'[142]

On 17 February 1920, the National Federation of Discharged and Demobilised Sailors and Soldiers wrote to the office of the British Prime Minister asking him 'to bear in mind that the Irish ex-servicemen has no friends capable of helping him in his own country, and he looks to the government for that assistance which he justly considers his right.'[143] Though accepting that the letter effectively conveyed their desperate plight, the Ministry of Labour advised Lloyd George's office not to reply. The department explained 'the trouble is due to a kink in the Irish brain.' It was decreed that regardless of any British intervention, 'it is not in our power, or for that matter, in the power of any department, or of the government as a whole to straighten out this kink.'[144] Such attitudes regarding a 'kink in the Irish brain' were long established.

Assessments of how Irish civilians viewed the British ex-serviceman during this period are hard to define. Research into the Irish War of Independence stresses the uneven violence and IRA activity throughout Ireland.[145] While severely compromising British authority in Ireland, the Dáil Éireann failed to get a firm hold on local militancy across Ireland. Sinn Féin also proved far more successful in urban areas during the Irish local elections in 1920. Recruitment returns and the national vote on the Anglo-Irish Treaty, which would decide the cessation or continuation of the Anglo-Irish War and Ireland's future relationship with Britain, were similarly dictated by regional attitudes.[146] These regional variations also impacted on the treatment of returning Great War veterans. Violence and hostility during the Anglo-Irish War varied by geographical region, as did reprisals against ex-servicemen. Employment discrimination was similarly area-dependent with the unemployability of returning veterans correlating with scanter enlistment trends.[147] The Ministry of Pensions often overlooked the importance of regionality.

Economic stagnation and an oversubscribed labour supply were further hampered by the Anglo-Irish War which dissuaded investment and new initiatives from facilitating employment.[148] One conservative estimate calculated that revolutionary hostilities could cost as much as £50,000,000 per year in damage and infrastructure. This figure amounted to over 30 percent of national output.[149] A combination of these factors made it inevitable that many ex-servicemen in South Ireland became unemployed. The economic situation in Ulster was not much better. Although industries such as linen making and shipbuilding had experienced a boom during the First World War, these industries struggled from 1920 onwards. This unstable period again discouraged investment and economic investment in the region ensuring widespread unemployment.[150] In the words of Richard Grayson, few Ulstermen 'found that the land to which they returned to was fit for heroes.'[151] It was, however, Catholic ex-servicemen who faced the most unfavourable post-demobilisation experience. While veterans of the UVF had a better likelihood of attaining employment, Catholics were in danger of being denied or removed from employment. Industries such as shipbuilding experienced sectarian discrimination and violence and intimidation. Many Catholics felt prevented from attaining work or were banished from their employment, such as on the Belfast shipyards, including men who had seen active service during the First World War.[152]

One Catholic Great War veteran in Belfast stated: 'If this is the thanks you get for serving your King and country no wonder people uphold Sinn Féin ideals.'[153] Catholic pensioners suffering from neurasthenia felt their religion led to discrimination being meted out by employers and Ministry of Pensions officials. In April 1921, one Catholic ex-servicemen, Michael Cunningham, wrote to the regional headquarters in Belfast: 'You must be aware that all Catholics (ex-servicemen included) has been deprived of the right to work and earn a living in this city of cowards, bigots and some knaves.' Of the Ministry of Pensions charged with helping him, Cunningham wrote: 'This establishment is not I am sorry to say the place where men of my religious and political beliefs may apply for justice.' Cunningham felt aggrieved that he only received a 20 percent pension for his mental disability. With Cunningham's confidential pension records describing him as a 'rabid Sinn Féiner', his feelings of persecution may have had merit, and further emphasises the subjective biases of Ministry officials.[154]

Writing about the difficulty in alleviating the unemployment experienced by ex-servicemen in South Ireland, Sergeant Humber Wolfe, an official at the Ministry of Labour, attested:

> The position as revealed by these men, is so serious and, indeed, so pitiful, that I do not feel we can any longer maintain the position that we will administer the regulations identically for England and Ireland. The feeling which I have in my mind is that we shall have to treat the Irish ex-service men in something the same way as disabled ex-service men in this country. We shall, in fact, have to say just as disability in England makes it impossible for a man to resume his old occupation so military service in Ireland itself disqualified a man for employment.[155]

Wolfe's view that able-bodied British ex-servicemen in South Ireland should be treated as disabled ex-servicemen were in Britain perfectly illustrates the unfortunate position of disabled veterans in the region. Disabled veterans were disabled twice via their literal war wounds *and* through their association with the British Army. By 1922, 3,194 disabled men awaited training in South Ireland while 855 were undergoing some form of Ministry of Labour training.[156] Despite the much higher enlistment figures, waiting list figures in Britain amounted to 4,806 men.[157] It was, however, placing these men in relevant employment after their training which proved most difficult.[158] Like Ministry of Pensions facilities, the five facilities aimed at training disabled men for future employment in South Ireland suffered a 'small amount of damage and loss of stores' as a result of nearby hostilities involving the British Army, the IRA and the Black and Tans during the conflict.[159] The Ministry of Labour described the training scheme for disabled ex-servicemen in Ireland as being of 'a most irregular nature' and 'very unsatisfactory.'[160] The lack of relevant positions to accommodate the newly trained ex-serviceman was especially detrimental to the training scheme.[161] Problems manifested in South Ireland as the training provided was largely industrial while such positions were at a premium in the region.[162]

In May 1919, the Ministry of Pensions appreciated that 'few facilities exist for disabled soldiers in Ireland such that exist in England and many of the men are really badly off.'[163] The Irish Federation of Discharged and Demobilised Sailors and Soldiers in Ireland wrote: 'The training of disabled men under the Ministry of Labour is admittedly a failure. The small number of men in Ireland who have received training have joined the ranks of the unemployed and are in the unhappy position of having received an elementary training in a capacity in which they see no prospect of employment.'[164] Hostility towards the Ministry of Labour's scheme was also in evidence: 'The hostile attitude of firms and employers appears to increase rather than diminish as time goes on … It need scarcely be added, that the political unrest does not tend to diminish the hostile attitude of both employers and their employees towards the discharged ex-service man.'[165]

Gordon Campbell, a Ministry of Labour official in South Ireland, cited the 'very special problem' of training disabled ex-servicemen: 'with such a surplus of labour it is extremely difficult to obtain employment for the four or five thousand disabled men in the country … There is little industry at the moment, little prospect of any developments.' This dearth was intensified by 'political considerations [which] add other and very serious difficulties.'[166] Even when employment for trained ex-servicemen was available, it remains doubtful how beneficial it proved to neurasthenic pensioners. The Regional Director for the West Midlands Ministry of Pensions region stated occupational treatment proved fruitless as 'difficulty is experienced with the employers, who are often unwilling to accept men after they had heard details of their disability.'[167]

Further difficulties arose in revolutionary Ireland as it did not implement the King's National Roll due to republican and trade union resistance.[168] The *Irish Times* deduced that this opposition largely stemmed from republicans positioned in trade union official quarters, who were largely socialist, and had previously opposed Irish involvement in an imperialist war as seen in their staunch and active support during the Conscription Crisis of 1918 in Ireland. The report also wrote there was little opposition to this position from the general public who felt it was 'justified.'[169] A malfunctioning training scheme and the absence of a King's National Roll thus provided a minimal practical benefit to the employment of disabled Great War veterans residing in revolutionary Ireland. The likelihood of attaining employment post-discharge from a training centre in England was held to be 'very dark.' [170] While accepting that physically and mentally disabled British ex-servicemen shared similar homecoming conditions in Ireland, the situation in South Ireland was darker still for those Irishmen suffering from neurasthenia.

Safety, danger and recovery from trauma

In addition to the IRA murdering serving RIC members, retired police officers feared for their lives during the guerrilla conflict due to their former British connections.[171] Despite the irregular spread of violence across revolutionary Ireland, British ex-servicemen averaged almost 50 percent of 'spies' assassinated by the IRA. In counties Kilkenny, Meath and Wexford, for example, British veterans constituted three-quarters and above of mortality figures.[172] There has been intense historiographical debate as to why British ex-servicemen were targeted for violent reprisal. Jane Leonard and Peter Hart argue that the IRA meted out violence to British ex-servicemen due to their former army service. By contrast, Paul Taylor re-evaluates the British veteran's status as a victim of republican militancy, emphasising that ex-servicemen shared with the wider adult male population the risk of suspicion and retribution.[173]

Historians of Ireland during the revolutionary period emphasise how society sketchily and fluidly defined populations within society as 'outsiders.' First World War veterans in nationalist Ireland often lived as a distinct class of people with potential British sympathies which seemingly increased their likelihood of being suspected of fraternising with agents of the British state. British ex-servicemen becoming more liable to interact with individuals connected to the British crown does not equate to their likelihood of being informers for the British state.[174] O'Halpin stresses the importance of this social ostracism, arguing that volunteering for British Army service and casual contact with serving British soldiers in Ireland increased the likelihood of violent retribution. The poor social standing of First World War veterans in Ireland contributed to republican suspicions. Many unemployed veterans also partook in seeking casual work by travelling across Ireland in search of it, which may have created further doubt as to their motives and distrust of their character amongst IRA officials. It has even been speculated that British ex-servicemen remaining in regular correspondence with agents of the British state, such as the War Office and the Ministry of Pensions, or traumatised ex-servicemen acting erratically, may have created further suspicion.[175] Brian Hughes theorises that it would have been easier for a militant republican to validate the assassination of ex-servicemen who had, in all likelihood, previously wounded or killed others themselves.[176] It was, therefore, the marginalised position of British ex-servicemen in Irish nationalist society which explains why they were excessively targeted, rather than specifically and universally besieged, by the IRA.

Regardless of the precise causality, the *awareness* of an increased threat to their livelihood would have been psychologically catastrophic to traumatised Great War veterans. The therapeutic importance of the post-war 'environment' and the need for a shell-shocked ex-serviceman to 'come out of his shell' and peacefully reintegrate in society is cited in wartime medical literature.[177] One medical publication, published in 1920, notes an appreciative recognition for 'past suffering' and 'the feeling of injustice' helped or hindered a pensioner's neurasthenic condition.[178] Neil Diamant reviews the existing literature on the homecoming of returning ex-servicemen of twentieth and twenty-first-century wars to argue that societal attitudes towards a conflict, and notions of its perceived worthiness, have been a constant factor in dictating the reintegration of veteran communities.[179] Jonathan Shay analyses the homecoming experience of traumatised combat veterans across three millennia to similarly argue that safety, acceptance, respect and being part of their country's future are crucial in the mental wellbeing of an ex-combatant.[180] This correlation is evidenced by Prisoners of Wars of the Vietcong's infamous 'Hanoi Hilton' who experienced lower rates of PTSD in comparison to GIs despite the brutal conditions of their captivity. By way of an explanation, their lower rates of PTSD have been attributed to their superior homecoming as they were celebrated and welcomed home like 'returning astronauts' with public meetings with President Richard Nixon and special homecoming parades.[181] These therapeutic measures also apply to wider traumatised communities. Judith Herman cites the establishment of safety as the foundational block allowing traumatised people to build their recovery. Once established, a regaining of their state of mind is achievable only when a traumatised individual reconnects with an ordinary life similar to the one they had experienced before the moment of trauma.[182] The fundamental building blocks of safety, recognition and the potential to peacefully reintegrate into a familiar lifestyle were absent in revolutionary Ireland.

Ex-servicemen in South Ireland were denied employment, including those disabled as a result of war service. Some GAA clubs even disqualified ex-servicemen from joining, and in Munster, an area which experienced intense activity during the fight for independence, local councils and poor law boards barred the enlistment of ex-soldiers with local post offices and railway companies being obliged to do the same.[183] A secretary of the Dublin War Pensions committee attested:

> A reaction took place in Dublin in this sense that these men went off amidst applause and god-speeds, but in the intervening period things happened in Ireland, and when these men came back disabled and broken down in some cases they found that their own relatives had changed their views on public affairs and matters were extremely uncomfortable for the unfortunate man.

The sacrifice of mind and body did not, therefore, protect an ex-serviceman: 'The public in its resentment is inclined to threaten the disabled man.'[184] There were even misgivings about insane Service Patients being differentiated in clothing or identification in the Irish asylum owing to 'the present feeling against the Army in many parts of Ireland.'[185] Elderly veterans would later recall instances of intimidation while out in post-Easter Rising Dublin on pass from Ministry hospitals in their distinctive 'Hospital Blues' uniforms.[186] Disabled British veterans shared with non-combatant veterans the ire of republicans and the existing anti-British sentiment. Former medical personnel also recounted their experience of intimidation, stigma and unemployment owing to the strength of hostility regarding former service for the British Army.[187]

Previous work into stigma and mental illness has recognised the highly fluid and interpersonal nature of stigma.[188] Interactions and perceptions of mentally ill British ex-servicemen in Ireland are similarly difficult to universalise. Evidence suggests that psychoneurotic veterans in Ireland were stigmatised by both their disability *and* British connections. Forward acknowledges that the neurasthenic pensioner was not exempt from 'the present hostile attitude which is directed collectively and individually against men who served in the late war.'[189] Wounded and disabled British ex-servicemen men lived in fear for their wellbeing. The discharge of servicemen under treatment at the King George V Hospital, a military hospital in Dublin, was compromised. The Ministry of Pensions was wary of 'the possibility of action being taken by their neighbours on their returning home, which may make them in a worse condition than they were when they were admitted to hospital.'[190] The department wrote: 'The difficulties in this connection explain largely the aggravation in their condition which frequently occurs after men have been discharged from hospital.' As a result of this situation, and the ensuing lack of assistance and employment available, 'the actual condition and the duration of stay in hospital' of a neurasthenic soldier was 'very much affected by the present situation in Ireland.'[191] Living in Donegal in July 1921, O'Ryan's condition was affected by the ongoing conflict in Ireland and the perceived hostility aimed towards British forces. Ministry officials during one meeting recorded that 'he confesses to being afraid of Irish rebels.'[192] It is, of course, difficult to determine from welfare records the 'true' causation of a man's disability, especially when it comes to psychological symptoms. As Jason Crouthamel argues: 'It is arguably more important to analyse how traumatised men perceived their injuries.'[193] Whether real, imagined or exaggerated, veterans of the First World War *perceived* a threat from militant republicans, as did medical staff at the King George V Hospital.

Ex-servicemen in the north were again adversely affected by broader sectarian divisions. One Ministry out-patient clinic in Belfast was shut for several weeks due to the volatile sectarian disturbances in 1920.[194] Neurasthenic Catholics in Ulster undergoing in-patient treatment in Craigavon Hospital suffered from intimidation via anonymous personal threats. A letter sent to one Catholic ex-servicemen published in the *Freemans Journal* reveals the sectarian and overtly hostile extent of the threats:

> [You] and all the others are known; so look out for what you get if any of you traitor dogs are got about the place in 3 days from now. Death to rebels and papists, red hand for ever. Don't blame men in hospital, but we won't have you among loyalists. You low bred swine. You and your sieeking [sic] dogs of papish – must go . £5 reward won't save yous, nor will Popes, Priests, Holy Water ... Time's up. Go or we will riddle every rotten Papish both in Craigavon and UVF., as you are a rotten lot of bastards.[195]

Colonel Spender, Secretary to the Cabinet, Northern Parliament remarked to Lionel Curtis, who worked for the colonial secretary on Irish affairs: 'Probably the threats are not really of a very serious character from a purely psychological point of view, but when conveyed to ex-servicemen suffering from shell-shock, they are of a most cowardly character and unfortunately produce a great effect on the individual.' There was at least one threat given to a Protestant ex-serviceman at the institution, but this was dismissed as merely a reprisal.[196] Seemingly at their own request or, at least, with their blessing, most Catholic in-patients were subsequently transferred to another unnamed hospital. While the location of their new treatment facility was not published, Leopardstown Hospital was the only facility in Ireland equitable to the treatment facilities afforded in Craigavon Hospital.[197] The treatment of mentally ill Catholic in-patients at Craigavon was the very antithesis of what the Ministry's secluded and scenic in-patient facilities were aiming to provide: complete withdrawal from the war and thoughts of conflict and danger.[198] The experience of Craigavon supports previous research which argues that, despite its deep respect for the British ex-service community, the dominant ideology of Protestant unionism in Ulster was enough to ostracise and persecute mentally disabled Catholic veterans.[199]

The societal isolation of British ex-servicemen in the predominantly nationalist South Ireland and of Catholic veterans in the broadly unionist Ulster should not be understated. One voluntary pensions worker assessed that the emotional and psychological benefits of sympathy and gratitude were far more valuable to a disabled veteran than a compensatory pension.[200] Comparison between the neurasthenic pensioner in South Ireland and the Vietnam War veteran in America suffering from PTSD is pertinent. As Bourke writes: 'psychological collapse was more frequent when servicemen were returning to a country vastly different from the place veterans had left.'[201] Any direct comparison, however, would underplay the atrocious homecoming conditions that mentally ill Irish veterans experienced. Their war service was not only unpopular but potentially viewed as treacherous. In addition to societal suspicion and ostracism, the perception of a threat against their person also existed.

Conclusion

One British ex-service journal wrote that there was 'no disillusionment like the disillusionment of returning' during a veteran's 'return to a world that does not want him of the man who knows he has saved it.'[202] The potential for disillusionment was manifested in revolutionary Ireland. Not only was homecoming daunting but it was also potentially dangerous and psychologically catastrophic. The treatment of neurasthenic pensioners in South Ireland suffered from several crucial factors distinct to the region. First of all, the Anglo-Irish conflict severely compromised the work of pension staff. Staff throughout the region were unable to visit, assess and transfer patients for treatment within Ministry facilities or even admit Service Patients into district asylums amid ongoing guerrilla conflict. Additional anti-British sentiment combined with the stigma of mental illness to further limit a neurasthenic pensioners' potential for employment in nationalist Ireland. Militant republicanism even added to the stresses and strains of psychoneurotic veterans who lived in fear of IRA reprisal because of their perceived British sympathies. The unfortunate position of pensioners in the region may have increased the likelihood of regional staff, given significant local autonomy thanks to the Ministry's decentralisation ethos, transferring men for treatment. This likelihood was not matched by available facilities, with the British Government reluctant to invest further finances in the region while its political future remained so precarious. These factors better explain the inflated waiting list figures in South Ireland. The region provided the most unsuitable homecoming conditions for mentally ill pensioners in the UK. Veterans discovered their government and society considered them to have fought for the wrong side.

Veterans returned to South Ireland having fought in an army now considered by many as the enemy, and in a conflict many began to see as an unfortunate reminder of an uncomfortable past. Ireland reflects similar complex ethnonational conflicts amongst combatant nations and their impact on returning veterans. Such a reversal of fortune could also apply to men from Alsace and Lorraine, who fought in the German Army, or men from Croatia, who had fought against the Serbs as a member of the Austrian Army and now found themselves living in the newly established Yugoslavia. The psychological implication of this reversal was catastrophic. To add insult to injury, Irish neurasthenic pensioners were blamed for their illness. Long-held and widespread assumptions amongst British officialdom permeated, allowing Baldie and Wallace to dismiss Irish waiting list figures as being a result of the widely assumed biological predisposition to mental illness.

The Ministry remained influenced by long-held discriminatory discourse despite the progressive compensation and innovative treatment it offered to neurasthenic pensioners. While the First World War has been cited as a clear demarcation line between the Victorian period and the modern era, and shell-shock as a huge contributory factor in the progress of mental-health treatment, a continuation of cultural discourse was also in evidence. Previous research into the homecoming of combat veterans assesses that psychoneurotic veterans expect and require an appreciation of their sacrifice of nerves, treatment to aid their recovery and financial compensation via pensions. In revolutionary nationalist Ireland, neurasthenic pensioners regularly just received the latter. Bourke is therefore right to assert that these mentally disabled Great War veterans' 'sacrifice of nerves did not end in 1918.'[203] This partial rehabilitation would continue into the 1920s and 1930s as Ireland was diplomatically split into Northern Ireland and the Irish Free State.

Notes

1. NA, PIN 15/56, Memorandum on Conference of Neurological D.Cs.M.S. held at Headquarters, 17 June 1921.
2. Ibid., Ministry of Pensions, Dublin, to Ministry of Pensions, London, 24 November 1921.
3. Ibid.
4. Ibid., Memorandum on Conference of Neurological D.Cs.M.S. held at Headquarters, 17 June 1921.

5 Ibid.
6 Ibid.
7 Bourke, 'Shell-shock, psychiatry and the Irish soldier', 159.
8 John Rylands Library, University of Manchester, GES/2, 'Race, Nationality and Character' (1918) by Grafton Elliot Smith.
9 Bourke, 'Shell-shock, psychiatry and the Irish soldier', 159; Bourke, 'Effeminacy, ethnicity and the end of trauma', 61; NA, PIN 15/56, Memorandum on Conference of Neurological D.Cs.M.S. held at Headquarters on Friday, 17 June 1921.
10 As Richard Evans argues, 'The gaps in a document, what it does not mention, are often just as interesting as what it contains'; Richard Evans, *In Defence of History* (London: Granta, 1997), 92.
11 NA, PIN 15/56, Treatment of Neurasthenia, 1921–1922.
12 As was the case in Britain, clearly physically unsuitable men were able to enlist in the British Army in Ireland. This was due to both inadequate medical checks during the enlistment process and the desperate desire for manpower; Michael Robinson, 'Broken soldiers: the chaos of enlistment in the British Army in the early months of the Great War', *History Ireland*, 24 (2016), 30–4.
13 This infamous quote was much derided by champions of disabled ex-servicemen such as James Hogge MP who helped establish the National Federation of Discharged and Demobilised Sailors and Soldiers; Cohen, *The War Come Home*, 24; Barham, *Forgotten Lunatics of the Great War*, 110–11, 392.
14 Bettinson, 'Lost Souls in the House of Restoration', 36.
15 Bourke, 'Shell-shock, psychiatry and the Irish soldier', 156.
16 NA, PIN 15/56, Memorandum on Conference of Neurological D.Cs.M.S. held at Headquarters, 17 June 1921.
17 NA, PIN 15/55, Ethnal Shakespeare to Director General of Medical Services, London, 12 December 1919.
18 NA, PIN 15/56, Ministry of Pensions, Dublin, to Ministry of Pensions, London, 24 November 1921.
19 Deborah Stone, *The Disabled State* (Basingstoke: Macmillan, 1984), 26–7; Paul Longmore, *Why I Burned My Book and Other Essays on Disability* (Philadelphia: Temple University Press, 2003), 58.
20 Smith and Pear, *Shell Shock and its Lessons*, 52; Jean Lepine, *Mental Disorders of War* (London: University of London Press, 1919), 193; HC Debates, 12 December 1922, vol. 159, cols 2694–855; HC Debates, 9 May 1923, vol. 54, cols 56–62; Bourke, *Dismembering the Male*, 118; Leese, *Shell-Shock*, 131; Mitchell and Smith, *Medical Services*, 341.
21 Stone, 'The Military and Industrial Roots of Clinical Psychology in Britain', 202–3.
22 NA, PIN 15/56, Ministry of Pensions, London, to Ministry of Pensions, Dublin, 21 December 1921.
23 Leese, *Shell-Shock*, 124; similar theories supporting the need for war neurotics to be engaged in employment to aid their recovery were supported in Germany by the

Weimar Government; Greg Eghigian, 'The German welfare state as a discourse of trauma', in Mark Micale and Paul Lerner (eds), *Traumatic Pasts: History, Psychiatry, and Trauma in the Modern Age, 1870–1930* (Cambridge: Cambridge University of Press, 2001), 107–8.

24   Bourke, *Dismembering the Male*, 118.

25   NA, PIN 15/56, Memorandum on Conference of Neurological D.Cs.M.S. held at Headquarters, 17 June 1921.

26   Mike Mantin, 'Coalmining and the national scheme for disabled ex-servicemen after the First World War', *Social History*, 41:2 (2016), 155–70.

27   Eghigian, 'The German welfare state as a discourse of trauma', 107–8; NA, PIN 15/4200, 'Extracts from the Report of a Conference held at Ottawa in December 1936 of a Board of Psychiatrists and Neurologists appointed by the Canadian Government', 136.

28   Noel Whiteside, 'Counting the cost: sickness and disability among working people in an era of industrial recession, 1920-39', *Economic History Review*, 40:2 (1987), 228–46.

29   Richard J. McNally and B. Christopher Freuh, 'Why are Iraq and Afghanistan veterans seeking PTSD disability compensation at unprecedented rates?', *Journal of Anxiety Disorders*, 27:5 (2013), 524–5.

30   Allan Young, 'Trauma and Harm', plenary presented to Cultures of Harm in Institutions of Care: Historical and Contemporary Perspectives, Birkbeck University, 14 April 2016.

31   There is debate as to whether PTSD represents a timeless and universal ailment or whether traumatic ailments are historically dependent, being shaped by the existing socio-cultural values in which they occurred; Paul Lerner and Mark Mikale, 'Trauma, psychiatry, and history: a conceptual and historiographical introduction', in Mark Micale and Paul Lerner (eds), *Traumatic Pasts: History, Psychiatry, and Trauma in the Modern Age, 1870–1930* (Cambridge: Cambridge University Press, 2001), 6–7; see, for example, the classic text on the history of trauma and the evolution of PTSD: Allan Young, *The Harmony of Illusions: Inventing Post-Traumatic Stress Disorder* (Princeton: Princeton University Press, 1995).

32   Millais Culpin, 'The problem of the neurasthenic pensioner', *British Journal of Psychology*, 1 (1921), 326.

33   NA, PIN 15/56, Ministry of Pensions, East Midlands, to Ministry of Pensions, London, 15 November 1921.

34   Bourke, 'Effeminacy, ethnicity and the end of trauma', 65.

35   NA, PIN 15/57, The Chronic Mental.

36   Jessica Meyer, *Men of War: Masculinity and the First World War in Britain* (Basingstoke: Palgrave Macmillan, 2009), 97; Jones and Wessely, *From Shell-Shock to PTSD*, 133.

37   Douglas McMurtrie, *The Disabled Soldier* (New York: Arno Press, 1919), 105.

38   C. W. Hutt, *The Future of the Disabled Soldier* (London: Bale & Co, 1917), 154–60.

39   NA, PIN 15/56, Memorandum on Conference of Neurological D.Cs.M.S. held at Headquarters, 17 June 1921.

40 NA, PIN 26/16836, Peter Fitzpatrick Pension File.
41 *Reveille*, 3 (February, 1919), 440.
42 The historiography of the Anglo-Irish War is extensive. A suitable overview is provided in Michael Hopkinson, *The Irish War of Independence* (Montreal: McGill University Press, 2004).
43 Steven O'Connor, '"It's up to you now to fight for your own country": Ireland's Great War veterans in the War of Independence', in David Swift and Oliver Wilkinson (eds), *Veterans of the First World War: Ex-servicemen and Ex-servicewomen in Post-War Britain and Ireland* (Oxon: Routledge, 2019), 104–20.
44 NA, PIN 15/56, Ministry of Pensions, Dublin, to Ministry of Pensions, London, 24 November 1921.
45 Arnold's Typescript Recollections, 128.
46 NA, MH 120/12, County Cavan Local Committee to Ministry of Pensions, Belfast, 8 November 1920.
47 NA, LAB 2/855/ED5412/7/1921, Meeting of the Minutes with the Parliamentary Secretary of the Ministry of Transport, 4 May 1920.
48 NA, PIN 15/2998, Ministry of Pensions, Dublin, to Ministry of Pensions, London, 21 February 1921.
49 Ibid., Commissioner of Medical Services, Dublin, to Ministry of Pensions, London, 4 March 1921; Ministry of Pensions, Dublin, to Ministry of Pensions, London, 23 March 1921.
50 Ibid., Ministry of Pensions, Dublin, to Ministry of Pensions, London, 7 February 1921.
51 NA, PIN 15/325, Claims for Compensation for Malicious Damage.
52 NA, PIN 15/2998, Ministry of Pensions, note, 10 March 1921.
53 One Medical Officer working for the Guinness Brewery in Dublin protested the personal threat to his safety carrying out his professional duties in the city; David Durnin, 'Ireland's British Army doctors and the treatment of Irish nationalists, 1916–23', in Ian Miller and David Durnin (eds), *Medicine, Health and Irish Experiences of Conflict, 1914–45* (Manchester: Manchester University Press, 2016), 98–9.
54 John Borgovono, 'Revolution, ex-servicemen and the Cork branch of the National Federation of Discharged and Demobilised Sailors and Soldiers, 1918–1921', in David Swift and Oliver Wilkinson (eds), *Veterans of the First World War: Ex-servicemen and Ex-servicewomen in Post-War Britain and Ireland* (Oxon: Routledge, 2019), 94.
55 NA, PIN 15/325, Claims for Compensation for Malicious Damage.
56 The heist occurred the day when the office had large amounts of money on the premises. The IRA cut the telephone wires in the office and had men placed in the street on observation, and a getaway car nearby. Ibid., Ministry of Pensions, note, 25 November 1920; Ministry of Pensions, Cork, to Ministry of Pensions, Dublin, 24 November 1920.
57 Hart, *The IRA and its Enemies*, 81.

58 Ibid., 72.
59 NA, T 161/24/2, Hospitals: Ireland – Buildings Maliciously damaged or destroyed, 26 May–22 February 1921.
60 Brian Hughes, *Defying the IRA?: Intimidation, Coercion and Communities during the Irish Revolution* (Liverpool: Liverpool University Press, 2016), 47–9.
61 Arnold's Typescript Recollections, 126–7; for more information on this and role of police during Revolutionary Ireland, see Richard Abbott, *Police Casualties in Ireland, 1919–1922* (Cork: Mercier Press, 2000).
62 Arnold's Typescript Recollections, 128.
63 NA, PIN 15/2998, Ministry of Pensions, Dublin, to Ministry of Pensions, London, 28 February 1923.
64 NA, LAB/2/522/TDS3949/2/1919, Ministry of Labour, Dublin, to Ministry of Labour, London, 5 May 1919.
65 Donnacha Seán Lucey, *The End of the Irish Poor Law?: Welfare and healthcare reform in revolutionary and independent Ireland* (Manchester: Manchester University Press, 2015), 21.
66 NA, PIN 15/2685, Letter from Sim, Ministry of Pensions, Dublin to Chrystal, Treasury, London, 27 August 1920.
67 Arnold's Typescript Recollections, 126.
68 NA, PIN 15/899, Provision of Employment for Ex-serviceman in Ireland; Bourke, 'Effeminacy, ethnicity and the end of trauma', 65.
69 NA, PIN 15/899, Provision of Employment for Ex-serviceman in Ireland, 11 March 1921.
70 NA, PIN 15/56, Ministry of Pensions, Dublin, to Ministry of Pensions, London, 24 November 1921.
71 Ibid.
72 Ibid., 13 December 1921.
73 Ibid., Ministry of Pensions, London, to the Regional Director, All Regions, 10 January 1922.
74 Ibid., Re: Facilities for Treatment of Neurasthenia in Ireland – South Ireland.
75 NA, PIN 15/55, Ministry of Pensions, note, 26 May 1921.
76 Bourke, 'Effeminacy, ethnicity and the end of trauma', 66.
77 NA, PIN 15/56, Ministry of Pensions, Ulster Region, to Ministry of Pensions, London, 14 November 1921; Ministry of Pensions, West Midlands Region, to Ministry of Pensions, London, 19 November 1921; Ministry of Pensions, Yorkshire Region, to Ministry of Pensions, London, 17 November 1921; Ministry of Pensions, Northern Region, to Ministry of Pensions, London, 23 September 1921; Bourke, 'Effeminacy, ethnicity and the end of trauma', 67.
78 NA, PIN 15/54, Unknown Author to the Earl of Derby, War Office, 29 May 1917.
79 Arnold's Typescript Recollections, 128.
80 NA, PIN 15/899, Ministry of Pensions, Dublin, note, 24 March 1921.
81 Taylor, *Heroes or Traitors?*, 122–3.
82 NA, PIN 15/899, Ministry of Pensions, Dublin, note, 24 March 1921.

83 Charles Townsend, *The Republic: The Fight for Irish Independence, 1918–1923* (London: Penguin, 2013), 125–7, 149.
84 This republican police force was part of the wider policy to overrule and replace the existing legal system in Ireland. The force originally enlisted many members of the Irish Volunteers; Townsend, *The Republic*, 133.
85 NA, PIN 15/899, Ministry of Pensions, Dublin, to Secretary Crown Agent, London, 20 September 1920; Director General of Medical Services: Certifying Cases of Lunacy, 1 January 1921; Ministry of Pensions, Dublin, note, 24 March 1921.
86 Ibid., Ministry of Pensions, Dublin, note, 24 March 1921.
87 Ibid., Richmond District Lunatic Asylum to the Inspectors of Lunatics, Dublin Castle, 12 October 1920; Townsend, *The Republic*, 235.
88 NA, PIN 15/899, Richmond District Lunatic Asylum to the Inspectors of Lunatics, Dublin Castle, 12 October 1920.
89 Ibid., Ministry of Pensions, Dublin, to Ministry of Pensions, London, 26 May 1920.
90 Ibid., 27 August 1919.
91 These difficulties are discussed throughout NA, PIN 15/899, The Treatment of Lunacy Ireland, 1919–1921. Indeed, one British ex-serviceman who was born and had lived in Dublin was refused transferral to Richmond from Clonmel Asylum. In the absence of any agreement, the Ministry of Pensions allocated a transferral at Farnham House, a private facility in Finglas, County Dublin; Taylor, *Heroes or Traitors?*, 124.
92 Durnin, *The Irish Medical Profession and the First World War*, 184.
93 NA, PIN 15/899, D.C.M.S. Note, Ulster Region, 14 March 1921; Ministry of Pensions, note, 15 March 1921; Inspector of Lunatics Office, Dublin Castle, to Director General of Medical Services, 11 May 1920.
94 Ibid., Ministry of Pensions, Dublin, note, 24 March 1921.
95 Ibid., Ministry of Pensions, Dublin, to Departmental Committee of Enquiry, London, 15 March 1921.
96 Ibid., Ireland South Region, Special Neurological Board to Commissioner of Medical Services, Ministry of Pensions, 15 March 1921.
97 Ibid., Ministry of Pensions, Dublin, note, 24 March 1921.
98 Ibid., Provision of Employment for Ex-servicemen in Ireland, 11 March 1921.
99 Myers, *Shell-Shock in France*, 139.
100 Bettinson, 'Lost Souls in the House of Restoration', 313–14.
101 NA, PIN 15/56, Memorandum on Conference of Neurological D.Cs.M.S. Held at Headquarters, 17 June 1921.
102 NA, PIN 15/899, Provision of Employment for ex-servicemen in Ireland, 11 March 1921.
103 NA, PIN 15/56, Memorandum on Conference of Neurological D.Cs.M.S. held at Headquarters, 17 June 1921.
104 *British Legion Journal*, 1 (March, 1922), 210.

105 Barr, *The Lion and the Poppy*, 122.
106 NA, PIN 15/56, Ministry of Pensions, note, 15 December 1921.
107 Ibid., Ministry of Pensions, note, 29 November 1921.
108 Ibid., Ministry of Pensions, Dublin, to Ministry of Pensions, London, 13 December 1921.
109 Ibid., Ministry of Pensions, London, to Ministry of Pensions, Dublin, 21 December 1921.
110 Ibid., Regional Directors - all Regions, 23 June 1921.
111 Ibid., Memorandum on Conference of Neurological D.Cs.M.S. held at Headquarters, 17 June 1921.
112 Ibid., Ministry of Pensions, London, to Ministry of Pensions, Dublin, 21 December 1921.
113 Bettinson, 'Lost Souls in the House of Restoration', 314; NA, PIN 15/134, Belfast Ministry of Pensions Minute Sheet, 16 July 1921.
114 NA, PIN 15/899, Provision of Employment for ex-servicemen in Ireland, 11 March 1921.
115 Ibid.
116 NA, LAB 2/855/ED5412/13/1921, Irish Federation of Discharged and Demobilised Sailors and Soldiers.
117 PRONI, D989/B/3/6, Ex-Service Men in Southern Ireland. Their Terrible Sufferings, 1.
118 NA, PIN 15/899, Provision of Employment for ex-servicemen in Ireland, 11 March 1921.
119 Ibid.
120 Ibid.
121 NA, LAB 2/522/TDS1636/1919, Memorandum by Mr Campbell on Certain Aspects of the Work of the Ministry of Labour in Ireland, 1–2.
122 Hughes, *Defying the IRA?*, 58.
123 Taylor, *Heroes or Traitors?*, 99.
124 'Service Men's Bureau: Advice for Soldiers and Sailors', *Weekly Irish Times*, 22 February 1919, 1.
125 HC Debates, 10 November 1919, vol. 121, cols 76–77; 'Soldier's Pensions: The Position in Ireland', *Weekly Irish Times*, 21 August 1920, 2.
126 Taylor, *Heroes or Traitors?*, 98.
127 Arnold's Typescript Recollections, 126
128 Brotherton Library, University of Leeds, INDEX/LIDDLE/GA/2012, Driver Wilfred Rhodes Correspondence.
129 NA, PIN 15/789, Report written by Office of the Representative of the Ministry of Pensions, Dublin, 22 January 1918.
130 Arnold's Typescript Recollections, 127.
131 NA, PIN 15/899, Provision of Employment for Ex-servicemen in Ireland, 11 March 1921.
132 Ibid.
133 NA, PIN 26/75, Lance Sergeant Henry Dale, Royal Irish Rifles, Pension File.

134 NA, LAB 2/855/ED5412/7/1921, National Federation of Discharged and Demobilised Sailors and Soldiers, Dublin, to David Lloyd George, 17 February 1920.
135 Ibid.
136 NA, LAB 2/522/TDS1636/1919, Memorandum by Mr Campbell on Certain Aspects of the Work of the Ministry of Labour in Ireland, 18 November 1919, 1.
137 NA, PIN 15/899, Provision of Employment for Ex-Servicemen in Ireland, 1; LAB 2/855/ED5412/7/1921, Internal Memo, Department of Application for Training and Employment in Ireland, 13 March 1920.
138 NA, LAB 2/855/ED5412/7/1921, National Federation of Discharged and Demobilised Sailors and Soldiers, Dublin, to David Lloyd George, 17 February 1920.
139 Hughes, *Defying the IRA?*, 50.
140 Leonard, 'Facing the finger of scorn', 62.
141 NA, LAB/2/522/TDS3949/2/1919, Gordon Campbell, Ministry of Labour, Dublin, to Ministry of Labour, London, 5 April 1919.
142 Ibid., Report on Industrial Training of Discharged Ex-service Men in Ireland, 4.
143 NA, LAB 2/855/ED5412/7/1921, National Federation of Discharged and Demobilised Sailors and Soldiers, Dublin, to David Lloyd George, 17 February 1920.
144 Ibid., Ministry of Labour to Prime Minister's Office, 24 March 1920.
145 Hopkinson, *The Irish War of Independence*, 200–1.
146 Taylor, *Heroes or Traitors?*, 85–8.
147 David Fitzpatrick, 'Militarism in Ireland', in Thomas Bartlett and Keith Jeffery (eds), *A Military History of Ireland* (Cambridge: Cambridge University Press 1996), 379–406.
148 Taylor, *Heroes or Traitors?*, 98.
149 Eoin McLaughlin, 'Economic Impact of the Irish Revolution.' [Online] Available at: www.standrews.ac.uk/media/deptofgeographyandsustainabledevelopment/pdfs/DP%202015%2013%20McLaughlin.pdf [accessed 1 September 2016].
150 D. S. Johnson, 'The Northern Ireland economy, 1914–39', in Liam Kennedy and Phillip Ollerenshaw (eds), *An Economic History of Ulster* (Manchester: Manchester University Press, 1985), 184–8; Jonathan Bardon, *A History of Ulster* (Belfast: Blackstaff Press, 2001), 518–23.
151 Richard Grayson, *Belfast Boys: How Unionists and Nationalists Fought and Died Together in the First World War* (London: Continuum, 2009), 148.
152 Johnson, 'The Northern Ireland Economy, 1914–39', 214–15; Grayson, *Belfast Boys*, 154; Hughes, *Defying the IRA?*, 151; Hart, *the IRA at War*, 249; for more information on Belfast and sectarian violence, see Jim McDermott, *Northern Divisions: The Old IRA and the Belfast Pogroms, 1920–1922* (Belfast: Beyond the Pale, 2001).
153 Jane McGuaghey, *Ulster's Men: Protestant Unionist Masculinities and Militarization in the North of Ireland, 1912–1923* (Montréal: McGill Queens University Press, 2012), 144.
154 Barham, *Forgotten Lunatics of the Great War*, 197–8.

155 NA, LAB 2/855/ED5412/7/1921, Meeting of the Minutes with the Parliamentary Secretary of the Ministry of Transport, 4 May 1920.
156 NA, LAB 2/528/TDS1181/1921, Ministry of Labour Report, 6 July 1923.
157 Ibid., Copy of Extract from Parliamentary Debates for 27 June 1923; between 1919 and 1924, 88,000 ex-servicemen in Britain were able to be retrained with the assistance of the Ministry of Labour; Julie Anderson, *War, Disability and Rehabilitation in Britain: 'Soul of a Nation'* (Manchester: Manchester University Press, 2011), 46.
158 Kowalsky, 'Enabling the Great War', 104.
159 NA, LAB 2/528/TDS1181/1921, Administration of training scheme in Northern and Southern Ireland as a result of the Government of Ireland Act 1920, 6 July 1923.
160 NA, LAB 2/522/TDS3949/2/1919, Ministry of Labour note, 8 January 1920; Ministry of Labour note, 30 January 1920.
161 NA, LAB 2/522/TDS3949/2/1919, Ministry of Labour report, 15 November 1919.
162 HC Debates, 19 February 1920, vol. 125, cols 1029–32.
163 Taylor, *Heroes or Traitors?*, 105.
164 NA, LAB 2/855/ED5412/7/1921, National Federation of Discharged and Demobilised Sailors and Soldiers, Dublin, to David Lloyd George, 17 February 1920.
165 NA, LAB 2/522/TDS3949/2/1919, Report on Industrial Training of Discharged Ex-service Men in Ireland, 1–2.
166 Ibid., Ministry of Labour, Dublin, to Ministry of Labour, London, 5 April 1919.
167 NA, PIN 15/56, Memorandum on Conference of Neurological D.Cs.M.S. held at Headquarters, 17 June 1921.
168 Leonard, 'Survivors', 216.
169 'Trade Unions and the Soldiers and Sailors', *Irish Times*, 20 February 1920, 5; Theresa Moriarty, 'Work, warfare and wages: industrial controls and Irish trade unionism in the First World War', in Adrian Gregory and Senia Paseta (eds), *Ireland and the Great War: 'A War To Unite Us All'?* (Manchester: Manchester University Press, 2002), 73, 76.
170 NA, PIN 15/34, The Future of the Permanently Subnormal Ex-Serviceman.
171 Hart, *The IRA and its Enemies*, 274.
172 Eunan O'Halpin, 'Problematic killing during the War of Independence and its aftermath: civilian spies and informers', in James Kelly and Mary Ann Lyons (eds), *Death and Dying in Ireland, Britain and Europe: Historical Perspectives* (Kildare: Irish Academic Press, 2013), 332.
173 Taylor, *Heroes or Traitors?*, 19–88; Hart, *The IRA and its Enemies*, 301, 312; *The IRA at War*, 136; Leonard, 'Getting them at last', 118–29.
174 Hughes, *Defying the IRA?*, 132; Joost Augusteijn, *From Public Defiance to Guerrilla Warfare: The Experience of Ordinary Volunteers in the Irish War of Independence, 1916–1921* (Dublin: Irish Academic Press, 1996), 293.
175 O'Halpin, 'Problematic killing during the War of Independence', 317–49; Borgovono, 'Revolution, ex-servicemen and the Cork branch of the National Federation of Discharged and Demobilised Sailors and Soldiers, 1918–1921', 96.

176 Hughes, *Defying the IRA?*, 132.
177 Gustave Roussy, Jean Lhermitte and William Turner, *The Psychoneuroses of War* (London: University of London Press, 1918), 164; A. J. Brook, 'The war neurasthenic', *The Lancet*, 23 March 1918, 436.
178 Bourke, 'Effeminacy, ethnicity and the end of trauma', 62.
179 Neil Diamant, *Embattled Glory: Veterans, Military Families and the Politics of Patriotism in China, 1949–2007* (Lanham: Rowan & Littlefield, 2009), 329–30.
180 Jonathan Shay, *Odysseus in America: Combat Trauma and the Trials of Homecoming* (New York: Scribner, 2002), 168, 245; Herman, *Trauma and Recovery*, 3.
181 D. A. Alexander and S. Klein, 'Combat-related disorders: a persistent chimera', *Journal of the Royal Army Medical Corps*, 154:2 (2008), 98; David Morris, *The Evil Hours: A Biography of Post-Traumatic Stress Disorder* (Boston: Houghton Mifflin Harcourt Publishing, 2015), 49–50.
182 Herman, *Trauma and Recovery*, 155.
183 Hart, *The IRA and its Enemies*, 312.
184 Bourke, *Dismembering the Male*, 70.
185 NA, PIN 15/897, Office of Lunatic Asylums, Dublin, note, 12 August 1918.
186 Leonard, 'Facing the finger of scorn', 62.
187 Durnin, *The Irish Medical Profession and the First World War*, 167–70.
188 Vicky Long, *Destigmatising Mental Illness: Professional Politics and Public Education in Britain, 1870–1970* (Manchester: Manchester University Press, 2014), 15–16.
189 NA, PIN 15/899, Provision of Employment for ex-servicemen in Ireland, 11 March 1921.
190 Ibid., Ministry of Pensions, Dublin, note, 24 March 1921.
191 Ibid., Special Neurological Board to Ministry of Pensions, Dublin, 15 March 1921.
192 NA, PIN 26/22244, O'Ryan Pension File.
193 Jason Crouthamel, 'Memory as a battlefield: letters by traumatized German veterans and contested memories of the Great War', in Joan Tumblety (ed.), *Memory and History: Understanding Memory as Source and Subject* (London: Routledge, 2013), 144.
194 NA, PIN 15/133, Durham Street Clinic, Belfast.
195 Durnin, *The Irish Medical Profession and the First World War*, 198–9.
196 PRONI, CAB/6/9, Letter from Colonel W. B. Spender, Secretary to the Cabinet, to Lionel Curtis, Colonial Office, 25 March 1922.
197 Durnin, *The Irish Medical Profession and the First World War*, 199.
198 W. H. Rivers, 'The repression of war experience', *Proceedings of the Royal Society of Medicine*, 11 (1918), 3.
199 McGaughey, *Ulster's Men*, 156–7.
200 A Voluntary Pensions Worker, *Pensioners of the Great War*, 22.
201 Bourke, 'Shell-shock, psychiatry and the Irish soldier', 167.
202 'Editorial', *The Comrades Journal*, 1 (July, 1919), 69.
203 Bourke, 'Shell-shock, psychiatry and the Irish Soldier', 155.

3

NEURASTHENIC PENSIONERS IN THE IRISH FREE STATE AND NORTHERN IRELAND

The Treaty and Civil War

By 1921, both Irish and British officials recognised the Anglo-Irish War constituted a military stalemate with a compromised settlement appearing imminent. The Ministry of Pensions foresaw a bleak future for ex-servicemen residing in South Ireland: 'Conditions in Ireland will improve in the near future, but it seems very questionable, even if the country becomes settled again, whether the ex-soldier will not be regarded still as an outcast and an undesirable by his fellow man.' This situation was likely 'owing to the present hostile attitude which is directed collectively and individually against men who served in the War.'[1] In early dialogue with the Dáil Éireann, proposing to arrange negotiations, the British Government cited the administration of war pensions as an important issue for discussion in any future transferral of power.[2] The Regional Director of the Ministry of Pensions in South Ireland remained concerned that any diplomatic change or transferral of power would have a detrimental impact on the Ministry's remit and function in the region. Ministry officials in the region were subsequently dissatisfied at not being represented during treaty negotiations to discuss these concerns.[3]

The establishment of the Free State would go on to cause much consternation amongst Ministry staff in the region, especially in the aftermath of an article in the *Irish Times* falsely reporting that the administration of the department would be transferred to the newly established government. The Regional Director subsequently wrote to the various Ministry branches and treatment facilities across the Free State emphasising that the organisation would continue to remain solely responsible to the British Government.[4] The correspondence did not mention the anxiety that this misinformation would have caused disabled ex-servicemen relying on their pension for survival.

Both the Ministry of Pensions and the Ministry of Labour operated as an autonomous 'Imperial Obligation' within the Irish Free State.[5] Under the Transfer of Function Order (1922), the Free State Government was legally obliged to provide amnesty and prevent discrimination against those who had previously served in British services, including Great War veterans.[6] In March 1922, W. G. Fallon, Secretary of the City of Dublin War Pensions Committee, unsuccessfully put forward proposals to Michael Collins TD, Minister of Finance, to transfer the British Ministry of Pensions to a newly established Irish Ministry of Pensions solely under the remit and function of the newly established Free State Government. Proposing that the new department could administer all pensions issues in the Free State, including disabled IRA veteran pensions, old age pensions and job-related pensions, Fallon held that any such transferral would have immense political value. In particular, Fallon suggested that it would enable the new government to distance itself entirely from any notions that it held British ex-servicemen as 'unfriendly persons.' Fallon also advanced his doomed proposal by advising that the large financial expenditure of the Ministry of Pensions provided by the British Treasury, which he estimated at no less than £3,000,000 per year, would afford ammunition to anti-Free State supporters.[7]

A continuation of hostilities ensued in Ireland following a split in the republican movement over the Anglo-Irish Treaty. Rejecting the compromised dominion status of the Free State and the partition of Ireland headed by Michael Collins, de Valera and anti-Treaty IRA units took up arms to oppose the Treaty. The anti-Treaty side's opposition to the diplomatic settlement was again associated with mental illness, with the popular *Punch* magazine equating them to a 'mad bull.'[8] Like the Anglo-Irish War, the Irish Civil War included armed insurrection from those opposing the state against those deemed to be agents acting on behalf of an illegitimate authority. Policemen again became targets of potential reprisal alongside government jurors, Free State soldiers, civil servants and politicians.[9] The Irish Civil War, lasting between June 1922 and May 1923, ensured further complications in establishing the infrastructure to train disabled ex-servicemen. Disabled men making applications to the Ministry of Labour for training, for example, were prevented from doing so with the suspension of postal facilities in June 1922. Correspondence sent to ex-servicemen on how to appeal Ministry decisions regarding pension applications was similarly compromised.[10] It was within this context that the treatment of neurasthenic pensioners would remain problematic. In October 1922, one Ministry official in the Free State, D. A. Carruthers, pleaded with colleagues in London to increase facilities for further out-patient clinics for neurasthenic pensioners in Dublin. He even enquired as to the possibility of holding sessions in nearby boardrooms due to the 'feeble' facilities which had been 'a matter of urgency for over a year.'[11] During a Parliamentary debate in December 1922, the Earl of Mayo referred to the unfortunate position of disabled ex-servicemen in Ireland resorting to 'grinding organs, singing songs, and playing bands in the streets' to make ends meet, decreeing that 'they had been left in the lurch.'[12]

With the destruction of bridges and railway stations, Arnold and his Ministry colleagues visited cities across the newly established Free State to inspect the operations of the Ministry in hazardous conditions, including one 24-hour-long journey on a steamboat from Dublin to Cork. On his arrival, anti-Treaty IRA men had occupied several post office buildings. Fearing that disabled veterans would starve without the allocation of their pensions, Arnold oversaw diplomatic relations with occupiers to obtain the necessary release of documents and funds to ensure the reimbursement to disabled veterans.[13] The period also impacted upon Leopardstown Hospital. The hospital's store was raided three times by anti-Treaty IRA brigades during the summer of 1922, with clothing and the hospital van being stolen. This thieving had a military objective rather than being driven by anti-British sentiment. A raider apologised to a member of the hospital's staff during one raid, explaining that 'it was necessary for his men to have changes of clothing and overcoats as they were away from their homes, being chased by the national troops.'[14]

The Free State Government quickly assembled an army of approximately 60,000 men to deal with the anti-Treaty IRA. It was this ex-service community, rather than British ex-servicemen, who would go onto receive prioritisation regarding government jobs, fulfilling promises made at recruitment.[15] Captain Redmond recognised that ex-National Army men experienced employment preference 'then come the civilians, included among whom are British ex-servicemen.'[16] Despite being a staunch advocate for the British ex-service population residing in the Free State, the SILA decreed that it was reasonable for the new government to prioritise ex-National Army men and fulfil promises made during enlistment.[17] Official estimates state that around 50 percent of the National Army consisted of British ex-servicemen. British Army veterans subsequently became a primary reason for the victory of the pro-Treaty Free State forces.[18] Arnold wrote of the economic opportunity that the new domestic conflict provided British Army veterans: 'The old days of the soldier of fortune blossomed again for a short season. Make hay while the sun shines was their motto. More power to them.'[19] Even Ministry officials in Dublin, often scornful of Free State governmental and societal assistance provided to Great War veterans, would recognise that these British Army veterans were subsequently able to benefit from preferential treatment provided to National Army ex-servicemen.[20]

Free State President, William Cosgrave, agreed: 'In so far as ex-servicemen are also ex-national army men, they share in the preferences accorded to the class.'[21] Neurasthenic pensioners, however, would have been reluctant to seize upon this redemptive chance and to re-enlist for military service due to their compromised mental state.[22]

British ex-servicemen were affected by their former comrades' enlistment in the Free State Army. A Ministry office in Cork was set ablaze by anti-Treaty IRA forces in March 1922. Their intention was 'the destruction of records [which] would cause serious difficulty and is believed to have been generated maliciously with intent to cripple the work of the Pensions Office.' An anonymous letter was received by the secretary of the branch the morning following the attack which read: 'Let M. Collins' bodyguard of ex-service men put it out this time, they will lose their bloody money for a bit as their records go with the flames. Dirty lot.'[23] The secretary of a local pensions committee in County Leitrim was also shot dead during the conflict.[24] The second domestic conflict in Ireland was short-lived with the eventual triumph of the Free State Government and its National Army. The resumption of peace in the Free State coincided with Ministry officials in London congratulating themselves on having educated and trained enough neurasthenic specialists and now being better able to increase in-patient and out-patient facilities and open enough rehabilitative facilities to finally cater to mentally ill pensioners.[25] Rather than experiencing an increase in facilities alongside Britain, however, the eventual resumption of peace Ireland would coincide with a significant reduction of state intervention in the treatment of mentally ill Great War veterans across the UK.

Declining state intervention and societal sympathy

The War Office Committee of Enquiry into Shell-Shock, often known as the Southborough Report, was convened in 1920 and published in 1922. The report set out to collate expert and first-hand witnesses knowledgeable and experienced with shell-shock to better inform military understanding of combat neurosis. Witnesses decreed that it was very tough to lay down 'a type', and that there was 'no characteristic common to all the individuals affected.' Previously capable and stable men could break down in the atrocious conditions prevalent during the First World War.[26] Long-held and prejudiced views of the mentally ill also continued to feature in the report.[27] Sir Hugh Sandham Jeudwine, General Officer Commanding of the 5th division, testified: 'Breakdown was purely a matter of "nerves" and that the nervous state might be temperamental and pre-existent or induced by worry, hardship, danger or bad health, though in all of these cases a temperamental predisposition probably existed in a dormant state.'[28] The Southborough Report asserted that many cases of mental breakdown included men with a congenital or biological disposition to neuroses. Such hypotheses were a continuation of views held during the war and were a transnational phenomenon.[29] Contradictory statements that some men were predisposed to shell-shock, yet still accepting that anyone could break down, reveal the ambiguities in medico-military discourse. One clear example of this discrepancy is evident in the report's conclusion which justified the labelling of shell-shocked soldiers as cowards while simultaneously asserting that cowardice was beyond an individual's control.[30]

Those with 'artistic temperaments', Jews, 'imaginative city-dwellers' and other such 'highly strung' people were deemed liable to suffer from war neurosis. The often-proclaimed innate cowardice of tentative conscripts also made them suspect to breakdown.[31] The assumption of an inherent Irish national mental weakness also emerged. Dr William Brown told the committee how he was struck by the fact that men from certain regiments were overrepresented in receiving care for war trauma.[32] Major Pritchard Taylor of the Royal Army Military Corps offered specifics: 'The typical Irishman does well, probably brilliantly up to a point, but will not stick it like the typical Scot.'[33] The committee concurred: 'Among general predisposing causes were racial characteristics, education and social conditions and environments.'[34] The remarks of the Southborough committee are highly suggestive of the fact that suspicions of the Irish temperament remained unmoved by the First World War and Britain's experience of shell-shock.[35] The report thus reflected existing social narratives. Numerous post-war literary depictions of fictional Irish characters also continued to display symptoms of a variety of mental illnesses. Memoirs, genealogical 'stud-books' and anthropologists continued to emphasise that emotional and fragile mental traits were hereditarily passed on between races and mostly remained confined between certain peoples – including the Irish.[36]

Ministry officials and Southborough committee members and witnesses were often members of the military or medical elite. Products of the British middle and upper classes, who had benefitted from a public school and university education, they would have been long exposed to theories regarding social Darwinism, eugenics and race.[37] The Southborough Report ironically concluded that a recruit's socio-economic and ethnic background played 'an immense part in the incidence of shell-shock.' This generalisation could equally apply to those on the committee who were predisposed to *formulating* theories on shell-shock.[38] The report would leave the causality of shell-shock unsolved and without a clear philosophy on how to treat the tens of thousands of neurasthenic pensioners living in Britain and Ireland. This contradictory and confused approach coincided with a significant reduction in Ministry after-care of the disabled ex-service population.

Ministry restrictions were an ingredient of the infamous 'Geddes' axe' which enforced a host of tax increases and economic cutbacks in the public sector.[39] The British Treasury wrote to all pensions departments in 1921 urging austere economic policies. In 1921, the outlay of medical costs stood at almost £15,000,000 with this annual figure shrinking to £1,017,000 by 1939. Overall spending for the department was reduced from £106,600,000 in 1921 to £39,400,000 eighteen years later. A reduction in medical facilities shaped the saving. While 332,000 disabled pensioners were undergoing Ministry funded treatment in 1921, this figure stood at just 4,739 by 1939. There was a similar decline in national staff from 21,685 central and local employees in 1921 reduced to only 3,071. General Practitioners took up the vast majority of war-related medical care of disabled pensioners with the Ministry covering the cost from the mid-1920s onwards.[40]

The Ministry's records subsequently referenced that their spending was being 'very carefully watched' by the Treasury.[41] For example, Sugar's request for Leopardstown Hospital in Dublin to be increased to 200 beds in the summer of 1921 was rejected by the Ministry of Pensions in London due to inadequate finances: 'although the provision of accommodation for neurasthenics is an urgent and indeed a vital one, still we have to balance this necessity with the economic and financial conditions of the country.'[42] Sugars' request seemingly reflected desires within the Ministry of Pensions to increase the availability of resources. Two years earlier, the Ministry had requested an increase of 7,000 beds to provide in-patient facilities for various disabilities and to accommodate the 9,797 pensioners awaiting treatment. The British Treasury declined the department's appeal to finance the policy because 'it is common knowledge that Civil Hospitals are urgently in need of funds and that wards are being closed in many parts of the country.'[43] It was the British Government's reluctance to set a precedent and initiate demands to increase and improve civilian medical facilities that prevented the increase of Pensions' facilities. The reply to the Ministry's request for an increase of in-patient facilities affirmed: 'In these circumstances it appears indefensible that any Government Department should acquire and equip new hospital accommodation of its own.'[44] The Ministry's demands led to a more modest increase in facilities to cater for a further 1,800 in-patients.[45] Such instances buttress previous research which concludes that Treasury control and underfunding fatally compromised Ministry facilities.[46] Public sentiment regularly regarded the Ministry of Pensions as bureaucratic, unsympathetic and miserly. Historians otherwise cynical of the

Ministry's liberality recognise that the department was delicately balanced between public ire for their inaction while being economically restrained by the Treasury.[47]

The reduction in Ministry liability and state intervention was aided by the lessening in societal concern for the disabled veteran as the British population became desensitised to their plight in a time of increasing austerity and employment scarcity.[48] Even the ESWS would doubt the extent to which the general public acknowledged and cared about mentally ill veterans by 1930.[49] This decrease in societal concern may have had a detrimental impact on the recovery of neurasthenic pensioners.[50] Reflecting this reduction in emotional weight and medical resources for mentally ill veterans, 'shell-shock' also slowly faded from the mainstream medical discourse.[51]

The Ministry restricted the potential for future state liability by introducing its 1921 War Pensions Act implementing a seven-year time limit on claims within seven years of a veteran's discharge, or from 31 August 1921, depending on which came sooner.[52] The Treasury advocated this measure, writing:

> [if] the pension system is to remain watertight this limit will have to be rigidly maintained. As the average age of the general body of pensioners approaches 50 their general level of health will decline in the normal course and an endeavour will undoubtedly be made to force the State to accept this normal physical deterioration as due to abnormal conditions experienced in the Great War.[53]

The Ministry, Parliament and Ministry of National Service were acutely aware of the apparent abuses within the American Civil War pensions system. By 1914, the liberal American system had become, to all intents and purposes, an old-age pension.[54] By 1914, 93 percent of union veterans, nearly 400,000 men, received a state pension for a war-related disability.[55] The British Legion unsuccesfully agitated for the removal of the time limit. The charity criticised the Ministry for emphasising cost-cutting over the personal wellbeing of disabled ex-servicemen, even describing it as using 'medieval methods.'[56]

The Ministry of Pensions may have compared unfavourably with Australia and Canada who had no time limits on pension claims, but it was more benevolent than the French and American system which had a four-year and two-year limit respectively.[57] Even the ESWS, as a staunch advocate on behalf of the neurasthenic pensioner, referenced the awkward position the Ministry was placed in, recognising that it was often difficult to trace the relationship between war service and mental illness over more than a decade.[58] Due to the Ministry's time limit, there was an increase in neurasthenic pensioners between 1921 and 1927, but a stillness to their numbers from 1928 onwards (Figure 8).

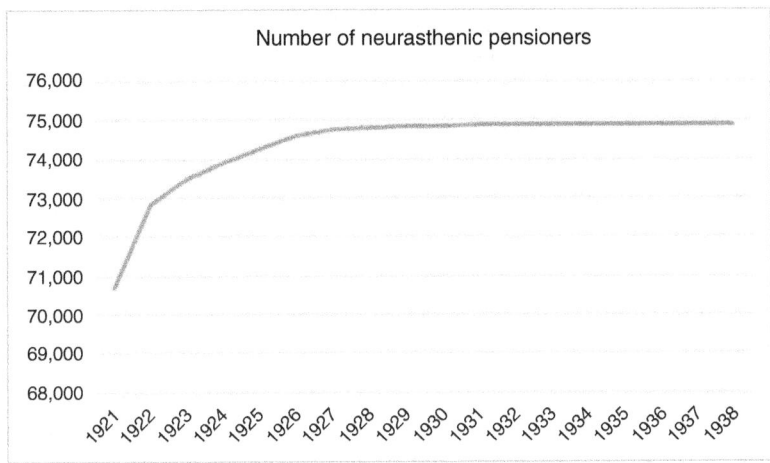

Figure 8 The number of neurasthenic pensioners throughout the UK, 1921–38. Calculated from Ministry of Pensions Fourth Annual Report to Twenty-Second Annual Reports; Annual Reports covering the period 1 April 1920 to 31 March 1938.

The 1921 legislation also introduced 'Final Awards.' Final Awards included pensions for life for those whose disability was diagnosed to have reached a point of permanency. Those in receipt of a 20 percent pension or less were provided with a final gratuity and removed from the Ministry's pensions list, reducing future liability. By 1925, almost half a million such awards were distributed, of which 240,000 included one-off gratuities for pensions graded at less than 20 percent. This permanency would help to reduce expenditure by removing the need for repeated medical boarding.[59] While over 1,250,000 disabled veterans were boarded from 1920 to 1921, only 47,500 boardings occurred between 1928 and 1929.[60] Peter Fitzpatrick was one such pensioner designated a Final Award in Ireland with his 20 percent expiring after seventy weeks.[61]

The Ministry's post-1921 austere outlook and restrictive policy ensured a significant scaling back of Ministry in-patient and out-patient treatment (Table 4).

The transferral of the Maghull Hospital, the foundational block upon which the Ministry's assessment and treatment of neurasthenic pensioners was built upon, to the Board of Control to be used as a high-security psychiatric hospital in the early 1930s provides a striking metaphor of the Ministry's dismissal of institutional treatment.[62] Just months before its closure, one Ministry official

Table 4 Numbers of neurasthenic pensioners receiving in-patient and out-patient treatment in the UK, 1921–36.

Year	In-patients	Out-patients
1921	2,951	6,975
1927	1,373	541
1928	1,066	359
1929	890	224
1930	867	218
1931	745	169
1932	674	94
1933	633	53
1934	426	49
1935	370	40
1936	364	40

Source: Jones and Wessely, *From Shell-Shock to PTSD*, 132–3.

reviewed the hospital, describing its chronic and long-term patient profiles 'for whom retention in hospital on purely medical grounds, is now doubtfully justified.'[63] Alongside a reduction in available facilities, the treatment outlook within Ministry in-patient hospitals would adopt a more vocational outlook at the expense of psychotherapy.

Hardening and Leopardstown

Relapses and re-admissions of in-patient patients were common, with the Ministry again citing the lack of employment in civil society: 'The anxiety condition does not entirely clear up so long as the uncertainty as to the future remains ... we consider that it will do them as much harm as good to keep them in hospital, the probability of relapse and further deterioration on discharge unless some employment is found for them is considerable.'[64] By the early and mid-1920s, veteran charities and even medical practitioners previously sympathetic to the plight of the shell-shocked ex-serviceman held that a large number of neurasthenic pensioners were unable to be successfully treated via psychotherapy. Employment became the fundamental issue to aid recovery.[65] This relationship between employability and neurasthenia had transnational reach. At a conference held in Ottawa in December 1936, which was attended by Ministry representatives, twenty-two psychiatrists and neurologists working for the Canadian pension authorities concluded that a 'social investigation' of a pensioner's or claimant's region was often crucial in inducing or aggravating neurasthenic symptoms.[66]

A philosophy of 'hardening' ensued in Britain and Ireland. 'Hardening' involved physically capable in-patients working for at least six hours a day at associated workshops acquiring new vocational abilities such as brush-making and basket-weaving.[67] George Chrystal, the Ministry's Director of Finance, summarised the change of philosophy as such:

> As time went on it became apparent that psychotherapy by itself afforded but a partial solution of the problem and much better and more lasting results are obtained by adding to its organised occupational treatment workshops, with special instructors, were attached to the neurasthenic hospitals, and efforts made to secure suitable employment for pensioners on discharge.[68]

The new focus on vocation led Hebb to advise that in-patients receiving hardening treatment should not receive more than the bare minimum of psychotherapeutic treatment.[69] The ESWS cited the benefits of curative work treatment for providing in-patients with a sense of meaning and resolution in the sheltered and working environment provided. Rather than having to hide anxiety neuroses from co-workers and employers, curative workshops supposedly benefitted veterans psychologically from 'the very certainty of tolerance' of their irritability and depression which, in turn, induced their reduction.[70] 'Hardening' at Leopardstown was also commented upon favourably by Sugars: 'considerable improvement has been manifested in many cases … [it has] displaced proportionately their mental preoccupation with their health.' A lack of infrastructure and staff, however, continued to permeate. Only 30 percent of Leopardstown's patients were able to participate in such continuous treatment at any one time.[71] Barham describes the Ministry's policy of 'hardening' as '"social reconstruction" at work – a form of community care that endeavoured to retain the pensioner as an efficient economic unit as an alternative to banishing him to an asylum.'[72] Psychotherapy remained largely confined to the First World War and in its immediate post-war years.

Leopardstown was one of six Irish hospitals run or funded by the Ministry in 1929 (Table 5).

The varying pension grades of in-patients in the sole surviving admission and discharge register for Leopardstown, 1930–31, attest to the fluctuating severity of mental illness amongst patients, ranging from 30 to 100 percent. There was also a variance in the length of pensioner residencies. While one patient discharged himself following a residency of just over a month, three pensioners remained at the hospital for eleven, twelve and sixteen years

Table 5 Ministry of Pensions' hospitals operating in Ireland, 1929.

Name and location of Institution	Nature of treatment provided	Total accommodation reserved
Ministry of Pensions hospital, Blackrock, Dublin	Limb-fitting (arms and legs), special surgical treatment	233
Ministry of Pensions hospital, Leopardstown, Dublin	Neurasthenic, neurological, psycho-therapeutic, curative workshops, general medical and surgical	88
UVF Hospital, Craigavon, Belfast	Neurasthenic, neurological, psycho-therapeutic	75
UVF Hospital, Galwally Branch, Belfast	General medical and surgical and surgical and special treatment	85
Shankhiel Hospital, Sundays Well, Cork	General medical and surgical and surgical and special treatment	87

Source: Twelfth Annual Report of the Ministry of Pensions, 1928–1929, 18.

respectively. The latter would remain in Leopardstown until his death in June 1941.[73] The case notes of Thomas Whelan, admitted into Leopardstown for in-patient treatment on three separate occasions between 1926 and 1930, describe a man blighted by recurring psychoneurotic symptoms. The symptoms could, nevertheless, be improved upon and stabilised under the sheltered conditions of the hospital:

> FIRST ADMISSION 2.9.1926: Pains in head and sleeplessness and depression. Complaints of frequent severe headache sometimes lasting as long as three weeks on end. Does not sleep too well. Feels depressed, run down, nervous, highly strung. Subdued, nervous, depressed, introspective, lacking in confidence and emotional unstable.
>
> 5.10.26: Complains of severe headache and appears as if suffering. Did not sleep well last night, Depressed and self-centred. Working in joinery. Apathetic to therapy.
>
> 14.10.26: Headaches come and go, but depression is there all the time and cannot shake it off. Is always depressed in appearance and in conversation from the impression, as if was on the verge of breakdown. Working in joinery.

27.1.26: Recently has appeared somewhat brighter and admits some response. Headaches easier. Sleeping better and feels a bit more cheerful. Appetite is very fair.

9.11.26: Variable, but on the whole better, headache not so frequently and not so miserable.

17.11.26: Improved. Retain for consolidation.

1.12.26: Progress has been slow. There is a considerable degree of depression which is not likely to respond to treatment.

24.12.26: Discharged.

In addition to soothing his mental state, Whelan's admission would improve the quality of his life. While initially being admitted into Leopardstown as a pensioner in receipt of a small disability pension for a gunshot wound to the head, it was during Whelan's first stay that the Ministry seemingly arranged a medical boarding to assess his neurasthenic condition. A 50 percent pension was subsequently awarded. Whelan would also go onto perform paid casual labour working on the grounds of Leopardstown Hospital after his first discharge, affording him a wage often unattainable in civil society. Highlighting how financial recompense or employment should not, however, be equated with recovery, Whelan was re-admitted to Leopardstown two years later:

SECOND ADMISSION 29.8.28: Complains of pains in head. Depression and sleeplessness. Feels run down.

21.9.28: Admits benefit and appears less on edge and brighter, though still very depressed, subdued, timid, seclusive, listless and preoccupied. Memory impaired, easily confused.

4.10.28: Not much change to date. Some days feel better while others is depressed and has severe headache. Working outdoor.

12.10.28: Possibly a little brighter otherwise much as on admission. Melancholic type, always appears miserable and is on verge of breaking down.

30.10.28: On admission [was] suffering from breakdowns very subdued, miserable ... Is somewhat better since admission, but appears to have deteriorated since previously here and I suggest assessment by next board. Condition is regarded as due to persistent effects War Service.

31.10.28: Discharged. Breakdown type.

Despite the lack of recovery during Whelan's second spell of treatment, his residency again proved beneficial. Large amounts of war debris were removed from Whelan's ear by Leopardstown's medical staff during his second residency.

This medical attention subsequently improved the pains in his ear. Whelan's final admission came in January 1930.

> THIRD ADMISSION 14.1.1930: Complaints as before.
>
> 3.2.30: Complains weakness in legs and that he is going paralysed. Looks depressed and very worried about himself.
>
> 12.2.30: Frequently complains of feeling bad. Headache, weakness ... obviously very concerned about himself.
>
> 7.3.30: In a very anxious condition still complains feeling weak all over today and appeared very much on edge. Excused work for today.
>
> 19.3.30: Frequently complains feeling bad and is genuinely anxious about himself. Looks depressed and worried and is subdued and emotional. No reference to any psychotic features. Still obsessed with the idea that his legs are going paralysed.
>
> 2.4.30: Somewhat brighter at present, and does not complain so often. No reference [to] voices.
>
> 14.4.30: Now seldom complains and seems brighter and more cheerful. Still complains of weakness in legs from knees down. No evidence of neuritis ... Discharged. Breakdown type likely to deteriorate further.[74]

This case study reflects Tyron's assessment of the wider in-patient population. Although a permanent and total cure would often prove elusive, Ministry in-patient care could prevent a deterioration of symptoms and a potential admission to a lunatic asylum.[75] Even after psychotherapy became increasingly marginalised during the inter-war period, Leopardstown Hospital and Ministry out-patient facilities in Dublin offered superior facilities unobtainable to Free State citizens who had not served in the British Army.[76]

Following the death of Gertrude Dunning on 27 June 1926, her husband revoked ownership of the Leopardstown country home, offering it as a gift to the Ministry of Pensions to remain as an exclusive facility for Great War veterans.[77] Craigavon Hospital also operated throughout the inter-war period due to Craig's generosity. It remains unclear whether the Ministry of Pensions would have provided the necessary finances without these generous donations, although it appears unlikely as the department pursued a policy of descaling and non-intervention post-1921. The Ministry's de-escalation of funding and facilities to help rehabilitate the disabled veteran would, nevertheless, have an immense impact on the remit and function of Leopardstown Hospital. The Ministry's Blackrock Hospital, the largest ex-service rehabilitative facility in Ireland, closed in 1931 due to the continuation of Ministry cutbacks. Leopardstown filled the subsequent void by incorporating limb-fitting, surgical treatment and orthopaedic care within its remit and function. Neurasthenic pensioners would thereafter constitute a minority of in-patients receiving care in the facility. Psychoneurotic pensioners constituted just 8 percent of admissions by 1938.[78]

The intrinsic relationship between the national economy, unemployment and disability returned in 1939. The Ministry brought special attention to the dire economic conditions in Leopardstown admissions, writing that it was the existing 'economic factors which lead pensioners in the Irish Free State being admitted to hospital in a state of extreme debility.'[79] Leopardstown's Medical Superintendent similarly noted the acute and chronic nature of its mentally ill residents who were unable to function in civil society and whose 'debilitated appearance' was obvious on admission.[80] The Medical Superintendent's annual report two years later describe the general pattern of neurasthenic admissions: 'Many of the Old War cases of the chronic type require permanent institutional treatment; a few are constantly in and out, and we have endeavoured to make their stay as short as possible.' The six mentally ill pensioners receiving in-patient care were described as requiring permanent institutional care with two remaining largely bed-ridden. Without the supervision, shelter and opportunity to work within Leopardstown, these pensioners were assumed doomed to regress outside of the Ministry facility. This thesis is verified by a resident for seven years discharging himself against medical advice and shortly afterwards requiring admission into a public mental hospital.[81]

The facilities at Leopardstown could only ever cater for a tiny fraction of the neurasthenic pensioner community in the Irish Free State. This imbalance reflected larger UK trends: 74,905 veterans in the United Kingdom were receiving a pension for neurasthenia in 1936, but only just over 400 neurasthenic pensioners were receiving in-patient or out-patient treatment.[82] It is possible that neurasthenic pensioners did not seek out treatment due to the stigma attached to mental illness regardless of the severity of symptoms and the location of medical care provided. It was even feared that mixing with fellow neurasthenic ex-servicemen would be psychologically damaging and could result in admission into a district asylum.[83] The majority of neurasthenic pensioners in Ireland would attempt to reintegrate back into civil society, alongside their former comrades, including those physically disabled, as best they could without undergoing Ministry treatment. This restoration was increasingly difficult in the Irish Free State due to the country's socio-economic, political and cultural context.

British ex-servicemen in the Irish Free State

Taylor suggests that Great War veterans were not discriminated against by the Irish Free State government or society.[84] His thesis aligns itself with the Report of the Committee of Enquiry into the State of Ex-servicemen published in 1928. Yet, the report also concedes that there may have been sporadic incidences of discrimination in the 'choosing of men locally' by 'foremen' regarding 'labour' opportunities.[85] Such instances should not be underplayed. The Ministry cites discrimination against the British ex-servicemen in government positions and public roles, particularly in western counties 'where officials with pronounced views allow their political prejudices to govern selection ... Such prejudices are openly displayed.'[86] One disabled ex-Irish Guardsman, Patrick Regan, complained that his war-induced disability did not favour his employment in the Free State civil service which it would otherwise have done had he been living in Britain.[87] Private employers also forwarded accusations of official discrimination against British ex-servicemen:

> I am a small employer of labour and lately upon giving work to a couple of ex-service British soldiers was on the following day waited on by an official of the Free State government who threatened me and warned me not to give 'on any account work to men who had served in the enemy army, and to reserve all employment for those who had served in the Free State army and especially those who had served prior to the treaty.'[88]

One Ministry of Pensions official in Dublin accepted that 'there are individuals on both sides who allow their personal official authority to be subordinated by their political leanings.'[89]

The British Legion in Northern Ireland conducted a review of conditions in the Irish Free State in November 1926, concluding: 'In many parts the men are afraid to identify themselves with the Legion, for to acknowledge themselves as ex-servicemen, means, speaking generally, unemployment.' The report asserted 'The position of ex-servicemen is pitiable in the extreme' and concluded that ex-servicemen in the south of Ireland were 'one of the greatest problems in the empire.'[90] The British Legion in the Free State similarly attested that no body of men had suffered from unemployment more in the country than British ex-servicemen.[91] In 1929, almost 60 percent of unemployed men in Britain were Great War veterans.[92] The situation facing the same group of veterans was even more difficult in the Free State as recognised by the SILA: 'It must not be assumed from above that the ex-serviceman in the Irish Free State is on parity with his fellows in Great Britain or Northern Ireland. Such is by no means the case ... he has to cope with a proportionally higher ratio of unemployment.'[93] Ex-servicemen in Ennis were labelled as being destitute and struggling for necessities such as boots and blankets.[94] Ex-servicemen living in the Irish Free State were described by G. Wolfe, TD as being in a 'very bad state' on 16 November 1927.[95]

Once again, the broader socio-economic context merits consideration. Often accusations of discrimination are more nuanced than a straightforward narrative of persecution suggests. In the 1930s, ex-servicemen in receipt of a pension were prejudiced against by employers who preferred employees who were solely dependent on their working wage.[96] One pensioner in Cork recalled: 'I got a job on a relief scheme for some weeks and there was an objection raised that I was a pensioner and I was dismissed. I reported to the City manager and he could not help me as there were others he said with nothing so that is the way we are treated here as a British Ex-Serviceman.'[97] Refuting allegations of the discrimination of British ex-servicemen, Seán Lemass TD, and Taoiseach between 1959 and 1966, argued in 1936:

> He is not entitled to unemployment assistance because he has means in excess of the limits laid down ... It is not because he is getting a pension. The only reason I am dealing with this is because the manner in which it has been referred to suggests that in some way we have discriminated against British ex-servicemen. That is not correct.

Lemass stated that ex-servicemen in receipt of pensions 'would similarly be debarred if the amount of money they got was derived from any other source, including a pension under our own Military Service (Pensions) Acts, or revenue from a farm, shop, house or boat. Because they are not entitled to unemployment assistance.' Thus, ex-servicemen in receipt of a pension 'are in no different position to any other members of the community', or 'to any other person having means of the same value', with regards to unemployment assistance.[98]

The Great War veterans shared with the wider population the privations of a weak economy, heavily reliant on agriculture, which accounted for more than half of the country's workforce, further hampered by an absence of industrialisation. A lack of qualifications also hampered Great War veterans in this economic climate.[99] Added to this economic deprivation were occasional prejudice and widespread apathy to the plight of British ex-servicemen. A Ministry of Pensions' report from Dublin in 1936 best summarised the predicament facing Irish Great War veterans living in the region, stating: 'In general, while there is no sympathy for the ex-servicemen as such, there is no boycott.' The same report concluded that their 'difficulties do not spring from his war service but are indigenous to the economic conditions of the country in which he lives and are shared by all other members of the same community.'[100] Ministry officials in Dublin also emphasised that 'while not discriminated against', ex-servicemen were 'not officially regarded as candidates for favours.'[101]

The economy in Northern Ireland was also desolate. By 1932, the official unemployment figures amounted to 72,000 people. Three years later, with an estimated 102,000 people unemployed, Northern Irish unemployment rates peaked at 30 percent which was higher than any comparable area in Britain. Reliant on a small range of exports, industry in Northern Ireland suffered from foreign governments raising tariffs on external produce to protect domestic production.[102] Returning veterans would share this austerity with the wider population. On 3 April 1928, the *Irish Times* reported: 'The dream of the ex-service men that they would live in a land "fit for heroes" has not come true so far as the Belfast contingent are concerned.' The Belfast Union housed 285 ex-servicemen designated as 'paupers' with a further 223 ex-servicemen relying on outdoor relief.[103] In contrast to the Free State, however, attempts were, at the very least, made to accommodate ex-servicemen in a tough economic context. The Northern Ireland Civil Service, for example, attempted to employ 1,000 veterans constituting around 50 percent of the workforce.[104] Great War veterans in Northern Ireland also benefitted from employment and fundraising schemes assisted by high-profile members of society, including the Prime Minister. One Free State veteran even wrote to the Northern Irish Prime Minister, James Craig, for assistance. The veteran received a personal gratuity from Craig as 'a little sign of his sympathy to an old comrade.' Such an incident provides an apt metaphor of the opposing views the Northern Irish and Free State governments attached to war service.[105]

A Great War pensioner in the Irish Free State remained eligible for British sponsored state assistance in the form of employment training provided by the British Ministry of Labour to assist their employability. There were five Ministry of Labour training facilities operating in the Irish Free State in 1925. Three were located in Dublin with one each in Tipperary and Clonmel. Courses provided included carpentry, blacksmithing, watch and clock repair, basket-making and motoring. These facilities catered for 650 men at a time. The Ministry of Labour clarified the reluctance of the Free State Government to become too involved with the scheme to alleviate the situation: 'The Free State Government have not displayed any hostility to the Training Scheme, but they have carefully avoided any open connection with it. They are glad that the British Government should spend money in Ireland, but they do not wish to be regarded as in any way responsible for their activities.' The department thus wrote that they had no choice but to proceed with the scheme 'quietly' with little likelihood of waiting lists being reduced.[106]

The same *laissez-faire* principle evident in the Free State applied to wider society, as is evidenced by the continued absence of the King's National Roll.[107] In Britain, 80 percent of all disabled men who benefitted from a war pension attained employment because of the scheme between the years 1921 and 1938, which was a significantly lower figure when compared to the non-disabled ex-servicemen population. An annual average of 26,000 employers in Britain took on 380,000 disabled Great War veterans between 1921 and 1938.[108] The Ministry of Labour in Northern Ireland also established and oversaw the King's National Roll. Local employment committees throughout Northern Ireland were noted as having taken 'energetic steps' to increase the number of enrolled employers and maximise the prospects of employment of disabled ex-servicemen. In February 1924, 505 firms had signed up, which was a dramatic increase on the 105 who had done so by 1921. The number of unemployed disabled ex-servicemen had also decreased from 1,183 to 636 during the same period.[109] By February 1924, the scheme was described as being 'heartily supported' by Belfast employers.[110]

On 11 February 1924, the Prime Minister made an appeal to local employers at the Belfast City Hall for the further employment of 700 disabled ex-servicemen in Belfast.[111] Teething problems persisted. Several employers signed up to the scheme but were never patronised by the National Roll and government officials.[112] Towards the end of the 1920s, the President of the King's National Roll in Northern Ireland admitted that the scheme had been beneficial to thousands of disabled Great War veterans in Northern Ireland, but stressed that 'much remains to be done.'[113] This shortcoming is in tandem with Britain where, as the memory of the war faded, and the economic insecurity and widespread unemployment of the 1920s and 1930s became fully realised, the sense of obligation to disabled Great War veterans in Britain became less of an imperative as men competed for limited opportunities to work.[114]

While no equivalent to the King's National Roll was implemented in the Free State, assumedly due to the lack of societal and government support and the trade union resistance previously cited, private employers were encouraged to provide preferential treatment to ex-National Army servicemen.[115] In 1924, the 'Council of the Unemployed' subsequently complained that 'the Government is doing nothing for civilians and everything for ex-army men.'[116] The disadvantages that ex-servicemen faced in returning home to a society where another group of veterans received preferential treatment again become evident. In June 1936, one Ministry official summarised the position of pensioners in the Free State, writing: 'The disabled ex-servicemen have not the general and wholehearted support which is enjoyed by their comrades in Great Britain. There is no King's Roll, no wide appeal to public sympathy backed by Church or State.'[117] The Ministry recognised the secluded position that many ex-servicemen experienced in the Irish Free State, avowing: 'He suffers from a sense of inferiority and helplessness born from his isolation from England and the apathy and lack of interest that surround him.'[118] The Ministry's report in June 1936 subsequently concluded:

> The Irish Free State refuses to regard itself as having participated as a nation in the Great War and has repudiated responsibility for the cost of its after affects. Every southern Irishmen who enlisted did so as a volunteer, and each individual must either bear responsibility for the results of his voluntary act or look to his employer, the British Government, for redress.

One particularly prophetic line specified: 'The Great War and its aftermath does not enter the ethical conscience of the Free State, with the result that those who suffered by volunteering their services excite neither interest nor sympathy.'[119]

Under such circumstances, an unspecified number of disabled Great War veterans in Cork resorted to pawning their pension books to make ends meet.[120] Daniel Mulcahy, in receipt of a pension for bronchitis, gunshot wounds and debility, lived in two rooms of a tenement house with his wife and seven children, including his disabled teenage son. He explained that he undertook such a measure when he was broke explaining 'that is the way we have to try and exist in this country.'[121] Accusations from Ministry officials and British politicians that Irish ex-servicemen such as Mulcahy were curators of their misfortune due to idleness persisted.[122] Living in an unsympathetic society, and in the absence of an interventionist government, the comradeship of British ex-servicemen in the Free State becomes understandable. For example, Arnold met with three illiterate and downtrodden disabled veterans in Limerick who complained about their treatment by the Ministry. After each pensioner articulated his case, Arnold described the moving solidarity between the men as each one was clapped by the other two following their speech.[123] While recognising instances of discrimination towards British ex-servicemen living in the newly formed state, apathy appears to have been the overriding emotion. The additional prejudice attached to their disability further compromised the ability of mentally ill veterans in the Free State to reintegrate back into civil society.

Mentally disabled pensioners

Recalling writing *Shell Shock and its Lessons*, Thomas Pear recognised that the treatment of mentally ill servicemen extended beyond medical intervention and that a cultural shift in legitimising and sympathising with traumatised ex-servicemen was equally necessary to facilitate their reintegration into the labour market and civil society.[124] This recognition was absent in both post-war

British and Irish society. Harold Ozzard, a neurasthenic veteran of the Royal Irish Fusiliers, repeatedly attested to his inability to attain employment due to his neurasthenic disability.[125] Ozzard would share this unfortunate position with similarly afflicted former comrades in Britain. T. H. Mills of the ESWS wrote in 1930: 'The blinded man is a tragic figure; the limbless man is a tragic figure, but the mentally disabled and the injured in mind is the greatest tragedy of all.'[126] Another British veteran, W. D. Esplin, similarly describes the neurasthenic veteran community's futile attempt to reintegrate back into inter-war society owing to the 'insuperable prejudice towards men who are known sufferers from "nerve-trouble". Employers will have none of us: we are as lepers in the labour market. The living dead.'[127] An ESWS fundraising appeal and an article in a journal for British expatriates similarly wrote that the nervy and unpredictable nature of psychoneurosis ensured little societal sympathy towards the neurasthenic pensioner in comparison to the physically disabled.[128] Ministry memorandums and ESWS reports similarly attest that local employers did not employ neurasthenic pensioners when they became aware of their disability due to their supposedly unpredictable and unproductive nature that required extra instruction and supervision.[129] Reflecting the disciplinarian and moral shift in their treatment and perception of the neurasthenic pensioners, the Ministry told its Medical Officers in 1931 that a veteran's psychoneurotic symptoms were often shaped by their innate inability to handle economic pressure and the trials and tribulations of everyday life.[130] Even medico-military staff conceded that they would not employ some of the supposedly erratic neurasthenic pensioners with whom they came into contact.[131] The ESWS recognised the difficulty of placing mentally ill Great War veterans in employment owing to societal perceptions, writing: 'It is obvious that with a large number of unemployed, employers will not take a neurasthenic ex-service man when a fit man is available. The unsuccessful question for work has a very definite depressing effect upon these men.'[132]

The mental fragility of neurasthenic ex-servicemen could induce their relinquishment of or removal from permanent employment due to periodic breakdowns or crises of confidence. It was not uncommon for them to assume a less stressful and often junior and less well paid position even when a neurasthenic did obtain employment.[133] Despite being described as intelligent and in possession of a university degree, O'Ryan's obsessions, introspection and inability to concentrate impaired his functioning and employability. He was eventually able to find employment as a part-time secretary at a local golf club in 1930, although the job was poorly paid with work involved being 'very light.'[134] O'Ryan's physical ailments improved dramatically by 1924; he was described as looking in a 'good physical condition' and able to play golf. His mental fragility, however, persisted. His pension board reports describe a man suffering from 'severe anxiety neurosis' with depression, reclusiveness, tremulous limbs, nervousness and religious obsessions blighting his daily life:

> Inclined to be reclusive and to avoid companionship and social intercourse ... quite unable to shoulder responsibility to any mental or even physical effort ... whole life governed by obsessions. The simplest actions arouse a chain of obsessions and resultant depressed state ... has to bring 'right' or 'wrong' with all his actions – even closing a door.

O'Ryan told pensions offices that he 'couldn't get his breath', which his doctor attributed to his nervous condition, suggesting that he also suffered from recurrent panic attacks.[135] O'Ryan's conduct reflects contemporary trauma theory which suggests that traumatised individuals restrict and compartmentalise their lives to create a sense of order and safety in their lives to combat persistent fear.[136]

Eustace Percy, MP for Hastings, and the future Parliamentary Secretary to the Ministry of Health, held that neurasthenic pensioners carefully avoided alerting contemporaries to their condition: 'Each becomes a *cause celebre* in his district ... Notoriety ... preys on his mind.'[137] Despite the severity of his psychoneurotic symptoms, O'Ryan was both keen and able to conceal his torment from wider society. On 1 September 1932, one Ministry official who assessed him wrote:

> [Dr] Graham, who sat with me on the Board, knows the Officer quite well socially, being a member of the same golf club. He was surprised and rather amused to find that the Officer was drawing a high pension for Neurasthenia as he had always regarded him as a thoroughly normal young man, though he knew that the right leg gave rise to periodic trouble.

O'Ryan was anxious to prevent his mental illness from being broadcast and had to be assured by the examining officer that the contents of the assessment would remain confidential. The assessment officer wrote: 'I did not regard his perturbation as significant of malingering but rather as indicating his fear that the barrier of reserve that he had built around himself was to be broken down.' The inspecting officer proved 'satisfied that he is in a highly unstable mental condition although his behaviour may appear quite normal. As regards actual Neurasthenia there are few signs.' O'Ryan was able to function effectively despite his condition as he was able to drive alone to one board meeting 'and was obviously quite accustomed to this sort of thing.'[138] O'Ryan's attempt to hide his psychoneurosis is verified by his niece, Ann O'Ryan, who spent annual summer vacations with the O'Ryan family in Sandycove, Ireland, during her childhood. Ann was knowledgeable of her uncle's physical disability pension for his gunshot wound but was unaware of the British pension he received for neurasthenia.[139]

Neurasthenic pensioners in Northern Ireland also struggled in their daily lives. Peter Fitzpatrick struggled to attain employment, remaining blighted by neurasthenic symptoms for much of the 1920s. Fitzpatrick's depression, nerves, tremulous limbs and feelings of ostracism from society persisted, and he was subsequently admitted into Craigavon Hospital for in-patient treatment in February 1926. In-patient therapy included staff discussing with Fitzpatrick his symptoms and attempts to reason a causality and remedy. This treatment was offered alongside light outdoor work on the grounds of Craigavon. Despite a slight improvement in his condition, Fitzpatrick discharged himself just under three months later pending the re-opening of his pension assessment award. Fitzpatrick told Craigavon staff that its distribution would provide a tremendous financial and psychological benefit to his wife and children. The Ministry's subsequent boarding notes on Fitzpatrick reveal his unfortunate mental state:

> Complains of confusion, is nervous, feels depressed. Pains in his head. Is easily excited and shakes all over. Is very religious, attends mass regularly. His sleep is disturbed. Worried about his household affairs and gets very irritable at the least thing. Has no interest in anything … facial expressions denotes worry and anxiety. Memory is fair, emotionally he is unstable and introspective. Inclined to be solitary. Worries about his health. Moderately severe effect on function. The difference in the condition is that the man is unstable, emotional, introspective and there is anxiety neurosis. It will not materially shorten the normal duration of life but prohibits him from taking up any form of manual labour.

Demonstrating that 'Final Awards' were not *always* final, Fitzpatrick's pension was increased to 40 percent following a specially assembled medical boarding to assess him in Belfast in December 1926.[140]

A deterioration in Fitzpatrick's condition, including persistent headaches, sleeplessness, emotionality and mental instability and distrust of people, was noted during a boarding assessment at the Ministry's regional office in Belfast in September 1931, leading to his readmission to Craigavon. His resulting admission notes describe a nervous man convinced that people were sneering and laughing at him, who had trouble with violent and murderous dreams, was unable to cope with the loud noises made by his young children and suffered from recurrent migraines. Fitzpatrick was provided sleeping sedatives and opportunities to work, although he showed little inclination for the latter. This reluctance, combining with his persistent thoughts that fellow in-patients were gossiping about him, led to his discharge just five weeks after his admission with staff assessing that no further treatment would be useful. His release was rushed through due to the disturbance Fitzpatrick was causing other patients by refusing to go to bed and his repeated demands for the attention of Craigavon staff during the early hours of the morning.[141] While continuing to provide treatment and assessments of Fitzpatrick, and even being willing to overturn a prior legislative decision at its own expense, the slight increase from a 20 to a 40 percent pension appears a miserly return for a man so blighted by service-related psychoneurotic symptoms. Similarly, Ministry and Craigavon staff seemingly displayed few qualms about prematurely discharging Fitzpatrick back into civil society, despite his evident and persistent mental health problems. The Ministry's treatment of Fitzpatrick provides another example of the Ministry's cold and dismissive treatment of mentally ill veterans existing alongside its progressive and liberal attempts to treat and compensate them.

It remains impractical to determine the extent to which O'Ryan's and Fitzpatrick's personal experiences correlated with the wider neurasthenic community in Ireland. While historians assert that Great War veterans 'retired into historical oblivion', O'Ryan was able to hide in plain sight by utilising a 'barrier of reserve' to obscure his mental debility. This 'tendency to concealment' was common amongst mentally ill Great War veterans.[142] Many neurasthenic pensioners in Britain successfully concealed their pension and the nature and severity of their disability from employers, colleagues and fellow citizens in the belief that knowledge of their mental illness would prejudice behaviour towards them.[143] The vast majority of neurasthenic pensioners endeavoured to recommence life in civil society without undergoing medical treatment.[144] Percy held that societal reintegration would prove hugely difficult, believing that these attempts by neurasthenic pensioners would be disturbed due to 'the almost invariably intermittent character of symptoms.' This inconsistency made it difficult for medical staff to assess pensioners accurately and recommend the appropriate treatment.[145] O'Ryan's experience verifies Percy's fears. Previous feminist conceptions of shell-shock, where sufferers were associated with 'powerless femininity', was apparent.[146] An assessment of O'Ryan in August 1932 describes him as displaying a 'complexion and appearance rather feminine.' Another report written six years later, however, conversely describes him as having a 'gentlemanly appearance.' A more composed O'Ryan told officials in March 1933 that his neurasthenic 'feelings come in cycles.' A board's report one year previous noted that his 'attention, intelligence concentration and memory [were] up to normal standard.'[147] The sympathetic approach shown towards O'Ryan and his substantial pension complicates the narrative forwarded by veterans that the Ministry's boarding of mentally ill veterans involved prejudice, bullying and tactlessness where a pensioner was treated akin to a criminal.[148]

Percy believed that the repeated medical board assessment of veterans to decipher pension rates hurt a pensioner's mental condition, arguing that 'the men feel that they are being suspected and analysed and investigated and re-investigated.'[149] Percy's criticisms are again evident in O'Ryan's pension reports. One report noted that he exhibited 'morbid flushing, which can be produced merely by looking steadily at him when questioning him.' During the final assessment before his death at the age of seventy-seven, O'Ryan 'broke down during examination and wept profusely.'[150] Ultimately, O'Ryan's and Fitzpatrick's pension records reveal men with little evidence of progress or recovery; Percy concluded that 'the state is spending large sums of money on these cases with no result whatsoever ... I believe that the Ministry's present policy is definitely wrong.' Yet, Percy had little idea as to what policy was 'definitely right' conceding that 'at the present the only common-sense treatment is to pension them off and leave them alone.'[151] The distribution of pensions to both physically and mentally disabled veterans in the Irish Free State proved to be both sustained and critical.

An imperial obligation

The SILA attested to the isolated position of Great War veterans residing in the Irish Free State:

> It has been said to me that Southern Ireland today is a self-governing Dominion, and that it is no concern of this country what happens over there. To some extent this statement is true, but these ex-service men are peculiarly England's responsibility; they volunteered to fight their battles, and she promised to look after them. Is it right for England to repudiate her promises just because she has thought fit to remove herself from Southern Ireland and throw that improvised country on her own slender resources, with the result that thousands of those who helped here are left to starve.

The report concluded 'surely the cry of the children will be heard in this still wealthy country.'[152] This narrative of the abandoned Great War veteran is ill-founded. In addition to the British Ministry of Labour's 'quiet' training scheme, five war pension committees continued to operate in the Irish Free State with the assistance of a further thirty-six sub-branches. In September 1927, over 3,600 Great War pensioners were seen personally by a pensions official with over 1,700 medical examinations.[153] Neurasthenia was just one condition provided for within a wide variety of ailments and disabilities catered for by the Ministry. By 1928, the annual expenditure of the department in the Irish Free State amounted to £2,080,000.[154] The Ministry of Pensions recognised that pension costs including treatment allowances in the Irish Free State were excessive with pension ratios accounting for 32 percent of enlisted men in comparison to 10 percent in Britain and 16 percent in Northern Ireland (Table 6).[155]

Table 6 Cost of pensions per enlisted man, 1926–27.

	England/Wales	Scotland	Northern Ireland	Irish Free State
Enlisted men	4,279,082	557,618	62,104	72,104
Amount paid to men	£21,994	£2,327	£619	£1,251
Cost per man	£5 2s 10d	£4 3s 7d	£9 19s 8d	£17 7s 6d

The figures can be extrapolated from data provided within NA, PIN 15/757, Commission to enquire into the condition of British ex-serviceman in the Irish Free State; Taylor, *Heroes or Traitors?*, 117.

Costs were continually on the rise in the Irish Free State while pension costs were decreasing in Britain between 1921 and 1930.[156] Treatment allowance costs, for example, quadrupled in the Irish Free State in comparison to Great Britain.[157] Veterans in the Irish Free State were also more likely to successfully appeal Ministry decisions in comparison to similar claims in Britain.[158] These figures contradict Lord John Danesfort who complained that 'so far as the British Government, I regret to say, has not made itself responsible for relieving the sufferings of these men.'[159] Similarly, Barham's evaluation that the Ministry of Pensions was particularly resistant to providing financial support to Irish Great War veterans is problematised.[160]

As had been the case in 1921, officials in Britain were unhappy at the fluctuations evident in Ireland, remaining sceptical as to assessment standards. It was considered 'far more difficult' to trust waiting list figures for treatment of a physical disability owing to war service as Irish medical staff would grant medical certificates for men to help attain financial assistance from the British Government.[161] The fact that charities and social support were comparatively inactive in the Free State may offer a fundamental explanation as to the inflated pension outlay in the state. The tough economic conditions and more flexible health insurance initiatives may have ensured that British governmental officials and Irish medical officials in the Free State were keener to assist ex-servicemen. The influence of individual Free State politicians and their manipulation of the Ministry of Pensions should not be overlooked. There was political and economic capital gained via the support of disabled ex-servicemen; this capital, as well as the continued autonomy of pensions officials, shaped the inflated outlay in the Free State.[162] With these comparative pension payments in mind, Jack Lawson, MP told the House of Commons: 'I think the House will agree that it is much better to be an ex-service man in Ireland than in England at the present time.'[163]

Barham described a disability pension as 'a survival kit in the barren environment of mass unemployment.'[164] This 'survival kit' was even more necessary in the Irish Free State, where employment was sparser than in Britain with the lack of societal support or governmental initiatives available to British ex-servicemen. The benefit of a military pension was further increased because the Ministry's pension scheme did not consider the generally lower cost of living in Ireland.[165] Fallon's rejected proposals in March 1922 for the newly-established Free State Government to establish an autonomous Irish Ministry of Pensions highlights the monetary worth of a British Ministry pension for disabled First World War veterans residing in the Free State. After taking over from the British department, Fallon specified that any subsequent pensions provided by a new Irish department would be lower than what had been previously afforded by British authorities.[166] The Ministry's financial distribution is further magnified when remembering the existing austerity of public spending and welfare in the Irish Free State. Free State civil servants were, for example, paid less than their counterparts in Britain. Free State welfare costs lessened with pensions for the blind and old-age pensions reduced by 10 percent in 1924, lagging behind other Western countries in value.[167] The Ministry lived up to its billing as an 'imperial obligation' in the Irish Free State. Arnold's recollection of the Ministry of Pensions also attests to the steadfast commitment of regional and local staff to the disabled British ex-servicemen in the newly formed state.[168]

Other wars and transnational comparatives

Placing the Ministry of Pensions' remit and function within a transnational and transconflict context further foregrounds the department's liberality and benevolence. Mentally ill veterans in France were regularly held by French society, including veterans themselves, as a detached and inferior community of disabled ex-servicemen. Mentally ill veterans were not provided a free consultation, examination and boarding to help demonstrate that their disability was attributable to war service. They received negligible state-aided medical and pharmaceutical care and faced almost insurmountable difficulties in proving to pension authorities that their psychoneurotic symptoms were due to war service. This treatment stood in stark contrast to their physically disabled former comrades.[169] Across the British Empire, Australia and Canada enabled mentally ill veterans to receive pensions and treatment under administrative infrastructures.[170] There were, however, no special treatment facilities for neurasthenic pensioners in the Union of South Africa. Instead, military hospitals providing negligible specialist psychotherapeutic treatment accommodated psychoneurotic veterans. Ex-servicemen suffering severer forms of mental illness were accommodated in nursing homes or underfunded, miserable and poorly run mental hospitals with little provision for treatment nor an expectation of recovery.[171]

The Weimar Government distributed generous pensions and rehabilitative programmes to its disabled veteran communities during the 1920s. By the mid-1930s, however, German mentally ill veterans were singled out by the Nazi regime through having their pensionable rights and status revoked. This retraction was due to Nazi ideology advocating a doctrine of degeneration and hereditary traits.[172] Mentally disabled veterans in the Soviet Union followed a broad trajectory akin to those in the Free State: participation in the First World War representing an imperial power, a revolution, civil war and establishment of an alternative state in opposition to the aims of the Great War. In contrast to neurasthenic pensioners in the Free State, however, mentally ill Russian veterans of the First World War would receive negligible attention and no state assistance as the solidifying of Marxist collectivist principles reigned supreme during the inter-war period.[173] The Balkan states and their separation from the Austro-Hungarian Empire negatively affected mentally disabled veterans. Many mentally ill ex-servicemen were unable to apply for medical and rehabilitative assistance and financial aid as no social insurance existed in the newly established nation-state of Yugoslavia.[174] Despite experiencing imperial diplomatic changes and the establishment of new territory, the Ministry's role and assistance in the Irish Free State remained sustained throughout the inter-war period, regardless of the bitter guerrilla conflict between paramilitary Irish republicans and British state forces.[175]

With regards to financial compensation and facilities, mentally disabled Great War veterans also surpassed the Irish veteran of the revolutionary conflicts. Psychoneurotic casualties arose as a result of active service in both the Anglo-Irish War and Irish Civil War.[176] Instances were brought up during Dáil debates stating that ex-National Army veterans were suffering from 'Shell-Shock' as a result of action during the Irish Civil War.[177] Writing about one ex-National Army man who was 'an absolute wreck', Mr A. Byrne wrote that 'It was a case of neurasthenia, caused, I think, by service in the Wireless Department of the Army.' He believed there to be 'many other cases of young men going up and down the country, sleeping in hay barns and wet blankets, and compelled to go for days together without any change of clothing.'[178] Nevertheless, President William Cosgrave stated that the inclusion of combat neurosis in the Army Pensions Act was not even considered.[179] There was no comparable care for mental disability under the legislation. The lack of such provisions led Lyons in the Dáil to deduce it was 'not an Army pension at all, but only a farcical sketch of a pension', complaining that 'the British Government, as bad as it was, treated their ex-servicemen who are living in the Saorstat well.'[180]

Different races from across the British Empire who served in the British Army during the First World War were paid on a different scale to British and Irish troops. For example, West Indian troops received a lesser payment for disabilities than those discussed throughout this study.[181] Research into war neurosis and the treatment of African Americans in conflicts from the American Civil War to the Second World War demonstrates that army medical and pensions staff advocated racist aspersions regarding disability and emotional volatility.[182] Psychoneurotic African American First World War veterans were treated apart or in separate facilities entirely in states such as Mississippi, Louisiana, Alabama, Texas and Georgia. The latter, for example, housed a large facility hosting 4,000 patients which was described by an American specialist in shell-shock and neurasthenia as 'very unsatisfactory'.[183] As a result of the substandard facilities and the prejudices attached, African American veterans sought in-patient treatment on a much lower scale than white veterans.[184] The Irish temperament was similarly doubted before 1914, during the First World War and throughout the inter-war period. Crucially, however, neurasthenic Great War veterans in Ireland were not denied financial compensation, and they shared equitable in-patient facilities with their former British comrades.[185] To the contrary, mentally ill Irish veterans appear seemingly better able to profit from state-funded recompense and, during the revolutionary period, more likely to seek in-patient treatment for neuropsychiatric symptoms than their former comrades in Britain.

Domestic care and charities

The treatment and experiences of disabled veteran communities should, of course, also extend *beyond* financial payment and medical treatment. The Ministry continued to co-exist with an active charity sector and substantial domestic and familial care. As Winter encapsulates: 'The Great War placed the disabled at the centre of civil society, but it was in homes and out of sight that their miseries were expressed.'[186] Thomas Whelan's wife told Ministry officials about her husband's insomnia where he would wander around the house all night, becoming very solemn, unapproachable and irritable during the day.[187] The Ministry of Pensions appreciated that the fate of mentally disabled pensioners depended heavily on their domestic setting.[188] While O'Ryan's medical reports denote that he was suitable for admission into a nursing home, with the Ministry of Pensions offering to provide his maintenance grant, this measure was avoided because of the assistance provided him by his wife, Mary Josephine O'Ryan. O'Ryan repeatedly told medical boarding officials of his wife's caregiving during the inter-war period: 'If it was not for his wife he couldn't carry on at all …

Cannot bear being left alone. Wife does everything for him.' In addition to spending long periods unable to leave his home, his wife dealt with O'Ryan's correspondence and finances including affairs related to his pension, and she even assisted with his secretarial occupation at his local golf club. As late as 1963, O'Ryan stressed: 'I am very dependent on my wife.'[189] The psychological benefit of this emotional support was as important as its practical effects. Despite his persistent and debilitating psychoneurotic symptoms, Fitzpatrick told Ministry staff that spending time with his wife and children was often the most effective remedy to soothe his psychoneurotic symptoms.[190] A dual approach to treatment was often on offer to neurasthenic pensioners in the 1920s and 1930s: first, the compensatory payment provided by the Ministry ensured financial relief to these men who could not always attain stable and well-paid employment.[191] Second, veterans' families assumed the large burden of responsibility with regards to their everyday emotional and physical needs.[192]

British charities would also provide integral assistance when British governmental schemes failed to meet the needs of disabled Great War veterans.[193] The British Legion was one such vocal and loyal comrade to the Great War veteran. They assisted with employment schemes, charitable donations, training opportunities, employment, pension payments and information on issues such as limb fitting. The organisation also represented men in their dealings with the Ministry of Pensions and provided financial assistance in particularly desperate times.[194] The Legion's functioning was, however, impaired in the Irish Free State. Hundreds of British ex-servicemen in Dublin sought relief from the British Legion which was unable to assist them, even running out of application forms.[195] The SILA criticised the work of the Legion in the Free State, and argued that 'it was apparent that in most districts it was found to be unsatisfactory.'[196] This view was reinforced by a British philanthropist, Elizabeth Whitman, in 1927, who observed that British Legion clubs in several areas of Ireland were 'a hopeless failure' with depressing, cold, and dirty facilities.[197] British Legion officials rarely attended Ministry committee meetings throughout the Free State despite their open invitation to attend.[198] Estimates as to how many veterans joined the British Legion in Ireland vary from between 3 to 10 percent. The percentage of ex-servicemen in the Irish Free State who enlisted in the British Legion thus remained the lowest in the United Kingdom.[199] While the British Legion has been described as a 'zealous advocate' of the neurasthenic pensioner, this thesis does not apply to the Irish Free State.[200] The 1928 Committee on the Claims of Ex-Servicemen suggested that they were consequently 'less well acquainted with their rights and were less liable to have pension regulations brought to their attention' as a result.[201] The fact that pension awards were inflated in the Free State would counter this assertion.

The SILA assumed a more prominent role in assisting the British ex-service community in the absence of a committed and well-organised Legion. While the original aim of the organisation was to assist loyalists who had suffered because of their political view, they chose to extend the scope of their work and accommodate all ex-servicemen regardless of their political allegiance. Many ex-servicemen came to depend on the charity. Situated in an upstairs office in central Dublin, the surge in applicants necessitated the employment of a non-commissioned officer to maintain order amongst waiting men.[202] Vast queues of ex-servicemen regularly trailed down the stairs which caused huge inconvenience to businesses sharing the building and was a serious health and safety concern.[203] The SILA described the poverty and emaciated appearance of ex-serviceman suffering from neurasthenia of which there were 'hundreds of such cases.'[204] The organisation provided basic relief to the entire British ex-service, including mentally ill veterans, in the form of food, fuel and clothing. However, assistance in finding and allotting employment was believed to be too difficult an area to get involved in: 'The question of unemployment among ex-servicemen … is so acute … one which the voluntary societies cannot touch.'[205] In contrast, the ex-service community in Northern Ireland had a committed British Legion lobbying on their behalf. The organisation forcibly lobbied for greater allocation of employment in Northern Ireland governmental departments such as the Civil Service throughout the inter-war period.[206] British Legion officials in Northern Ireland observed that the prominence of the charity, its clubs and ability to foster camaraderie amongst veteran communities were severely lacking south of the border, writing: 'The position of the clubs and branches in southern Ireland is entirely different to that prevailing in this country.'[207]

The British Legion was a mixed veteran organisation comprising able-bodied and disabled ex-servicemen incorporating the entire ex-service population ensuring that the Legion's remit remained broad. The ESWS was a composite charity incorporating neurasthenic and insane veterans within its remit.[208] With the reduction of Ministry intervention from 1921 onwards, the ESWS became a more vocal and active body in the rehabilitation and assistance of neurasthenic veterans.[209] The charity established three in-patient facilities: Kent (thirty beds), Wandsworth (twenty-eight beds) and Surrey (sixty beds). Like Ministry in-patient facilities, these institutions provided occupational training and vocational therapy alongside medical care incorporating qualified nurses and visiting psychiatrists to consult with neurasthenic pensioners.[210] Forty-two consultants worked for the ESWS throughout Britain and Ireland to mediate between individual ex-servicemen and the charity's headquarters in London to decipher the appropriate course of action, including making representations to the Ministry of Pensions on their behalf.[211] The recession of the memory of the war in the public consciousness combined with the Ministry's seven-year time limit and wider economic austerity in driving more desperate veterans to turn to the ESWS in the 1930s.[212] In 1932, 45,000 people subscribed to the ESWS funds with close to 40,000 being in England, over 3,000 in Scotland, almost 1,000 in Wales, but just 349 in Ireland.[213]

The ESWS stressed that its assistance to neurasthenic veterans in Ireland also included cooperation with the British Red Cross Society and the SILA.[214] Tellingly, and again foregrounding the unique socio-political conditions in Ireland, it was only when discussing its operations in Ireland that the ESWS felt the need to emphasise that the charity was apolitical.[215] Like the British Legion, there was a contrast in the charity's remit and function in the Irish Free State in comparison to Britain. In 1928, the ESWS wrote of the particularly dire position in Ireland: 'A great number of applications for help have been received from Ireland from those ex-servicemen who fought for the Empire, but who are now existing in abject poverty. Apart from financial help, 269 grants for food have been made.'[216] The organisation recognised the increased problems in the reintegration of mentally ill Great War veterans in the Irish Free State two years later:

> Cases from Ireland have again this year been very numerous, due, no doubt, to the distress in the country. Before any financial help is given, however, the case is investigated by the SILA or the British Red Cross Society. The ex-soldier and sailor appears to be finding it very hard to obtain work in the Irish Free State, hence we have a tremendous lot of them coming over to England.[217]

Despite these difficulties, the Chairman of the ESWS praised the charity's efforts in the Free State, and the 'financial assistance [which] has been given to a number of ex-servicemen in Ireland who fought for the Empire and who are now living under dreadful conditions.'[218] Indeed, one veteran in the territory wrote to the ESWS in gratitude for their assistance:

> For your great kindness to me which your Committee sanctioned and all what the Society has done, in many ways, to recover in body and mind, I do not know how to thank you. Words fail me – but gratefulness is here. I can see brighter times ahead, now a home of my own and nothing I desire more is that renewed happiness and health will continue. I hope to succeed in business, a big hope, then perhaps as time goes on, I can make the effort to return to what has been done for me, so as some other unfortunate brother may reap the benefit of the Society's kindness. It's a great Society, a human Society which judges with sympathy – and, as I know, helps, not impedes, we who have suffered from these awful brain spasms. I am sure the loads of years have gone, and I pray earnestly not to return. Here I can start afresh, in a new house and a new peace – at least clean.

May the work of the Society prosper. I know it has THE greatest blessing behind it. Again thanking you from the bottom of my heart.[219]

Even if ESWS' homes were not available in the Irish Free State, the charities could help veterans attain in-patient treatment. One former private of the Irish Guards in need of medical treatment for his psychoneurotic condition was admitted into Leopardstown Hospital for in-patient care in 1936 thanks to the intervention and representation of the charity.[220]

The ESWS helped over 25,000 mentally ill veterans with medical assessments, care, treatment or financial assistance during the inter-war period. The ESWS thus congratulated itself on being 'a potent representative of the mentally disabled ex-serviceman.'[221] Nevertheless, as the memory of the war faded, and the economic insecurity and widespread unemployment of the 1920s and 1930s became fully realised, the sense of obligation to disabled Great War veterans in Britain became less of an imperative as men competed for scant opportunities to work.[222] The situation for veterans in the Free State was even more precarious. While sympathy for the disabled veteran had receded in Britain by the 1930s, there was negligible sympathy in the Irish Free State from its inception. The psychological impact of both domestic and philanthropic assistance during an era when masculine ideals rested heavily on economic self-sufficiency should not be underplayed.[223] Nevertheless, the Ministry, domestic carers and charities attempted to assist disabled veterans throughout the inter-war period even in the most testing of conditions. Their intervention was important and deserves recognition. The Ministry's contrasting descriptions of O'Ryan include his inability to function and being plagued by mental torment coinciding with evidence of a life lived with meaning, marriage and having children, while also playing golf and attaining employment. This intricacy illustrates the complex and interchangeable adversity, tragedy and triumph often evident in the post-war lives of disabled First World War veterans. Not all mentally ill veterans were able to salvage such meaning.

Walking arguments

The chairman of the ESWS wrote in 1938 that many 'broken victims of shell-shock drift through life in despair and destitution' unable to reintegrate back into society.[224] Similar instances were visible in Free State society.[225] Men would recall similar instances in the Dublin tenements during the 1930s. Paddy Mooney, for example, recollected:

> There was a lot of cripples around and men that had come back from the war shell-shocked. They used to go around in threes and fours playing music, playing

instruments, through the streets and people would throw them a penny or ha'penny. There was one man used to go around with a stick and he'd roar 'Eeeeow' ... There was another one and Christ almighty it was terrible looking at him, sometimes he'd go mad and start bashing the metal rails along Whitefair Street School with his fist and you'd want to see the blood gushing out of him. That's the way he was affected by the war.[226]

Stephen Mooney also recollected his memories of the late 1930s:

There was one fella and that'd come down Marrowbone Lane and we'd call him names and he used to run after us and froth at the mouth. He'd chase us and actually beat you if he got hold of you. Then there was Jembo-no-toes. Jembo was shell-shocked but a very fine cut of a man. He lost some of his toes in the Great War and his balance wasn't perfect. He was inclined to waddle along. But he used to periodically go off the handle roaring and shouting.[227]

Harry Mushatt recounted similar experiences:

You got men coming back after the First World War with malaria and shell-shock and many of them got very fond of the drink. And they'd do anything for drink ... There was a fella, Cal was his name, and he was a character. He was in the army and shell-shocked and he'd go around mumbling and shouting and sometimes he would go off the deep end and come in with a cut across his forehead.[228]

Such emotionally scarred men reflect Winter's assertion that some mentally ill veterans became 'walking arguments against the view that demobilisation came to an end when the last serving soldier in a combat unit left the service.'[229] These 'walking arguments' are often difficult to centre. As one medical practitioner wrote in 1931, periodic episodes of mental illness amongst ex-servicemen would have frequently occurred but remained unrecorded.[230]

The relationship between criminality and combat neurosis has become an accepted feature in contemporary research.[231] Examples of shell-shocked Great War veterans being involved in illegality were also prevalent in British and Irish press reports in the aftermath of the First World War.[232] One of the ESWS' most labour-intensive duties was to deal with neurasthenic ex-serviceman arrested and charged for criminal activities.[233] A traumatised veteran could also harm himself as well as others. On 20 March 1932, the *Sunday Independent* reported on the increasing numbers of suicides which were a transnational phenomenon:

The reason is more likely to be found in new and difficult post-war conditions. The war itself left human wrecks by the million over the surface of the globe. Some of these shell-shocked, nerve broken, mentally-unhinged victims of the great tragedy took the quickest road leading away from their troubles.[234]

As suicide rates experienced an increase in Britain in the aftermath of the First World War, Irish rates also displayed an uptrend.[235] While it is impossible to determine the extent to which war service could drive an ex-serviceman to suicide, an examination of newspaper reports reveal the mental torment that drove Irish Great War veterans to take their own lives. George O'Sullivan, a captain during the conflict, took his own life in 1927 by drowning in the River Nore, Kilkenny, at the age of thirty-three. An inquest into his death cited that he had suffered from neurasthenia as a result of war service. His sister revealed that he had been sleeping poorly and was depressed. His doctor also testified that he had previously recommended that O'Sullivan receive treatment in a specialist hospital 'having suffered from neurasthenia since 1918.' One ex-serviceman killed himself by putting his head in a gas oven with the coroner at his death concluding: 'He had been in France for two and a half years ... suffered from shell-shock. He had never been the same since.' Another Great War veteran, a successful landowner, shot himself on his farm in County Wicklow in 1927. The man's medical attendant described him as 'a highly nervous and neurotic kind of man. He suffered from shell-shock as a result of his experiences in the war.' Another unemployed Great War veteran committed suicide with the inquest attributing grief, alcohol and insomnia as contributing to his suicide. The man left a suicide note lamenting: 'broken hearted and weary and long to find oblivion. Good night.' Another veteran of Gallipoli committed suicide by shooting himself in the head on the twentieth anniversary of his landing on V Beach in Turkey.[236]

The position in which British ex-servicemen thus found themselves in the Irish Free State contradicted the British Legion's ethos that 'every man that left Ireland was a volunteer and that was a thing they should all be proud of.'[237] The impact of societal apathy on the psychological state of mentally fragile Great War veterans in the Free State merits further consideration. 'Purification rights' in the form of societal appreciation and commemoration have been cited as being significant in the rehabilitation of mentally ill ex-servicemen.[238] An authenticated official memory of the war prevalent in Northern Ireland was absent in the Free State.[239] The commemoration of the conflict became circumscribed in the Irish Free State alongside respect for the disabled Great War veteran's sacrifice of body and mind.[240] Remembrance ceremonies commemorating Ireland's involvement in the Great War remained hostile occasions throughout the 1930s in Dublin. Even disabled veterans felt unsafe to sell poppies without fear of republican reprisals. Oral accounts also attest to the children of veterans placing razorblades inside their poppies to give painful injuries to agitators who would try and snatch them off the observer's clothing. During one Remembrance Day ceremony in Dublin in 1925, smoke bombs were set off during the ceremonial two minutes silence. While other cities in the Irish Free State were witnesses to similar instances of hostility, activity in Dublin was the most prevalent. 'Renegade Republican' attacks against those associated with the British army continued in the inter-war period. In 1927, the British Legion Hall at Inchicore was set ablaze. It was rebuilt only to have its roof and wall blown off in 1929. Pettier measures included Limerick's British Legion hall being broken into to destroy the premises and instruments of Irish veterans held in the property. The latter also received aggressive correspondence regarding their upcoming participation in an Armistice Day parade, and research has argued that it was only impressive police intelligence which prevented further incidents throughout the Free State.[241]

The compromised memory of the conflict is perfectly exemplified in the troubled history of the National War Memorial in Islandbridge. A proposal to erect a national memorial in Merrion Square, in central Dublin, was rejected by the Irish Senate in 1927. Kevin O'Higgins TD remonstrated: 'It is not on their sacrifice that this State is based and I have no desire to see it suggested that it is.' The difficulty for ex-servicemen trying to establish a rallying point of sacrifice, as was afforded veterans in Britain with the Cenotaph in London, is further reinforced when remembering that O'Higgins' brother died in the Great War.[242] The Dublin memorial was finally completed in 1938. The *Irish Times* claimed its location was a 'distant backwater'; yet, it was 'the nearest site that is considered politically expedient, and the protection of which can be reasonably assured.' The park was left in a dilapidated condition and was not officially opened until 1988.[243] The Free State Government also proved unwilling to patronise and observe Armistice Day ceremonies officially; its neutrality during the Second World War justified its scaling down of commemorative events.[244] In contrast, while Northern Ireland did not have a national equivalent to the Cenotaph, sixty-two public war memorials were erected by 1939 as the First World War became a central pillar of unionist mythology.[245] Like the impact of fearing IRA reprisal during the Anglo-Irish War, the inability of neurasthenic pensioners to peacefully commemorate their war service during the 1920s and 1930s may have had a catastrophic psychological impact.[246]

Conclusion

Disabled veterans in Northern Ireland broadly shared the same homecoming conditions evident in Britain. Wider society largely appreciated war service with assistance provided in the form of voluntary employment schemes such as the King's National Roll. By contrast, disabled Great War veterans in the Irish Free State returned to a society which placed little value on their war service and sacrifice. In Britain, Northern Ireland and the Irish Free State societal prejudice and Ministry reductions would magnify problems for the mentally ill pensioner by reducing their likelihood of attaining employment and receiving medical treatment. It was, however, only in the Irish Free State that mentally ill British ex-servicemen had to overcome *two* forms of stigma: namely the disputed and unpredictable nature of their mental disability and ostracism due to their former service in the British Army. The sustained efforts of the Ministry of Pensions to accommodate Great War veterans in the Irish Free State, at the continued expense of the British Treasury, became critical. The SILA's portrayal of ex-servicemen as being abandoned children is inaccurate.[247] At the very least, Irish neurasthenic pensioners had a benevolent uncle in the form of the Ministry of Pensions. The discourse of orphanage would be more apt for describing those not in receipt of military pensions and who did not go on to enlist in the National Army, the disabled 'old time serving soldier' who served before 1914, mentally disabled veterans of the revolutionary wars or even the mentally ill British Army veteran of the First World War whose claim for a pension came *after* the Ministry's seven-year time limit.

Due to Ministry restrictions and its streamlining of policy and infrastructure, departmental officials in the Free State noted a 'heavy and continuing decline in the volume of work' by 1934.[248] Officials at the Cork branch complained that 'it is hardly worth attending' committee meetings due to the absence of input required from staff.[249] The five advisory committees in the Free State were subsequently subsumed into one committee in Dublin from 1937. This national committee comprised seventeen members representing regional interests with meetings occurring four times per year.[250] In 1938, the British Treasury and Ministry of Pensions discussed the possibility of transferring financial responsibility of British ex-servicemen onto the Irish Free State Government. With an annual outlay of £1,435,000 for administration, medical treatment and payment of pensions in the region, the Free State Government rejected the proposition.[251] With no change in the pension infrastructure, the Ministry of Pensions estimated that the cost of expenditure with regards to Great War pensioners would continue well into the second half of the twentieth century.[252] Mentally ill pensioners would continue to be admitted into Leopardstown even as the hospital began to be dominated by those physically disabled and wounded veterans who had participated in the Second World War.[253] The individual case study of O'Ryan centres the continued support offered to mentally disabled Great War veterans. He saw out his final dying days in Leopardstown Hospital before passing away at seventy-seven years old on 6 August 1975. O'Ryan was still in receipt of a military pension for neurasthenia attributed to his war service in France six decades earlier.[254]

Notes

1. NA, PIN 15/899, Provision of Employment for ex-serviceman in Ireland, 11 March 1921.
2. NA, PIN 15/2701, Ministry of Pensions, note, 12 December 1921.
3. Ibid.
4. Ibid., Ministry of Pensions, note, 20 January 1922; Ministry of Pensions, note, 27 July 1922; Regional Director, Ministry of Pensions, London, to heads of all sections of Areas, Administrators and Medical Superintendents, 2 March 1922.
5. NA, LAB 2/528/TDS1181/1921, Ireland: Position of Industrial Training Scheme; PIN 15/2701, Changes in Government of Ireland Effect on the Ministry of Pensions, of the Constitution of the Irish Free State, Memo, 4 February 1922; DO 35/331/1, Claims of UK ex-servicemen in the Irish Free State; 'Victims of the War', *Irish Times*, 10 June 1924, 5; PRONI, AUS/3/13, Irish administration, information re: Ministry of Pensions, 1921.
6. Taylor, *Heroes or Traitors?*, 94.
7. NAI, FIN/1/216, Proposal for establishment of Ministry of Pensions in Ireland.
8. This cartoon was published on 15 February 1922; [Online] Available at: http://Punch.photoshelter.com [accessed 12 April 2016].
9. Michael Laffan, *Judging W. T. Cosgrave* (Dublin: Royal Irish Academy, 2014), 270.
10. Bourke, 'Shell-shock, psychiatry and the Irish soldier', 166; HC Debates, 19 February 1919, vol. 125, cols 1029–32; Taylor, *Heroes or Traitors?*, 114.
11. NA, PIN 15/133, Letter from D. A. Carruthers, CMS, Dublin to London, Ministry of Pensions, 22 October 1922.
12. HC Debates, 12 December 1922, vol. 159, cols 2694–855.
13. Arnold's Typescript Recollections, 128–9.
14. NA, PIN 15/325, Malicious Damage in Ireland; Ministry of Pensions, note, 30 May 1923.
15. Taylor, *Heroes or Traitors?*, 196; Dáil Éireann, vol. 3, 23 April 1931, 'In committee on finance – vote no. 3 – Dept of the President of the Executive Council.'
16. Dáil Éireann, vol. 21, 16 November 1927, 'Motion by Deputy Redmond: Disabilities of British ex-servicemen.'
17. PRONI, D989/B/3/6, Ex-Service Men in Southern Ireland. Their Terrible Sufferings, 6.
18. Taylor, *Heroes or Traitors?*, 212.
19. Arnold's Typescript Recollections, 129.
20. NA, PIN 15/758, Ministry of Pensions, Dublin, to the Ministry of Pensions, London, 19 June 1936.
21. Bernard Kelly, *Returning Home: Irish Ex-servicemen after the Second World War* (Dublin: Merrion Press, 2012), 23; Fitzpatrick omitted British ex-servicemen as 'losers' of the revolutionary period but, instead, included anti-Treaty republicans in the Free State and nationalists living in the north; David Fitzpatrick, *The Two Irelands: 1912–1939* (Oxford: Oxford University Press, 1998), 205.
22. Bourke, 'Effeminacy, ethnicity and the end of trauma', 68.

23 NA, PIN 15/325, R. G. Collins, Great Smith Street London, to His Majesty's Stationary Office, Westminster, 9 July 1923.
24 Ibid., Ministry of Pensions note, 30 May 1923.
25 Departmental Committee of Inquiry into the Machinery of Administration of the Ministry of Pensions Report to Ian Macpherson, MP, Minister of Pensions, 1921, 98; Fifth Annual Report of the Ministry of Pensions, 1921–1922, 12.
26 H. C. Marr, *Psychoses of the War* (London: Hodder & Stoughton, 1919), 48; Mosse, 'Shell-shock as a social disease', 105; The Southborough Report, 27, 62.
27 Ted Bogacz, 'War neurosis and cultural change in England, 1914–1922: the work of the War Office Committee of Enquiry into Shell-Shock', *Journal of Contemporary History*, 24:2 (1989), 249.
28 Reid, *Broken Men*, 83.
29 Read, *Military Psychiatry in Peace and War*, 5, 16; Henderson, 'War Psychoses', 174, 245; Woods Hutchinson, *The Doctor in War* (Boston: Cassel and Co, 1918), 368–70; Fenton, *Shell-Shock and its Aftermath*, 51–2; M. D. Eder, *War-shock. The psycho-neuroses in war: psychology and treatment* (London: William Heinemann, 1917), 142; Roussy, Lhermitte and Turner, *The Psychoneurosis of War*, 153; Reid, *Broken Men*, 97.
30 The Southborough Report, 140; Bogacz, 'War neurosis and cultural change in England', 246–7.
31 The Southborough Report, 13, 23, 26, 40, 72, 83, 165–70; Loughran, 'Shell-shock in First World War Britain', 67–8; Read, *Military Psychiatry in Peace and War*, 2; W. A. Turner, 'Neuroses and psychoses of war', *The Lancet*, 9 November 1918, 617; Frederick Mott, 'The neuroses and psychoses in relation to conscription and eugenics', *The Eugenics Review*, 14 (1922), 15, 19.
32 The Southborough Report, 43.
33 Ibid., 87.
34 Ibid., 96.
35 As Ted Bogacz concluded: 'Every pre-war English prejudice was mobilised to explain away all those crack-ups at the front'; Bogacz, 'War neurosis and cultural change in England', 249.
36 Curtis, *Anglo-Saxons and Celts*, 20–1, 53–5; Malcolm, 'Ireland's crowded madhouses', 315.
37 Bogacz, 'War neurosis and cultural change in England', 237; Chris Feudtner, '"Minds the dead have ravished": shell shock, history, and the ecology of disease-systems', *History of Psychiatry*, 31:4 (1993), 389.
38 The Southborough Report, 148.
39 Meyer, *Men of War*, 101; Andrew McDonald, 'The Geddes Committee and the formulation of public expenditure policy, 1921–1922', *The Historical Journal*, 32:3 (1989), 643–74.
40 These reductions were not solely due to Ministry streamlining. The death or recovery of pensioners, the remarriage of widows and the maturation of dependent children also eased financial costs; NA, PIN 15/2601, Expenditure of the Ministry

of Pensions; Nineteenth Annual Report of the Ministry of Pensions, 1935–1936, Part Two, 37; Bettinson, 'Lost Souls in the House of Restoration', 70–7, 91, 224.
41 NA, PIN 15/2601, 'Expenditure of the Ministry of Pensions.'
42 NA, PIN 15/56, H. S. Sugars to George Chrystal, 13 July 1921; PIN 15/55, A. L. Webb to George Chrystal, 27 May 1921; Kinsella, *Leopardstown Park Hospital*, 89.
43 NA, T 136/4, Letter from the Treasury to the Ministry of Pensions, 26 June 1920.
44 Ibid.
45 Fifth Annual Report of the Ministry of Pensions, 1921–1922, 12.
46 Bourke, *Dismembering the Male*, 122.
47 Cohen, *The War Come Home*, 25, 57.
48 Bourke, *Dismembering the Male*, 31, 54–6, 251.
49 Combat Stress Archive, Surrey, Annual Report for 1930, 18.
50 A Voluntary Pensions Worker, *Pensioners of the Great War*, 35.
51 Loughran, *Shell-Shock and Medical Culture in First World War Britain*, 212–13.
52 Graham Wootton, *The Official History of the British Legion* (London: Macdonald and Evans, 1956), 79.
53 NA, T 161/270, Notes on powers and policy of the Ministry of Pensions.
54 Bettinson, 'Lost Souls in the House of Restoration', 86–7.
55 For more information, see Theda Skocpol, *Protecting Soldiers and Mothers: The Political Origins of Social Policy in the United States* (Cambridge MA: Harvard University Press, 1992), 102–53.
56 *British Legion Journal*, 2 (August, 1922), 45; *British Legion Journal*, 12 (April, 1933), 349.
57 Bettinson, 'Lost Souls in the House of Restoration', 77.
58 Combat Stress Archive, Surrey, Annual Report for 1932, 12; Annual Report for 1936, 11.
59 Bettinson, 'Lost Souls in the House of Restoration', 76–9; Andrew Latcham, 'Journey's End: Ex-Servicemen and the State during and After the Great War' (PhD Thesis, University of Oxford, 1996), 361; Barr, *The Lion and the Poppy*, 122; Wootton, *The Official History of the British Legion*, 79.
60 Mitchell and Smith, *Medical Services*, 312.
61 NA, PIN 26/16836, Fitzpatrick Pension File.
62 The facility still operates with this function today; Jones, 'Shell shock at Maghull and the Maudsley', 393–4.
63 Ibid., 394.
64 NA, PIN 15/58, Special Investigation of Saltash Cases.
65 Stone, 'The Military and Industrial Roots of Clinical Psychology in Britain', 20–3; British Legion, 4 (February, 1925), 265; Combat Stress Archive, Surrey, ESWS Chairman's Report for 1927, 11.
66 NA, PIN 15/4200, 'Extracts from the Report of a Conference held at Ottawa in December 1936 of a Board of Psychiatrists and Neurologists appointed by the Canadian Government', 136.

67 Additional Ministry facilities dedicated to 'hardening' were established at Saltash (450 beds) and Harrowby Camp (230 beds); Jones and Wessely, *Shell-Shock to PTSD*, 133; NA, PIN 15/2946, Director General to all regions, 28 September 1923.
68 NA, PIN 15/2502, Letter from George Chrystal to E. C. Price, The Charity Organisation Society, ESWS, 9 May 1927.
69 Barham, *Forgotten Lunatics of the Great War*, 274–5.
70 Combat Stress Archive, Surrey, ESWS Annual Report for 1929, 17–18.
71 NA, PIN 15/2946, Ministry of Pensions, Dublin, to Ministry of Pensions, London, 27 October 1923.
72 Barham, *Forgotten Lunatics of the Great War*, 316–17.
73 Leopardstown Hospital Archive, Dublin, Leopardstown Park Hospital Admission register, 1930–36.
74 NA, PIN 26/17150, Royal Naval Reserve, Thomas Whelan Pension File.
75 NA, PIN 15/2502, G. C. Tyron Letter to El Hadfield, 5 September 1927.
76 The lack of scientific and progressive treatments and facilities to give advice on psychoneurotic ailments in the Irish Free State was, for example, lamented by the prestigious *Irish Quarterly Review*; Kelly, *Hearing Voices*, 131.
77 NA, PIN 38/529, Ministry of Pensions Hospital, Leopardstown Park, Dublin. Surrender by Mr Bernard Dunning of his revisionary interests in the property of the crown.
78 Leopardstown Hospital Archive, Dublin, Admission Register – Disability Patients – 1914–1918.
79 NA, PIN 15/4200, Report by Director of Medical Services, 1936/1937, 79.
80 Leopardstown Hospital Archive, Dublin, Leopardstown Hospital Annual Report, 1938–1939.
81 Leopardstown Hospital Archive, Dublin, Leopardstown Hospital Annual Report, 1940–1941.
82 Nineteenth Annual Report of the Ministry of Pensions, 1935–1936, Part Two, 14.
83 Bettinson, 'The Lost Souls in the House of Restoration', 323; Jones and Wessely, *From Shell-Shock to PTSD*, 133.
84 Taylor, *Heroes or Traitors?*, 244–5.
85 Ibid., 195.
86 NA, PIN 15/758, Summary of the Report from Dublin, 22 June 1936.
87 NA, DO 35/330/9, Letter from Patrick Regan to Land Settlement, 1 March 1928.
88 PRONI, D989/B/3/6, Anonymous author to the Duke of Northumberland, SILA, London, 16 December 1924.
89 Such incidents were described as 'exceptions' and 'not a very potent factor' when considering the entirety of the Irish Free State; NA, PIN 15/758, Ministry of Pensions, Dublin, to the Ministry of Pensions, London, 19–22 June 1936.
90 PRONI, D4246/2/3, British Legion Review of Clubs and Branches, 30 November 1926.

91 British Legion Annual, Irish Free State, 1937, 30.
92 Peter Leese, 'Problems returning home: the British psychological casualties of the Great War', *Historical Journal*, 40:4 (1997), 1058–60.
93 NA, PIN 15/758, D.C.M.S, Dublin, Private Report for Dominions Office, London, Regarding the General Attitude Towards, and Treatment of, Imperial Ex-Servicemen in the Irish Free State, 22 June 1936; PRONI, D989/B/3/6, Ex-Service Men in Southern Ireland. Their Terrible Sufferings, 1.
94 PRONI, D989/B/3/6, Major White's report of SILA meeting on 30 October 1929, 5.
95 Dáil Éireann, vol. 21, 16 November 1927, 'Motion by deputy Redmond: Disabilities of British ex-servicemen.'
96 Dáil Éireann, vol. 48, 14 July 1933, 'In committee on finance – vote 56 – industry and commerce.'
97 NA, PIN 15/2487, Statement of Daniel Mulcahy, 27 May 1937.
98 Dáil Éireann, vol. 61, 30 April 1936, 'Vote 61 – unemployment insurance and unemployment assistance.'
99 Myers, *The Great War and Memory in Irish Culture*, 32–3; PRONI, D989/B/3/6, Report by SILA, 30 October 1929; NA, PIN 15/758, Summary of the Report from Dublin, 22 June 1936; H. T. MacDonald, *What is Due to Me?: A Handy Compendium of Information on Pensions* (London: Daily Herald, 1919), 57; PRONI, D989/B/3/6, Ex-Service Men in Southern Ireland. Their Terrible Sufferings, 6.
100 NA, PIN 15/758, Summary of the Report from Dublin, 22 June 1936.
101 Ibid., Ministry of Pensions, Dublin, to the Ministry of Pensions, London, 19 June 1936.
102 Johnson, 'The Northern Ireland economy, 1914–39', 190–1; Bardon, *A History of Ulster*, 526–9.
103 'The Plight of Ex-Servicemen', *Irish Times*, 3 April 1928, 11.
104 PRONI, CAB/4/224, Employment of ex-servicemen in the Northern Ireland Civil Service.
105 PRONI, PM/2/20/166, Secretary to the Cabinet, 21 June 1924.
106 NA, LAB 2/528, Ireland: Position of Industrial Training Scheme, 6 July 1923; Taylor, *Heroes or Traitors?*, 107–10.
107 Some companies including the Guinness brewery factory and Jacobs biscuit factory incorporated the ethos of the King's National Roll by re-employing former employees following their discharge and giving preferential treatment to ex-servicemen and their children; Taylor, *Heroes or Traitors?*, 229–30.
108 Ibid., 92–3; Kowalsky, "This honourable obligation', 573.
109 PRONI, CAB/9/C/8/1, National Scheme for the employment of disabled ex-servicemen in Northern Ireland, 1923–1926.
110 'The Week's News of Ireland', *Weekly Irish Times*, 16 February 1924, 13.
111 PRONI, CAB/9/C/8/1, National Scheme for the employment of disabled ex-servicemen in Northern Ireland, 1923–1926.

112 PRONI, ED/13/1/744, Employment of Ex-Servicemen by Education Authorities, Ministry of Finance to All Departments, 15 October 1925.
113 'Plight of ex-Service Men', *Irish Times*, 3 April 1928, 11.
114 Bourke, *Dismembering the Male*, 31, 54–6, 251.
115 Taylor, *Heroes or Traitors?*, 196.
116 Ibid., 197.
117 NA, PIN 15/758, Ministry of Pensions, note, 19 June 1936.
118 Ibid., D.C.M.S, Dublin, Private Report for Dominions Office, London, Regarding the General Attitude Towards, and Treatment of Imperial Ex-Servicemen in the Irish Free State, 22 June 1936.
119 Ibid., Report from Dublin, 22 June 1936, 1.
120 NA, PIN 15/2487, Ministry of Pensions, note, 29 April 1943.
121 Ibid., Statement of Daniel Mulcahy, 27 May 1937.
122 NA, PIN 15/758, 'Report From Dublin', 22 June 1936, 1; HC Debates, 12 December 1922, vol. 159, cols 2694–855.
123 Arnold's Typescript Recollections, 131.
124 Jones, 'Shell shock at Maghull and the Maudsley', 384.
125 NA, PIN 26/22252, Temporary Lieutenant James Vincent Owens, Labour Corps, Pension File.
126 Combat Stress Archive, Surrey, ESWS Annual Report for 1930, 25.
127 NA, PIN 15/2502, Transcript by W. D. Esplin.
128 Phillip Gibbs, 'Wounded Souls: A Plea for Nerve-strained Victims of the War', *Overseas* (January 1927), 39; Combat Stress Archive, Surrey, ESWS Appeal, 1938.
129 Combat Stress Archive, Surrey, ESWS Chairman's report for 1927 9; NA, PIN 15/57, Mental and neurasthenic cases for supervision; PIN 15/2503, Ministry of Pensions Minute Sheet, 29 October 1929.
130 NA, PIN 15/2947, Neurasthenia and Allied Disabilities: Memorandum for the Guidance of Medical Officers, 1931.
131 Shephard, *A War of Nerves*, 149.
132 Combat Stress Archive, Surrey, ESWS Annual Report for 1933, 10.
133 Ibid., ESWS Annual Report for 1929, 7; Meyer, *Men of War*, 112.
134 NA, PIN 26/22244, Pensions Appeal Tribunal: P. J. O'Ryan.
135 O'Ryan's 'extreme scruples' continued beyond the inter-war period, with one medical board report in 1972 noting that he sought confession with his priest five times in just a few days; NA, PIN 26/22244, O'Ryan Pension File.
136 Herman, *Trauma and Recovery*, 46.
137 NA, PIN 15/1632, Lord Eustace Percy MP to Ministry of Pensions, London, 19 December 1922.
137 NA, PIN 26/22244, Pensions Appeal Tribunal: P. J. O'Ryan.
139 Interview with Ann O'Ryan and John O'Ryan, 23 February 2019.
140 NA, PIN 26/16836, Fitzpatrick Pension File; as the ESWS pointed out, even with a seven-year time limit, the Ministry promised to provide special machinery and due consideration to neurasthenic claims which arose after the limit which could

be indisputably proven to be attributable to war service; Combat Stress Archive, Surrey, ESWS annual report and balance sheet for 1928, 4.
141 NA, PIN 26/16836, Fitzpatrick Pension File.
142 Smith and Pear, *Shell-Shock and its Lessons*, 81.
143 Meyer, *Men of War*, 107–8.
144 Jones and Wessely, *From Shell-Shock to PTSD*, 134.
145 NA, PIN 15/1632, Lord Eustace Percy MP to Ministry of Pensions, London, 19 December 1922.
146 Joanna Bourke, *An Intimate History of Killing* (London: Granta Press, 1999), 253.
147 NA, PIN 26/22244, O'Ryan Pension File.
148 MacDonald, *What is Due to Me?*, 51–2.
149 NA, PIN 15/1632, Lord Eustace Percy MP to Ministry of Pensions, London, 19 December 1922. Such a problem had been previously recognised by the Irish Federation of Discharged and Demobilised Sailors and Soldiers in Ireland: 'A certain amount of worry is caused to a pensioner because of what may eventually happen to his pension, and this worry in many causes an aggravation of the disability'; NA, LAB 2/855/ED5412/7/1921, National Federation of Discharged and Demobilised Sailors and Soldiers, Dublin, to David Lloyd George, 17 February 1920.
150 NA, PIN 26/22244, Pensions Appeal Tribunal: P. J. O'Ryan.
151 NA, PIN 15/1632, Lord Eustace Percy MP to Ministry of Pensions, London, 19 December 1922.
152 PRONI, D989/B/3/6, Ex-Service Men in Southern Ireland. Their Terrible Sufferings, 7–8.
153 Taylor, *Heroes or Traitors?*, 112.
154 NA, PIN 15/2702, Estimated annual expenditure in respect of Great War pensioners in Eire.
155 NA, PIN 15/757, Ministry of Pensions, note, 29 February 1928; Taylor, *Heroes or Traitors?*, 116.
156 NA, PIN 15/757, Ministry of Pensions, note, 27 February 1928.
157 Taylor, *Heroes or Traitors?*, 120.
158 Michael Robinson, '"Nobody's children"?: the Ministry of Pensions and the treatment of disabled Great War veterans in the Irish Free State, 1921–1939', *Irish Studies Review*, 25:3 (2017), 323–5.
159 HL Debates, 25 June 1930, vol. 78, cols 162–74.
160 Barham, *Forgotten Lunatics of the Great War*, 196.
161 NA, LAB 2/528/TDS1181/1921, Administration of Training Scheme in Northern and Southern Ireland as a result of Government of Ireland Act 1920, Internal Memo, 6 July 1923.
162 Taylor, *Heroes or Traitors?*, 122; Robinson, '"Nobody's children"?', 318–26.
163 HC Debates, 'Army Supply Estimate, 1922–1923', 12 December 1922, vol. 159, cols 2694–85.
164 Barham, *Forgotten Lunatics of the Great War*, 366.
165 Taylor, *Heroes or Traitors?*, 121.

166 NAI, FIN/1/216, Proposal for establishment of Ministry of Pensions in Ireland.
167 Laffan, *Judging W. T. Cosgrave*, 173–4; Walter Korpi, 'Welfare State and Development in Europe since 1930: Ireland in a Comparative Perspective.' [Online] Available at: www.esri.ie/pubs/GL23.pdf [accessed 22 August 2016].
168 Arnold's Typescript Recollections, 130.
169 Should a French veteran's mental illness be so severe as to require institutionalisation in an asylum, a meagre pension was provided to cover their treatment; Marie Derrien, '"Entrenched from life": The impossible reintegration of traumatized French veterans of the Great War', in Jason Crouthamel and Peter Leese (eds), *Psychological Trauma and the Legacies of the First World War*, (Cham: Palgrave Macmillan, 2017), 193–214; Gregory Thomas, *Treating the Trauma of the Great War: Soldiers, Civilians, and Psychiatry in France, 1914–1940* (Louisiana: Louisiana University Press, 2009), 85–126.
170 For case studies of Australia and Canada, see, for example, Marina Larsson, 'Families and institutions for shell-shocked soldiers in Australia after the First World War', *Social History of Medicine*, 22:1 (2008), 97–114; Mark Humphries, 'War's long shadow: masculinity, medicine, and the gendered politics of trauma, 1914–1939', *Canadian Historical Review*, 91:3 (2010), 503–31.
171 NA, PIN 15/2611, Report on the General Administration of War Pensions in the Union of South Africa and on the payment of Pensions made in the Union on behalf of the Ministry of Pensions.
172 Philipp Rauh, 'Violence and starvation in First World War psychiatry: origins of the National Socialist "euthanasia"', in Jason Crouthamel and Peter Leese (eds), *Psychological Trauma and the Legacies of the First World War* (Cham: Palgrave Macmillan, 2017), 261–86.
173 Paul Wanke, *Russian/Soviet Military Psychiatry, 1904–1945* (London: Frank Cass, 2005), 112.
174 Heike Karge, 'Making sense of war neurosis in Yugoslavia', in Jason Crouthamel and Peter Leese (eds), *Psychological Trauma and the Legacies of the First World War* (Cham: Palgrave Macmillan, 2017), 227–30.
175 Robinson, '"Nobody's children"?', 316–35.
176 Bourke, 'Effeminacy, ethnicity and the end of trauma', 68.
177 Whilst ineligibility of diseases in the pension act ensured that any request for these men to receive pensions was turned down, it is interesting that the term 'shell-shock', despite being dismissed as a useful term by the Southborough Commission, was used to describe the condition of those mentally affected by service in the Irish Civil War. Clearly, the term had caught the Irish public and political imagination despite it being problematic as a medical diagnosis; Dáil Éireann, vol. 13, 11 November 1925, Volunteer's pension claims; Dáil Éireann, vol. 7, 16 May 1924, Clare soldier's pension.
178 Orduithe An Lae, vol. 18, 25 January 1927, Orders of the day – Army Pensions (no.2) Bill, 1926.
179 Dáil Éireann, vol. 7, 20 May 1924, Adjournment Debate – Position of ex-servicemen.

180 Ibid.
181 Carden-Coyne, *The Politics of Wounds*, 345.
182 Jefferson 'Enabled courage', 1105.
183 Indeed, even when housed together in interacial facilities, disabled white veterans often refused to work alongside African American in-patients which compromised the purpose of occupational therapy and their recovery; Jessica Adler, *Burdens of War: Creating the United States Veterans Health System* (Baltimore: Johns Hopkins University Press, 2017), 152–3.
184 Out of every thousand white veterans, 5.1 was admitted, in comparison to 1.5 of every thousand black veterans; ibid., 153.
185 This study stands in stark contrast to previous research into Irish veterans of the American Civil War who, on average, were considerably under-represented in successfully applying for a disability pension; Peter Blanck and Chen Song, 'Civil War pensions for native and foreign-born Union army veterans', in Larry Logue and Michael Barton (eds), *The Civil War Veteran: A Historical Reader* (New York: New York University Press, 2007), 224.
186 Winter, 'Families', 59.
187 NA, PIN 26/17150, Whelan Pension File.
188 NA, PIN 15/57, Mental and Neurasthenic Cases for Supervision.
189 NA, PIN 26/22244, Pensions Appeal Tribunal: P. J. O'Ryan.
190 NA, PIN 26/16836, Fitzpatrick pension file.
191 Barham, *Forgotten Lunatics of the Great War*, 316.
192 Winter, 'Families', 60–1; Meyer, *Men of War*, 118; Cohen, *The War Come Home*, 107.
193 Their intervention helped to pacify Great War veterans helping to prevent them from becoming revolutionary as had been the case with various ex-service communities in Europe; Cohen, *The War Come Home*, 17; Anderson, *War, Disability and Rehabilitation in Britain*, 42; Leese, 'Problems returning home', 1056.
194 Reid, *Broken Men*, 123; Anderson, *War, Disability and Rehabilitation*, 48–9; Cohen, *The War Come Home*, 50; the League of Irish Ex-Servicemen became affiliated with the British Legion in 1925 forming its southern Irish branch; Taylor, *Heroes or Traitors?*, xiv.
195 PRONI, D989/B/3/6, SILA, London, to SILA, Dublin, 19 November 1925.
196 Ibid.; Major White's report of SILA meeting on 30 October 1929, 1–2.
197 Taylor, *Heroes or Traitors?*, 238.
198 NA, PIN 56/15, Ministry of Pensions, Area Advisory Committees, 15 June 1936.
199 In addition to an inactive Legion, ex-servicemen existed in comparatively small numbers and were dispersed over wide geographical areas ensuring that many did not join ex-servicemen groups; NAI, FIN/1/216, Proposal for establishment of Ministry of Pensions in Ireland; Barr, *The Lion and the Poppy*, 62; British Legion Annual, Irish Free State 1937, 19; Taylor, *Heroes or Traitors?*, 235; Leonard, 'Survivors', 218.
200 Barham, *Forgotten Lunatics of the Great War*, 336.

201 Bourke, 'Shell-shock, psychiatry and the Irish Soldier', 166; however, as the Ministry of Pensions recognised, such a disadvantage was not unique to those in Ireland as pensioners residing in the remote highlands of Scotland, parts of Wales and England would also have suffered from the same problem; NA, PIN 15/757, Observations of the Ministry of Pensions on the Report of the Committee on Claims of British ex-servicemen in the Irish Free State.
202 PRONI, D989/B/3/6, SILA, London, to SILA, Dublin, 10 February 1925.
203 Ibid.; Memo from Major White, 10 February 1925.
204 Ibid., Ex-Service Men in Southern Ireland. Their Terrible Sufferings, 1–8.
205 Ibid.; SILA, London, to SILA, Dublin, 15 January 1925.
206 The British Legion showed great annoyance when their requests were not met with a speedy response; PRONI, CAB/9/Q/12/1, Employment of ex-servicemen in the Civil Service in Northern Ireland.
207 PRONI, D/4246/2/3, British Legion Review of Clubs and Branches, 30 November 1926.
208 Gerber, 'Disabled veterans, the state, and the experience of disability in Western societies', 902; Jones and Wessely, *Shell-Shock to PTSD*, 127.
209 Combat Stress Archive, Surrey, ESWS Annual Report for 1936, 18.
210 Bettinson, 'Lost Souls in the House of the House of Restoration', 151; Jones and Wessely, *Shell-Shock to PTSD*, 54.
211 Combat Stress Archive, Surrey, ESWS Chairman's Report for 1926, 4; ESWS Chairman's Report for 1927, 6; ESWS Annual Report for 1937, 10.
212 Combat Stress Archive, Surrey, Annual Report for 1931, 19; Annual Report for 1933, 10; ESWS Appeal 1938.
213 Ibid., ESWS Annual Report for 1932, 25; ESWS Annual Report for 1935, 15.
214 Ibid., ESWS Annual Report for 1930, 13.
215 Ibid., ESWS Chairman's Report for 1927, 9.
216 Ibid., ESWS Annual Report for 1928, 7.
217 Ibid., ESWS Annual Report for 1931, 12.
218 Ibid., ESWS Chairman's Report for 1927, 9.
219 Ibid., 9–11.
220 Ibid., ESWS Annual Report for 1936, 12.
221 Ibid., ESWS Chairman's Report for 1926, 10; ESWS Annual Report for 1939, 17.
222 Ibid., ESWS Annual Report for 1933, 17; Bourke, *Dismembering the Male*, 31, 54–6, 251; Cohen, *The War Come Home*, 148.
223 Meyer, *Men of War*, 98.
224 Combat Stress Archive, ESWS Appeal 1938.
225 Richardson, *A Coward if I Return, A Hero If I Fall*, 306.
226 Kevin Kearns, *Dublin Tenement Life* (Dublin: Gill and Macmillan, 2006), 97–100.
227 Ibid., 150.
228 Ibid., 104.
229 Jay Winter, *Remembering War: The Great War between Memory and History in the Twentieth Century* (New Haven: Yale University Press, 2006), 60.

230 Coplans, 'Some observations on neurasthenia and shell-shock', 960.
231 Shay, *Odysseus in America*, 27.
232 Fiona Reid, 'Distinguishing between shell-shocked veterans and pauper lunatics: the ex-services' welfare society and mentally wounded veterans after the Great War', *War in History*, 14:3 (2007), 356.
233 Combat Stress Archive, Surrey, ESWS Annual Report for 1931, 11; ESWS Annual Report for 1932, 11.
234 'The Recent Rapid Rise in the World's Suicide Figures', *Sunday Independent*, 20 March 1932, 5.
235 Irish suicide figures provided by Vital Statistics Section, Central Statistics Office, Cork, via personal correspondence on 16 January 2015.
236 Suzie Grogan, *Shell-Shocked Britain: The First World War's Legacy for Britain's Mental Health* (Barnsley: Pen & Sword, 2014), 105–6; Leonard, 'Survivors', 213; 'Ex Officer Drowned', *Irish Times*, 20 January 1927, 8; 'Victim of Shell-Shock', *Freeman's Journal*, 13 February 1923, 6; 'Found Shot Dead', *Irish Independent*, 15 August 1927, 2; Leonard, 'Survivors', 213; Dungan, *Irish Voices of the Great War*, 46–8.
237 Tom Burke, '"To Hell With The Free State": Remembrance of the First World War in Ireland, 1924–1936', 5. [Online] Available at: www.greatwar.ie/wp-content/uploads/2016/03/To-Hell-with-the-Free-State.pdf [accessed 4 September 2016].
238 Dave Grossman, *On Killing: The Psychological Cost of Learning to Kill in War and Society* (Boston: Littlebrown, 2009), 265–6; Bourke, 'Shell-shock, psychiatry and the Irish Soldier', 166–7.
239 However, the emphasis on the role that the Great War played in warranting partition, with accompanying jingoism including the prominent use of the Union Jack, ensured that the position of nationalist veterans remained ambiguous and they were not necessarily made to feel welcome at such commemorative occasions; Myers, *The Great War and Memory in Irish Culture*, 79–88.
240 Jeffery, *Ireland and the Great War*, 115–16.
241 Tom Burke, '"Poppy Day" in the Irish Free State', *Irish Quarterly Review*, 92 (2003), 349–58; Myers, *The Great War and Memory in Irish Culture*, 69, 106; Leonard, 'Facing the finger of scorn', 66; Jane Leonard, 'The twinge of memory: Armistice Day and Remembrance Day Sunday in Dublin since 1919', in Richard English and Graham Walker (eds), *Unionism in Modern Ireland* (Basingstoke: Macmillan, 1996), 104.
242 Fergus D'Arcy, *Remembering the War Dead* (Dublin: Stationary Office, 2007), 176.
243 Jeffery, *Ireland and the Great War*, 118–21; Myles Dungan, *They Shall Not Grow Old: Irish Soldiers of the Great War* (Dublin; Four Courts Press, 1997), 203.
244 Myers, *The Great War and Memory in Irish Culture*, 74, 206.
245 For an insightful study into these memorials, see Catherine Switzer, *Unionists and Great War Commemoration in the North of Ireland, 1914–1939* (Dublin: Irish Academic Press, 2007).

246 Bourke, 'Shell-shock, psychiatry and the Irish soldier', 167–8.
247 PRONI, D989/B/3/6, Ex-Service Men in Southern Ireland. Their Terrible Sufferings, 7–8.
248 NA, PIN 56/15, Ministry of Pensions, note, 25 October 1934.
249 Ibid., Ministry of Pensions, note, undated; this change in treatment philosophy is evident within the Ministry of Pensions' annual reports covering the United Kingdom. While its second annual report, 1918–1919, consisted of ninety pages, the report covering 1933 included just ten; Second Annual Report of the Ministry of Pensions, 1918–1919; Seventh Annual Report of the Ministry of Pensions 1933–1934.
250 NA, PIN 56/15, Ministry of Pensions, note, July 1936.
251 NA, PIN 15/2701, Note by the Minister of Pensions on Cabinet Paper 300; PIN 15/2702, Malcolm MacDonald to Herwald Ramsbotham MP, 21 January 1938; Expenditure in respect of Great War Pensioners in Éire.
252 For example, due to the passing away of many Great War pensioners, it was estimated that the annual outlay in would equate to £353,500 in 1965; NA, PIN 15/2702, Estimated expenditure in respect of Great War pensioners in Eire.
253 Leopardstown Hospital Archive, Dublin, Admission Register – Disability Patients – 1914–1918.
254 NA, PIN 26/22244, O'Ryan Pension File.

4

THE WAR HOSPITAL IN IRELAND

Introduction

The UK's available bed space for the medical treatment of wounded servicemen amounted to 365,000 by the cessation of the First World War. Thirty-six affiliated auxiliary hospitals catered for war-related ailments in Ireland.[1] Voluntary charities and philanthropists ran numerous facilities, there was an expansion of existing military hospitals, building of new military hospitals, and the creation of military hospitals and wards within public institutions such as schools, workhouses and, of particular relevance to this study, asylums.[2] Twenty-four war hospitals were established on asylum property across the UK by 1919.[3] Fourteen facilities on asylum grounds catered exclusively for physical ailments, seven were specialised mental facilities for nervous and mental disorders and three facilities accommodated both physical and mental patients.[4] Mental casualties were put on a par with physical injuries with clothing, attire, entertainment and overall treatment equal for both sets of patients.[5] External pressure influenced this initiative, as was the case with the establishment of the Ministry of Pensions.[6]

War hospitals would treat 483,000 soldier-patients in total. Some facilities displaced the district asylum while others shared the complex of existing asylums. Some 15,750 asylum patients were transferred in England and Wales, and just over 400 patients in Ireland, to allow 21,000 beds to be made available for the treatment of servicemen. Remaining asylums received the dislodged patients ensuring an overcrowding of around 10 percent or about five extra patients per ward.[7] Approximately 4,470 asylum beds were available for the treatment of servicemen's mental and nervous injuries. This figure equated to around 14 percent of the accommodation provided on asylum property. Military admissions were allotted a maximum treatment time of nine months for staff to decipher whether they should be discharged from the army or if they required transferral to a public asylum.[8] As will be demonstrated, this time limit was not adhered to in Ireland due to the aforementioned delay of the Service Patient scheme and the reluctance of district asylums to admit insane British ex-servicemen during the revolutionary period. This delay would compromise the RWH and Belfast War Hospital's (BWH) remit as observational facilities.

Conditions that were previously good enough for asylum patients were no longer appropriate for mentally and physically injured servicemen. There was an alteration of locks on almost all doors to negate the use of keys, a renewal and repairing of furniture and bedding, a deep cleaning and disinfection of vacated buildings to ensure the best sanitary conditions and an improvement in the lighting and heating conditions.[9] Even previous asylum medical staff operating in war hospitals were given an official military rank with remaining nurses now dressed in military attire.[10] The Board of Control's replacement of 'asylum' with 'war hospital' was also designed to negate the 'pathetic reminder of stigma which still clings to mental diseases and institutions for their care in England.'[11] Soldier-patients receiving treatment for mental and nervous injuries were dressed identically to physically injured servicemen. Known as 'Convalescent Blues', patients were provided with a distinct blue pyjama-like uniform. The issuance of 'Hospital Blues' (Figure 9) assisted numerous purposes, including a propagandistic use by identifying the individual as wounded as a result of war service.[12]

The Belfast and Richmond District Asylums provided the War Office facilities for the treatment of nervous and mental casualties in Ireland.

Establishing Richmond and Belfast war hospitals

W. R. Dawson, Inspector of Lunacy in Ireland, was appointed by the War Office as its specialist in nerve injuries in Ireland in mid-1915.[13] Dawson immediately recognised that facilities to treat such casualties were inadequate. The War Office subsequently registered a request for accommodation to the Richmond Asylum authorities in January 1916.[14] Acute overcrowding in Irish asylums may help to explain why the first enquiry to establish a war hospital in Ireland occurred a full twelve months after the scheme began in Britain. Suggesting a deficiency in available bed space, the RWH became the smallest facility within the war hospital network providing just thirty-two beds.[15]

Situated in a northern suburb one kilometre outside of central Dublin, the RWH was ideally located to provide an opportunity for rest and recuperation; it had useful railway links to Dublin port which received 16,000 evacuated British and Irish servicemen between August 1915 and February 1919. It was also adjacent to the King George V Hospital, which was a distribution hospital

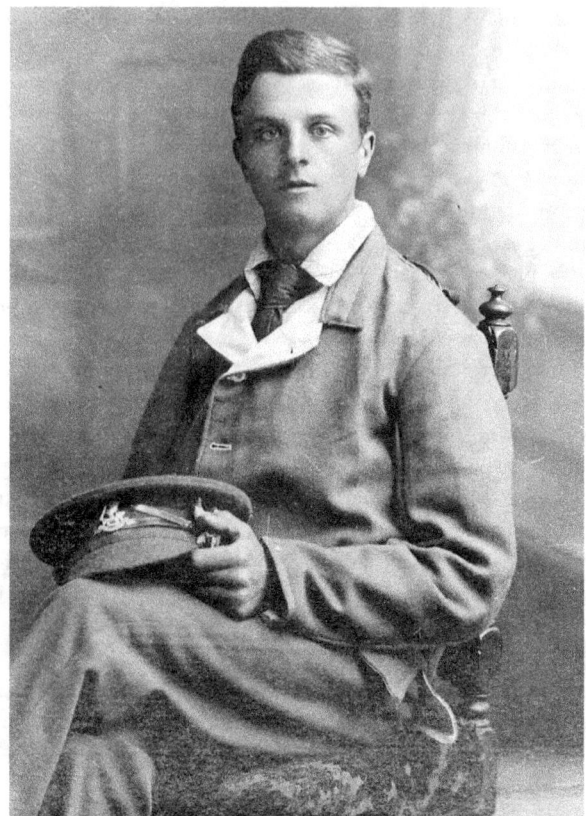

Figure 9 A soldier-patient dressed in Hospital Blues.

catering for a host of combat-related injuries and ailments and which would go on to forge intrinsic links with the RWH.[16] The Lunacy Inspectorate's annual report for 1916 notes the establishment of the RWH: 'A small separate block was placed by the committee of management at the disposal of the War Office for the use of mentally affected soldiers and has been freely availed of.'[17] 'Number 12 Block' was detached from the main asylum building.[18] The adjoining asylum accommodating 1,808 patients dwarfed the RWH. The RWH thus constituted less than 2 percent of the asylum population.[19]

Dawson described the RWH as 'small but well-equipped' indicating that the process of conversion was a relatively straightforward process. With the British Army paying the asylum committee 21 shillings per week per bed, in comparison to the 13s 2d weekly cost for an asylum patient, Richmond Asylum's committee approved the British Army's control of the facility as it provided a significant fiscal advantage.[20] The necessity for such a facility is evident in the number of admissions on its opening, with bed space quickly filled. There were 362 admissions from the RWH's foundation on 16 June 1916 until its closure on 23 December 1919.[21] Patients admitted to the RWH were institutionalised for observation without being certified insane and were cared for by the staff of the Richmond Asylum. The head night attendant objected to treating British Army servicemen on political grounds as a result of the pervading anti-British army sentiment. As Forde told the joint committee of the asylum: 'He is the only employee lay or medical who has hesitated to assist in relieving the sufferings of those brave soldiers who have risked their lives and sacrificed their health in their country's service.' It was decided that the attendant should not be involved in the RWH.[22]

Patients remained under the control of the War Office. Richmond Asylum staff were given twenty-four hours' notice in writing or via telephone about the impending admittance of a patient with seemingly little option for refusal.[23] The military also had full authority to discharge men. For example, in a letter sent to the RWH in November 1917, one mother enquired as to whether her son could be released. Donelan directed her question to Major Dawson as he had full jurisdiction on such matters.[24] Donelan would even become frustrated at the military authorities who transferred patients from the RWH before he deemed them as recovered.[25] Following dialogue between the asylum's committee, the Irish Inspectorate of Lunacy and the War Office, the latter assumed control of Belfast District Lunatic Asylum on the Grosvenor Road in April 1917 (Figure 10). The current asylum population of around 400 people was transferred to the Corry-Kerr buildings annexed to the Belfast Workhouse. A subsequent rearrangement of staff occurred with some attendants remaining at the facility to undertake responsibility at the BWH with others transferring to the workhouse.[26] In comparison to the more isolated RWH, the BWH was located near the Falls Road and was surrounded by houses, which sometimes led to interaction between patients on top of the high walls with nearby residents.[27]

The establishment of the BWH was not seamless with noted delays in acquiring and establishing equipment.[28] Its first admission did not occur until 15 May 1917. The former Resident Medical Superintendent's house allowed room for forty men, thus becoming the only war hospital in Ireland to treat mentally affected officers exclusively. There were 1,215 admissions into the BWH until its closure on 17 November 1919.[29] In addition to its size and segregation of officers, the BWH also diverged from the RWH in its everyday

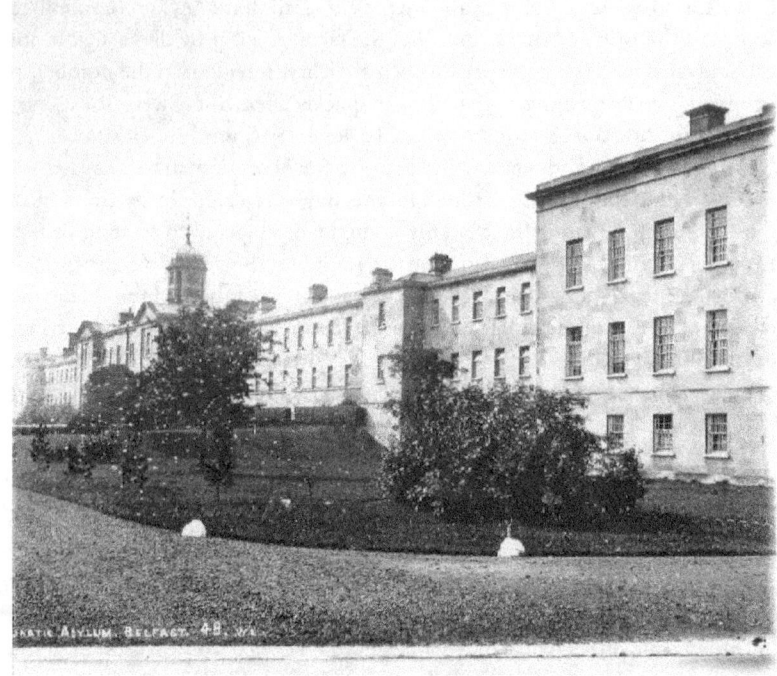

Figure 10 Belfast District Lunatic Asylum, c. 1890–1900.

running. The committee of the Belfast Asylum initially assumed control and responsibility for BWH and its patients. After the death of its Resident Superintendent, the War Office took command of the facility on 1 April 1918 until its closure.[30]

Admission

Dawson inspected and diagnosed patients under treatment across Irish military facilities. Men exhibiting prolonged symptoms of acute mental or nervous ailments were regularly transferred to the RWH for treatment. One transferral from the Dublin Red Cross Hospital wrote: 'This man is suffering from acute melancholia, and is suicidal. He should be transferred to the RWH without delay, as he requires constant supervision.'[31] Similar transferrals under the direction of Dawson occurred at the Lucan Red Cross Hospital and the Dublin VAD hospital in Mountjoy Square.[32] Two hundred transferrals to the RWH came from the King George V Hospital and 133 men were relocated from a military or war hospital in Ireland or Britain.[33]

Transferrals from the King George V Hospital thus constituted the most significant contribution. This included F. F. admitted to the RWH on 10 April 1917, with the explanation for this transferral as follows: 'Abusive tonight to orderly on duty – threatens to destroy him ... angry and violent ... a day or two after admission he can become rowdy and unmanageable on the ward ... He threatens to kill one of the wardens and man several times recently during the night.'[34] Corporal M. was also transferred having spent the night before transferral in similar facilities within the hospital: 'Violent. Kept in padded cell all night at King George V Hospital. Walked about all night in cell with hand grasping slashing throat. Has not spoken since admission.'[35] Leading medical officials interacting with shell-shocked patients denote a tendency to violence as a characteristic of the condition.[36] A lack of improvement could also prompt transferral. Private M. was admitted to the RWH with accompanying information provided by the King George V Hospital: 'I am sending the above man to you for observation ... he has been here for about two months ... is still in the same condition as on admission.'[37]

The RWH was not an exclusively Irish institution, treating British servicemen alongside a handful of Australian and Canadian servicemen.[38] The lack of bed space for mental casualties throughout the UK and the chaotic wartime system which catered for mental and nervous casualties ensured that war hospitals could not exclusively cater to servicemen according to nationality and birthplace.[39] Such attempts do appear to have been made: 133 patients were transferred from war hospitals in Britain and Belfast to the RWH. These transferrals included E. K., a forty-three year-old of the South Lancashire Regiment, who was transferred from the Warrington War Hospital to the BWH and then onto the RWH. The motivation for his transfer was that the patient wanted to be near his relatives living in Dublin.[40] Patients included nineteen Lance Corporals alongside four Corporals, thirteen Sergeants and two Captains. Like Ireland's district asylums, the RWH accommodated both Protestant and Catholic patients.[41] Patients served, on average, less than forty-eight months before admission with a mean of fourteen unbroken months with the field force. An estimated 10 percent had served for less than twelve months before admission. While there were huge contrasts in how long individual patients underwent treatment, the average length of residency in the RWH amounted to 102 days. This relatively short period is indicative of post-traumatic reactions to combat rather than an underlying mental illness. With regards to the 308 patients with a diagnosis on admission, melancholia was cited in eighty-four records, delusional insanity was referenced for thirty servicemen (10 percent) and mania (9 percent) accounted for twenty-seven citations.[42] The accuracy of such diagnoses remains suspect; understaffed and overworked medical staff, working in imperfect circumstances, often ensured very basic inquiries with previous medico-military personnel before transfer. Such diagnostic patterns, nevertheless, reflected wider patterns in the war hospital network.[43]

Causation

Speculation regarding causative agents in a servicemen's mental condition remains flawed.[44] Prior historical research into combat stress contends that some servicemen were predisposed to mental illness including those experiencing previous residency in an asylum before their enlistment.[45] It is possible that some soldier-patients may have had a mental illness separate to or worsened by war service. A minority of casebook files state that individuals had been previously certified as insane or had experienced neuro-psychiatric symptoms before they enlisted in the British Army.[46] Such instances were also apparent in British war hospitals.[47] Dawson held that RWH patients experienced a wide variety of symptoms which contrasted in duration and severity.[48] Individual soldier-patients discussed within the RWH's casebook verify an array of subjective symptoms. These symptoms include headaches, insomnia, bad dreams, depression, loss of memory, mental confusion and hallucinations.[49] As one British military doctor at a psychiatric unit assessed: 'The symptoms themselves are hardly ever the same twice over.'[50] The casebook's first entry was J. B., transferred from King George V Hospital on 11 October 1918 with 'Delusional Insanity':

> Physical: Heart and lungs clear. Tongue tremulous. Fine tremor of limbs. Sears on left forearm. One on back and one on front.
>
> Mental: He is very dull and confused and has delusions of persecution arising out of sight and hearing. He is so confused that he does not really know where he is and speaks at times as if he was in France. He states a whole crowd of them were following him all day and that they did the same last night. When questioned more closely he asked 'the guns are coming out of action aren't they? Aren't they coming up for a rest?' He states he hears everyone talking about him but cannot tell what they say. When questioned if he was in France he said 'yes' then said 'no I remember now. I'm in France aren't I? I think I am.'
>
> 12 October 1918: He remained quiet and slept through the night.
>
> 18 October: He is much improved. He states he does not now hear voices. His memory is much clearer. He is, however, dull at times ... he is very quiet and gives no trouble. Sleeps and eats well.

25 October: This man is very much improved. He is, however, rather giddy and silly in his manner is undoubtedly somewhat weak minded ... He is, however, well conducted.

11 November: This man is very much improved. He is bright and cheerful, gives no trouble. He states his head is now all right.

11 December: This man is now rational. He is bright and cheerful. Sleeps and eats well.

Discharged recovered to his home on 21 January 1919.[51]

J. B.'s example appears broadly typical of many men within the casebook who were suffering from cognitive disorders of rationality and memory but with no distinguishable incidents necessary to cause a man to require mental treatment.

Lieutenant Harold Tronson's pension records provide rare insight into a soldier-patient of the BWH. Tronson was transferred from the King George V Hospital following a breakdown on the Western Front:

18.9.17: On admission patient was in a restless excited condition, resisting anything being done for him. He was very noisy at night – shouting and singing. Next day he was still restless and excited and resented being visited or spoken to. He ordered everyone to leave the building and go to hell and that his orders must be carried out. Also had peculiar delusion about receiving help from the sun.

23.9.17: Remained much the same for a few days gradually getting more calm and quiet although his conversation was not quite coherent. He appeared somewhat nervous and shaky as the after-effects of some acute mental excitement. Slept fairly well.

24.9.17: Next day said he was tired and did not get up: lay in bed all day – feeling dull and depressed.

25.9.17: Was much brighter and felt better; conversation more rational. Slept well.

26.9.17: Appears to be quite normal again. Talks well and rationally and seems to have quite recovered. In talking about himself he says he was always nervous and self-conscious. He had no shell-shock in France, but says it was the constant strain that told on him.

Tronson was subsequently discharged from the hospital and the British Army before re-entering society.[52]

Frederick Mott, a leading neurologist who always held a strong belief as to the importance of organic and predisposition factors to explain shell-shock, recognised that the daily grind of trench life could lead to an attritional psychological collapse.[53] Depressive or melancholic states appear a common feature of RWH patients and reflect the wider war hospital network.[54] 'Melancholia' accounted for 27 percent of admissions to RWH.[55] References to 'depression' featured in the records of forty-two (41 percent) patients included within the casebook. For example, M. B. was admitted on 28 March 1919 with a year's service as a Gunner on the Western Front. Admitted with a diagnosis of 'Melancholia', his mental condition on admittance noted: 'Headaches at times was feeling nervous when he reported sick and his case was marked debility. He goes on to say he feels depressed and not as well as he used to feel or should feel but is better than he has been for some time. He says things of past worry him now and then.' M. B.'s mental condition improved; his penultimate casebook entry on 28 April 1919 recorded: 'Much improved. He is brighter and more cheerful. He states he is not so much worried now over the events of his past life.' He was discharged to his mother one week later.[56] Thirty-one RWH patients, almost three-quarters of the casebook's soldier-patients, displayed depressive states but then showed a recovery or improvement during their residency.[57]

One hundred and eight patients in the BWH had a physical wound owing to war service, one hundred and one patients had been blown up, buried or otherwise shell-shocked, sixteen patients had been gassed and a further sixteen had been torpedoed. Dawson wrote of such patients: 'These figures are not mutually exclusive, but they are sufficient to render it probable that a considerable amount of the insanity treated as to a greater or less extent brought about by the casualties of active service.'[58] American research similarly attests that the nearby explosion of shells, being buried alive or being under prolonged fire or physical stresses were prominent in causing the mental state of mentally afflicted soldiers.[59] Utilising this barometer for assessing causation, the RWH casebook described fifty-two men, more than half of the casebook's clientele, as having a single combat experience diagnosed as triggering their psychosis. These triggers included physical wounds, wounds and gassing, burial, and being under shell fire and shell shock; the latter of which appears to have been in the literal sense of suffering from shock as a result of shell fire.[60]

Purser described several patients whose mental condition was severely affected by having been buried alive as 'the most pitiable cases I have seen … it is my opinion that being buried adds to the intensity of trouble.' Such instances were apparent throughout specialist military facilities including the RWH.[61] Admitted on 11 October 1918, A. T. had served for two and a half years, and his mental condition was due to the 'hardship of war: buried by shell fire.' His casebook records note:

Physical: Weak and Emotional. Tongue tremulous … fine tremor of limbs.

Mental: He is dull depressed and confused and replies mostly by the motion of his head; in this way he indicates he had pain and noises in his head and that he hears voices and that something is following him. He after some time told me verbally on my questioning him more closely that he was blown up by a shell behind the lines. He seems rather nervous and apprehensive.

12 October: He remained quiet and slept fairly well during the night.

18 October: Much improved ... brighter and more communicative and seems less nervous. He sleeps fairly well.

25 October: Continues to improve. He is bright and cheerful in his manner but still complains of feeling nervous. His headache is much less and he is not now troubled by voices.

11 November: States he is now feeling all right. He states he has not felt as well for a long time.

11 December: Now perfectly rational. He is bright and cheerful. Gives no trouble.

Discharged 23 December 1918.

The fact that A.T. revealed more information when 'questioned more closely' indicates that Forde was flexible and responded to each patient subjectively.[62] Private M. entered the RWH on 30 October 1918 with his admission notes recording that he had previously been blown up by shell fire. His condition on admission was described as 'Dull and apathetic and seems depressed. He complained of pain and dizziness in his head and some noises that of calling ... insomnia and disturbing dreams. During which he wakes up in a fright.' His condition substantially improved within a month and he was discharged home on 30 October 1918.[63] 'Post-concussional injuries', where men continued to suffer from the after-effects of head trauma, were prevalent during the First World War and have remained a feature in subsequent conflicts.[64]

Thirty-six patients within the RWH casebook displayed a variety of hallucinations and delusions while under treatment, eight of which were war-related.[65] F. F. was admitted on 19 December 1918 following three years' service with visual hallucinations: 'He tells me he sees Germans everywhere he goes.' His hallucinations subsided before being discharged to his wife on 9 April 1919.[66] E. M. exhibited similar visual delusions on admission: 'He sees Germans at night. They stand with their hands up.'[67] Gunner G. was admitted with his mental condition depicted as 'dull and somewhat depressed. He complains of pains and bursting noises in his head and insomnia ... drops off to sleep wakes up in a fright and fancies someone is about his bed ... complains much of perspiration.' Gunner G. told RWH staff that he was 'caught in the middle of a field under shell fire but kept on and then broke down completely' before being sent to Ireland for treatment. His condition improved while receiving treatment in the RWH with his next casebook entry on 8 November 1918 recording: 'Very much improved in appearance and mentally. He seems to be getting more control over himself ... he states his head is less troublesome.' He was discharged from the RWH on 23 December 1918.[68]

Not all hallucinations and delusions were related to war service; twenty-eight patients experienced non-war-related symptoms.[69] For example, M. M. was admitted on 24 April 1919 following three years of service. Despite being noted as 'Bright and cheerful in manner', he heard voices: 'He states it can hardly be imagination and asks "could it be telegraphy? I take no notice of them. I pass them by."'[70] P. L. was admitted on 31 March 1919 suffering from 'vague persecutory delusions.' His condition remained much the same, and while he was awaiting discharge home he told Forde 'that he was going around to recruit for heaven.'[71] These states could cause alarm to the families of patients who were able to correspond with loved ones during their treatment. A letter addressed to Forde from the sister of one RWH patient with a diagnosis of delusional insanity, noted: 'I have received many strange letters from him at this hospital address, and I cannot understand what is the matter with him as there seems no sense in his letters.'[72] Regardless of speculation regarding causation, the majority of witnesses who attested to the Southborough Committee held that most mental and nervous casualties were a result of 'exhaustion' and 'prolonged strain.' The prognosis for recovery was not only good but speedy.[73] This pattern is also evident for the majority of patients recorded in the RWH's surviving casebook.

Treatment

While the treatment on offer at the various war hospitals in Britain and Ireland differed, a dual approach was often emphasised:[74] an environment conducive to fostering a patient's confidence and distraction from the war via recreational activities complemented by rest, recuperation and isolation.[75] Isolation and calmness were considered to benefit the treatment of neurasthenia before the outbreak of the First World War, and their use was still regarded as beneficial in the specialist war hospitals including the RWH.[76] Patients were thus able to enjoy the facility's grounds with family members able to visit patients to go out for walks on hospital grounds.[77] The Southborough Report supported such tranquillity as important to the recovery of servicemen: 'rest of mind and body is essential in all cases.'[78]

Nightmares were frequent amongst shell-shocked servicemen.[79] In *Conflict and Dream*, published in 1923, Rivers believed that traumatised and emotionally shattered servicemen resisted sleep in the hope of avoiding nightmares.[80] Read commented on mental patients under his care at 'D-Block' at Netley War Hospital who 'showed very vividly how the extreme limit of exhaustion had been reached, and yet with a few day's rest all was well.'[81] Purser similarly wrote of Irish cases: 'Bad dreams are constantly complained of. They are real, deafening and choking – nearly always about the war.' Purser held that 'cessation of bad dreams may be looked on as a favourable sign, for they appear to cease once the patient's condition begins to definitely improve.'[82] Reflecting the conservative and traditional approach of RWH staff, there appears to be little psychoanalysis of soldier-patient's dreams. Nevertheless, having experienced the physical and mental drain of trench life, just a few night's sleep in a safe and secluded war hospital could be hugely beneficial in the treatment of soldiers who were suffering from acute fatigue.[83] This pattern is evident within the RWH.

Difficulties in sleeping were recorded in twenty-two casebook records. An improvement in sleep was registered in all such instances. Private D. entered the RWH experiencing nightmares: 'He can see shells bursting about he states he wakes up very frightened at night.' Very quickly, however, his sleeping improved within the facility with one entry one week later recording: 'States he is feeling much better' before being discharged as recovered to his home on 3 February 1919.[84] F. C. was detailed on admittance as: 'dull and confused ... never gets a night's sleep.' Once again, the man's sleeping habits and mental condition improved in tandem during his residency at the RWH.[85] Located outside of central Dublin, the suitability of the hospital's location aided sleep. A. T. was described on admission as experiencing 'troublesome dreams of death and murder' which quickly dissipated. One week later his file logged: 'states he has much improved owing to the quietness of this place.'[86] Private F. slept badly on admission. However, having been given bromide on his first night in the RWH, he slept well.[87] As Purser wrote, such cases are 'happiest, and their condition improves most quickly in circumstances where they are warm and quiet and not bustled. As a rule these cases do well.'[88] The treatment and improvement of Private F. and Private E. appear to have been commonplace throughout the war hospital network and its treatment of exhausted and emotionally shattered soldiers.[89]

Medication was not solely restricted to inducing sleep; a wide variety of medication was implemented throughout the war hospital network including the RWH.[90] A meeting of the 'Irish Division' of the Medico-Psychological Association in 1917 recounted:

> Dr Forde, who had had many opportunities of treating these cases, gave the meeting the benefit of his experiences ... There was marked tremulousness of the musculature and shakings of the body, with profuse perspiration of the skin of the head. He had found a mixture of the bromides, together with antipyrine, and citrate of caffeine, gave great relief where headaches existed, and when the

mixture was discontinued the men begged for its repetition. Fletcher's syrup of the hydromates was useful and hastened recovery in some of the cases he had treated.[91]

Antipyrine was a painkiller which helped lessen inflammation and stabilise body temperature.[92] Private E. was described on admission as such: 'He hears voices speaking in German to him at night and the voices come back to him in dreams.' E.'s complaints of headaches continued during his first night under treatment, and he was subsequently provided antipyrine which reduced his symptoms.[93]

As was the case throughout the war hospital network, the poor physical condition of RWH patients on admission was referenced on admittance.[94] For example, F. K. was 'pale, thin and worn looking.' Another patient was described on admission as such: 'Skin is dirty. Much in need of a bath.'[95] These patients made substantial improvements in their physical condition while in the facility. For example, Gunner G.'s left arm on admission was 'badly torn' and 'septic', but both his mental and physical state showed clear improvement; his arm 'healed' just over a month later.[96] A. F.'s physical improvement was recorded just two weeks after admittance with his casebook noting that he was 'looking much stronger.' Even when a patient's mental condition did not improve, a development in physicality was achieved. P. F. was 'demented' requiring spoon-feeding. Nevertheless, his casebook records denote that he had 'improved much physically but very little mentally' in the seven months since admittance.[97] The resting, recuperation and bathing of patients very much aligned itself with pre-1914 practices of the Weir–Mitchell treatment of neurasthenic men and women.[98]

In addition to rest and recuperation, the military establishment advocated more active forms of therapy.[99] P. G. had tremulous limbs and facial muscles, and was subsequently transferred to the King George V Hospital for 'Electric Treatment.'[100] This form of treatment was again long-established in civilian medical practice and was used by several combatant nations during the First World War.[101] Despite modern perceptions that electrical treatment of 'faradism' was draconian and barbaric, it could prove effective in removing or improving the symptoms held by mentally ill soldier-patients including, for example, men who suffered from involuntary muscle movements, who could be effectively cured.[102] Indeed, the records of P. G. indicate progress in his condition, being subsequently discharged as recovered.[103]

Occupational therapy was evident in both the RWH and throughout the war hospital network, including working on war hospital grounds, kitchens and associated workshops as well as occupations outside of the asylum in nearby schools and farms.[104] Such facilities enabled what has been recently termed as

'Cure by Functioning' by providing an 'active and behavioural approach' for patients to experience a semblance of civilian life.[105] The opportunity to work had been longstanding in Irish asylums.[106] Patients within the Richmond Asylum were encouraged to work for incentives such as extra food provisions and payment while under treatment. Employment included decorating, tailoring, carpentry, laundry and bakery work.[107]

Entertainment was also arranged for servicemen under treatment throughout specialist mental facilities. Participation in these activities was believed to be a soothing distraction from the war.[108] The Irish Automobile Club took RWH patients out for drives, and brass bands, singers and drama groups provided productions for the patients and staff which greatly improved in the care and comfort offered to servicemen.[109] RWH patients experienced short-term parole which was again commonplace throughout the UK.[110] Sixteen patients within the casebook of the RWH were granted a short-term pass and parole.[111] This privilege was conditional on whether a soldier-patient's mental condition had suitably improved.[112] Sergeant. H, for example, was only allowed out on pass after his mental state was substantially enhanced in the ten days since his admittance.[113] The granting of parole appears to have been enjoyed by the patients as there are no references to men refusing to partake in the programme.[114] If a patient's family lived nearby, then it was possible to visit them within the system of parole. One patient was granted three days leave to attend his mother's funeral.[115] Male pauper lunatics similarly enjoyed pass and parole. Asylum patients were able to venture outside of the grounds and visit local picture house and theatre productions. Unlike the RWH, however, asylum patients were only allowed outside the grounds of the asylum under supervision and charge of accompanying attendants.[116] This difference in observational policy illustrates the contrasting views held towards the supposedly recovering shell-shocked soldier-patient in comparison to the permanently unpredictable lunatic.

The unsupervised nature of the parole system in the RWH could prove problematic. One patient's parole was revoked due to prior misconduct: 'Allowed out on pass ... took some drink and went to King George V Hospital accompanied by another soldier and tried to get admission there. He was brought back by an escort.' The withdrawal of parole was not welcomed by the patient whose records note: 'Demands pass every day despite constant refusal' with Forde explaining: 'I am sure he would drink and misconduct himself.' His subsequent casebook entry demonstrates a definite improvement in conduct over the previous month which was rewarded in his return of parole: 'He has recently improved and has become more docile and respectful in his manner. He has improved in every way ... he is now allowed out on pass every day.'[117] As was the case in other medical facilities, the granting and revocation of parole became a disciplinary measure within the RWH.[118]

Life at the RWH was not idyllic despite the emphasis on rest, recuperation and recreation. Staff and patients of the RWH endured physical and verbal abuse from unruly patients while working or receiving treatment at the facility. Such behaviour led to rebukes including placing troublesome patients within isolated observation wards.[119] R. F. was transferred to the observation ward with padded cells located in the adjoining Richmond Asylum one week after admittance with his records noting he was quarrelsome and had got into a physical fight with another patient.[120] The records of one Sergeant similarly note that he 'attacked orderly in charge of work. Had to be restrained in a padded cell. Very violent at times.'[121] It was also for a patient's protection that they were placed within isolated observation wards. Five RWH patients were suicidal, including Private D. who was placed under surveillance on account of his apparent suicidal tendencies.[122] This supervision was again frequent within both the war hospital network and the adjoining Richmond Asylum.[123] Less drastic instances of isolation occurred. One patient was removed to a separate single room after becoming 'very troublesome', illustrating that patients shared rooms, and that single rooms existed within the RWH.[124]

Such issues were not always the inevitable by-product of dealing with mentally ill patients. As previously mentioned, the Service Patient system was not introduced in Ireland until August 1919 which was over two years after the scheme's introduction in Britain. Twenty-nine of the thirty-one patients transferred to an asylum were relocated during the last three months of 1919. This further delay in the implementation of the Service Patient scheme was due to the aforementioned reluctance of asylums to receive Service Patients during the Anglo-Irish War due to local authorities in Ireland refusing to recognise the British Government and submit their accounts for audit. Chronic cases under treatment at the RWH and BWH were withheld from district asylums, ensuring that a significant number of incurable cases accumulated at both observational facilities.[125] This community continued to suffer from delusions, were confused, untidy, had a poor memory and were incoherent conversationally throughout their treatment. They even resorted to physical violence towards asylum staff.[126] M. O., for example, exhibited persistently threatening behaviour throughout his residency with his case notes for 16 October 1919 stating: 'restless and inclined to be violent. He has threatened me on one or two occasions.'[127] Working in Mercer Military Hospital in Dublin, which treated neuropsychiatric casualties alongside other physical ailments, Purser wrote that squabbles, disorder and noise could cause its mentally ill patient population to experience a 'return of all symptoms which patient treatment and time have caused to disappear', indicating that the chronic patients could have had a detrimental impact on other patients.[128] The delaying of the Service Patient scheme in Ireland, and the resulting continued stay of chronic soldier-patients, had a damaging influence on shell-shocked soldier-patients within the RWH. War hospitals were initially set up for nine months to observe whether a man was suitable for asylum treatment. The delay of the Service Patient scheme in Ireland undermined its remit as an observational facility. This feature was unique to Ireland, providing another instance of how its unique socio-political context shaped its particular experience of shell-shock.

Discharge

Purser had a favourable prognosis for the majority of soldier-patients treated at a war hospital.[129] The available RWH discharge data reveals 118 men released to friends, family or a general military hospital, 106 transferred to another war hospital for specialist treatment with 31 relocated to a district asylum.[130] For example, Private C. joined the British Army in January 1902, and he subsequently served on the Western Front with the Royal Dublin Fusiliers. He was admitted to the RWH from the BWH on 25 January 1919 diagnosed with 'chronic mania':

> On Admission: nervous and fidgety ... he states he heard voices in 'the other place' (Belfast) and was more or less under their influence.
>
> 31 January 1919: Rambling and incoherent in conversation ... dirty unnatural habits drink urine and puts it on his head. He is very careless ... seems more or less demented.
>
> 7 February: Puts urine on the face.
>
> 25 February: Slightly improved in habits he has ceased to put urine on his head. He is, however, eccentric in his manner and more or less irrelevant in his replies to questions and answers.

His records describe a continuation of these symptoms, with an unsuccessful escape attempt in April before he was transferred to the Richmond Asylum on 1 November 1919.[131] P. F. was admitted to the RHW on 1 February 1919, having served for over a year with the 1st Connaught Rangers. P. F.'s behaviour was similarly described as such:

> Mental: Dull apathetic and unable to give an account of himself. His memory is very bad. He suffers from hallucinations of hearing. He hears voices speaking to him but can't say what the voices say.
>
> 8 February 1919: Has to be fed with a spoon at times ... he is unable to carry on a simple conversation. Memory gone. He occasionally passed remarks to himself as if hearing voices. He stands about in the same position for long periods.

15 February: Babbling incoherently to himself ... demented.

1 September: Has improved much physically but very little mentally. He is however more communicative and his memory is improved but not normal. He is more jovial in mood ... he is very untidy in habits.

P. F. was subsequently transferred to Ballinasloe Asylum.[132] With such instances remaining a minority, the War Office concluded in 1919: 'Over half of whom were successfully treated and enabled to return to their homes without the blemish of having being certified as being insane.'[133] However, even Purser felt uncertain as to the future of those who were diagnosed as insane and transferred to a lunatic asylum, maintaining: 'I know no way of judging, at the outset, how any given case will do.'[134]

The fact that just two RWH admissions returned to duty is unsurprising. The initial letter from the War Office to Donelan stressed that the soldier-patient remained under the auspice of the War Office until they were '*invalided*' from the army, suggesting a general presumption that these men would not be returning to the front line.[135] In addition to those discharged to friends and family, Dawson specified the Belfast patients deemed as recovered also included those discharged to a less specialised military hospital and that such men were 'either recovered wholly or sufficiently improved to be treated as ordinary sane individuals.'[136] It appears as though transferrals to another military hospital facilitated a continuation of treatment for a patient's physical ailment or weakness.[137]

Regarding transferrals to another war hospital for specialist treatment, the mental condition of patients varied. Within the RWH casebook, of those later transferred to the BWH, eleven patients showed an improvement in their mental condition while in the RWH.[138] However, such a trend was not consistent: three patients showed no improvement in their mental condition before transferral to the BWH.[139] The records provide little information on these transferrals; it is possible that they were being moved to be closer to their friends and family. With regards to the BWH, of the 1,215 men whose discharge data is available, 865 were discharged to friends, family or another military hospital, 306 being sent to specialist mental hospitals or district asylums, 18 returned to duty while 21 men died while under treatment.[140] This Irish data is broadly comparable to analyses of discharges in English and Welsh war hospitals.[141]

Unsurprisingly, incorporating Richmond Asylum staff within its function, the majority of treatment methods employed at the RWH were a continuation of conservative civilian treatment practices. Donelan was an 'unimaginative clinician' who had a somatic interpretation of shell-shock. The experience of shell-shock at the RWH thus brought little in the way of unique or innovative treatment of the mentally ill, as was apparent of practitioners like Rows in facilities like Maghull.[142] Yet, despite the RWH's conservatism, the soldier-patients it hosted benefitted from being elevated above the lunatic patient in the adjoining asylum. Mortality rates intensified in the former during the war period. By contrast, with care in the RWH remaining decent, deaths in military facilities were negligible. Shell-shock and insanity historians point to the extreme difficulty in assessing stigma and public and medical opinion.[143] Comparing the standards of treatment and mortality rates centres the vital introduction of designating soldier-patients special status during the First World War which elevated their standing and care in comparison to the insane lunatic.

Comparisons with lunatic asylums

In 1921, an infamous memoir published by Montagu Lomax recounted his experience of working in Prestwich Asylum, Manchester, between 1917 and 1919. The work detailed scathing criticism of the British asylum network and its treatment of insane patients during the First World War:[144] 10,085 deaths occurred in English and Welsh asylums between 1905 and 1914, figures for 1917 and 1918 totalled 37,463.[145] By comparison, there were just 164 deaths in the war hospital network during the same period.[146] The annual death rate in English asylums rose by over 20 percent from pre-1914 averages.[147] J. L. Crammer's case study of Buckinghamshire County Asylum, 1914–18, foregrounds the inferior treatment facilities available and subsequent increased patient death rates.[148] This work has been added to by additional research into Yorkshire and Essex-based public asylums.[149] Over 140,000 asylum residents in Germany also passed away during the war, with these deaths being attributable to war-induced rationing and cutbacks.[150] A similar trajectory would occur in Ireland.

In 1919, 10,720 male patients received treatment within Irish asylums. Their recovery rate amounted to 38 percent.[151] The recovery rate of the RWH shows that 46 percent of patients were discharged as 'successfully treated.' Belfast Asylum had a recovery rate of 21 percent in comparison to the BWH's recovery rate of 71 percent.[152] Army medical staff argued that comparisons between military servicemen and lunatics in the civil asylum were 'practically valueless.'[153] The contrasting recovery rates between public asylums and military facilities are better understood when considering two key factors: first, they were two very different types of facility. The RWH and BWH were only in operation for three and a half years and two and a half years respectively. Military installations operated as observational facilities whereas Irish patients had already been certified as insane before admission. Myers held that 'the prognosis in cases of "shell-shock" is generally good' and his positive outlook was reflected in the RWH.[154] This prognosis was rarer amongst asylum patients. In the second half

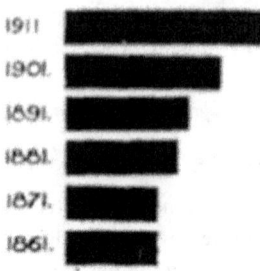

Figure 11 The age distribution of Irish lunatic patients, 1861–1911. Annual Report of the Inspectors of Lunatics, Ireland, 1913, xv.

of the nineteenth-century, the majority of patients were middle-aged, with a dramatic increase in the number of patients over the age of seventy admitted between 1861 and 1901.[155] The Lunacy Inspectorate's final annual report before the outbreak of the First World War notes the older patient profile of the asylum population (Figure 11). In contrast, army recruitment regulations allowed men from 18 to 45 years old to enlist. The average age of patients under treatment at the RWH was twenty-five years old, and only sixteen patients were forty-five years old or over.[156]

The Richmond District Asylum was more likely to house older and long-term patients. There was little chance of discharge once a residency surpassed twenty-four months. With regards to the rest of the asylum population, the vast majority of the patient population appeared chronic, remaining a patient until their death. Figure 12 provides evidence of this thesis. Medical officials conceded that some stable men became mentally ill purely as a result of war service. Such instances, however, were described by two witnesses as 'transitory' in duration.[157] A good percentage of patients admitted to a war hospital exhibited a mental illness of a 'temporary nature' of the 'mildest type.' The district asylum mostly held 'more advanced cases.'[158] It is more appropriate to compare the standard of treatments on offer rather than the pathologies of the two patient profiles.

As previously mentioned, the establishment of the war hospitals could only be accomplished via emptying existing asylum facilities, often inducing a transferral of patients to another asylum. Between 1914 and 1919, there was a

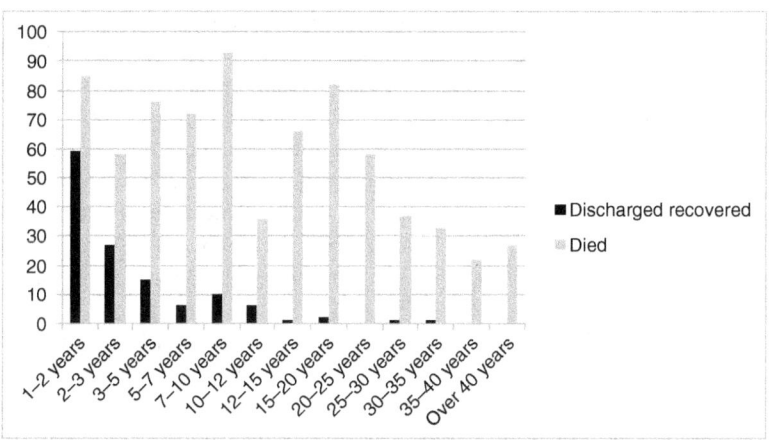

Figure 12 Length of residence of male patients in Irish asylums who were discharged recovered and those who died in 1919. Annual Report of the Inspectors of Lunatics, Ireland, 1919, 9.

decrease of 2,602 patients throughout the whole Irish district asylum network which averaged an annual reduction of 520 patients per year.[159] In 1915, the Board of Control argued that the need for public buildings for military purposes led to a shortage of institutional beds and the subsequent 'unavoidable limitation of admissions to cases most urgently needing treatment.'[160] The authority also held that the overcrowding of district asylums throughout the UK to make way for war hospitals ensured that friends and family were more likely to discharge a patient and care for them themselves. Families also became increasingly reluctant to send patients to more distant institutions if their nearby asylum had been vacated for the treatment of soldier-patients.[161]

Large numbers of asylum staff enlisted in the British Army during the First World War. Consequently, patients were attended to by fewer and less-trained replacement staff.[162] Irish asylums similarly lost prestigious and qualified staff during the period. The Belfast District Lunatic Asylum, for example, lost two senior medical officers in the summer of 1914. In 1915, the Resident Medical Superintendent of Armagh, Ballinasloe and Castlebar asylums enlisted as did the senior medical officers at Ballinasloe, Letterkenny, Londonderry and Sligo asylums.[163] The increase in the cost of supplies and foodstuff also led to growth in the cost per patient during the war.[164] This eventuality again reflected the British experience.[165] Irish asylums subsequently adjusted dietary arrangements, which included reducing the consumption of eggs and potatoes, sugars, rice, replacing cocoa for tea and margarine for butter.[166] The inflation of food prices and the decrease in imports of foodstuffs, alongside everyday commodities like medicines and coals, impacted the whole of Irish society.[167] Richmond and Cork Asylums were under strict economic controls ensuring that unsuitable items were still in use which would have been replaced in peacetime.[168] There was also an acute shortage of coal for use in the running of the Cork Asylum from 1917 due to the sinking of cargo ships by German submarines.[169] A further detriment to the patient experience came via the amusement and entertainment of patients becoming more limited than it had been hitherto.[170] Its reduction came despite the Medical Superintendent of Richmond explaining its therapeutic importance.[171]

In addition to the implementation of these 'war economies', a lack of financial assistance hampered asylum accommodation. Around 150 patients overcrowded Castlebar Asylum, and a plan to erect accommodation for 250 patients was subsequently postponed. Overcrowding existed at the Ballinasloe Asylum with recent plans to establish additional accommodation to address the problem being abandoned. In the absence of this extra bed space, some of the more severely ill patients were found sleeping on straw without adequate blankets while others slept on wet mattresses and several sheets covered with faeces.[172] With the lack of finance available to help projects that were 'not absolutely required in the interest of public health', asylum accommodation continued to be disadvantaged.[173] In 1917, Killarney, Sligo and Armagh asylums were overcrowded, utilising old and unsuitable wards and furniture with soiled bed clothing and unhygienic toilet facilities.[174] The Lunacy Inspectorate described the year 1918 'as undoubtedly the most trying within modern times to all concerned in the management of the District Asylums.'[175] Thus, in comparison to the conditions available to civilian patients at the adjoining Richmond Asylum, the RWH offered far better facilities to its soldier-patients.

The BWH offers a slightly more complicated narrative, with Belfast's insane population split between the old asylum building on Falls Road and a recently established villa colony system at Purdysburn. The new villa colony system at Purdysburn was described in favourable terms by the Lunacy Inspectorate due to the picturesque and scenic surroundings, describing it as the best public asylum in the UK.[176] The old asylum on Grosvenor Road and the location of the BWH received less favourable reviews by comparison:

> At each succeeding visit one is more and more struck by the great contrast between the accommodation provided in the old building in the City and the new Villa colony at Purdysbyrn. I need not dwell on the gloomy and prison-like character of the former, as has so often been done in previous reports, and which, notwithstanding every effort to brighten it ... cannot but prejudicially affect the chances of recovery.

The Lunacy Inspectorate summed up the comparative inferiority of patients placed in the old asylum facility: 'These patients are certainly much to be commiserated, when their lot is compared with that of their more fortunate fellow-patients located at Purdysburn.'[177] Reports on the old Grosvenor Road facility described the asylum as 'antiquated' with 'very evident signs of dilapidation' as the asylum committee were reluctant to commit the necessary finances to a facility that was soon to be abandoned.[178] The War Office recognised the imperfect condition of the old asylum on which the BWH was established:

> The building is a very old one, 100 years old and cannot be regarded as by any means up to date, the Belfast Corporation, having built a new Asylum already in occupation at Purdysburn, had spent very little of later years on upkeep of the old Building, which has suffered in consequence.[179]

In comparison to the 400 asylum residents of the facility on Grosvenor Road relocated to the Belfast Union workhouse, however, ex-servicemen experienced more favourable treatment. Unclean and staffed by a skeleton union workforce, the workhouse facility provided poor sleeping facilities, was cramped and overcrowded. The Lunacy Inspectorate wrote: 'the patients did not look so robust as could be desired, while their general health is stated not to be so good as in the asylum.'[180] The BWH thus took up a unique position within the UK war hospital network. Like most other military facilities, the BWH offered superior conditions than those offered to civilian lunatics who had been transferred to accommodate them. However, the BWH remained an anomaly in that a nearby civilian facility, the Purdysburn Villa Colony, was superior to the conditions hosting soldier-patients.

The fluctuations between the war hospital and district asylum impacted upon more than just everyday experiences of institutionalisation; they could also dictate survival. The proportion of patients who died within Irish district asylums were higher than was the case in the two Irish war hospitals.[181] The annual number of deaths in Irish asylums between 1913 and 1919 demonstrates the augmentation of fatalities during the war years (Table 7).

The influenza was the direct cause of 234 deaths across the Irish asylum network and was potentially attributable for another 236, representing over one-fifth of all asylum deaths in 1918. Mortalities expanded beyond the asylum. Previous estimates assess that the 'Spanish Flu' influenza of 1918 and 1919, for example, was responsible for over 20,000 deaths in Ireland.[182] While the increase in death rates in Irish asylums was on the rise from the late nineteenth century, the years covering 1915 to 1919 saw a definite augmentation in asylum death rates over quinquennial periods (Figure 13). British and Irish asylum death

Table 7 Annual number of deaths in Irish asylums, 1913–1919.

Year	Number of deaths	Comparison to previous year
1913	1,535	Increase of 111
1914	1,475	Decrease of 60
1915	1,676	Increase of 201
1916	1,743	Increase of 67
1917	2,191	Increase of 448
1918	2,243	Increase of 52
1919	1,796	Decrease of 447

Calculated from Annual Reports of Inspectors of Lunatics, Ireland, 1913–1919.

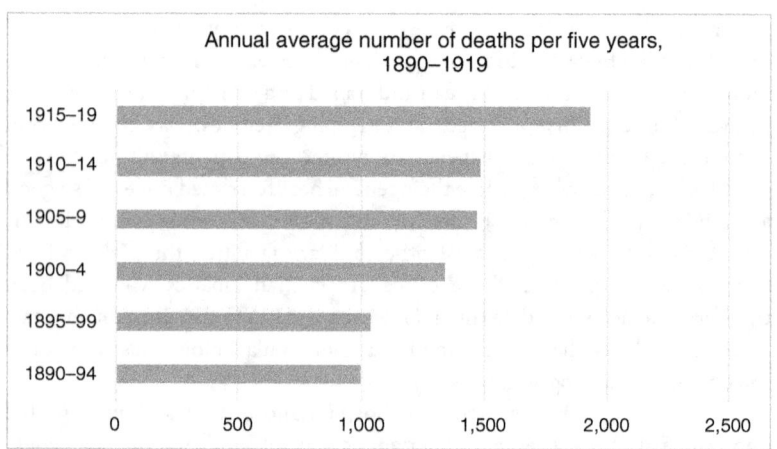

Figure 13 Average annual number of deaths in Irish asylum. over five-year periods, 1890–1919. Annual Report of the Inspectors of Lunatics, Ireland, 1919, xiv.

rates began to resemble pre-war averages when improvements in the standard and quantity of food increased during 1920.[183]

Not all deaths were unavoidable. British asylum authorities conducted an enquiry in 1918 to explain the spike in mortality rates. The report concluded that the reduction of finances, the quality of the diet provided and qualified staff as well as overcrowding and poor hygiene standards led to unmatched mortality rates.[184] Following an in-depth analysis of the increased mortality rate in the wartime asylum, the Board of Control cited the following explanations:

'The lowering of the weight of patients and general loss of nutrition due to food restrictions, the diminution of the care and attention they normally receive resulting from the calling up for military service of a large proportion of the skilled attendants.'[185] Analysis into a district asylum in Essex concludes that the number of deaths from respiratory tuberculosis increased during the period which led to the district asylum being 'a devastating arena of ill health and death.'[186]

Reductions were implemented to ease the workload of asylum staff. These included record-keeping duties and post-mortem examinations. Their reduction may have had a direct impact on the increase of deaths during the war years as these duties helped supervise and improve medical care and patient wellbeing. Numbers of post-mortem examinations, for example, decreased by 41 to 177 in 1914. Asylums at Armagh, Castlebar, Monaghan and Waterford did not conduct any post-mortems, and only one or two were carried out at Carlow, Sligo, Killarney and Letterkenny asylums during the war. The decrease in post-mortem examinations continued with only 104 examinations being carried out in 1918 which was a reduction of 52 from 1917 figures. In 1919, the Lunacy Inspectorate noted that only 63 deaths out of 1,976 were verified by a post-mortem, adding: 'The marked decrease in the number of these examinations which has continued for several years is to be regretted.' Letterkenny asylum staff also failed to keep the casebook entries up to date for its oldest patients, potentially contributing to the asylum's death rate. In the following year's Lunacy Inspectorate report, there were seventy-eight deaths in the Letterkenny Asylum. Despite having the twelfth largest asylum population, out of a possible twenty-four, it had the fourth highest death rate, surpassed only by the much larger facilities in Belfast, Dublin, Cork and Ballinasloe.[187] The conflict overshadowed the treatment of the civilian mentally ill. The Resident Superintendent of Belfast Asylum, William Graham, wrote in 1916: 'These are days in which annual reports have little interest for anyone unless the subject reviewed is glimpsed in the light of the present world conflict.'[188] In 1923, the editor of the *Journal of Mental Science* predicted that 'many years will go before the public will generally shed tears over dead lunatics.'[189] Tragically for Irish fatalities, there were no similar measures to investigate and understand their plight as was the case in Britain.

There were significant differences in the treatment of lunatics in the district asylum in comparison to the treatment of soldier-patients in the RWH and BWH. The latter were not diagnosed as insane, were segregated from asylum patients, wore a military dress akin to physically wounded servicemen when undergoing treatment, had better recreational facilities, and were provided greater liberality with regards to parole. It was, however, the standard of care on offer in each type of facility which best exemplifies the contrast in treatment.

The RWH provided a decent standard of care and attention, albeit in an orthodox and conservative way, while the standard of care plummeted in the district asylum during the war years. Nowhere was this recession more evident than in the increased number of fatalities. One US observer poignantly reflected upon these tragic deaths as such: 'one's thoughts turn to the helpless insane, never too well provided for, who were turned out of their hospitals and whose comfort as well as chance for recovery must have been seriously impaired by the change.'[190] Crammer argues that British asylum patients who died in the wartime asylum were 'casualties without any war memorial.'[191] Many Irish asylum patients who passed away between 1914 and 1918 deserve to share this epithet.

Conclusion

In further contrast to the wartime district asylum, Dawson spoke of the 'great kindness' afforded patients at the RWH with Forde's conduct adjudged to be 'beyond all praise.'[192] Dawson repeated his acclaim of the RWH and its staff in 1925:

> Small as it was, this hospital which was opened on June 16 1916, did excellent and indeed indispensable work, thanks to the interest and support of Dr Donelan, the Resident Medical Superintendent, and of the staff concerned in its management, but especially, I feel justified in saying, of the late Dr MJ Forde, at that time Senior Assistant Medical Officer in charge of the male department, who devoted himself con amore to looking after these cases.[193]

The War Office echoed similar approval:

> A letter was read from the Secretary of the War Office stating that, in connection with the closing of the RWH, Dublin, he was commanded by the Army Council to express their thanks to the joint committee of the Richmond District Asylum, Dublin, for their great efforts, upon which from June 1916, until December last this hospital has been dependent. The council deeply appreciate the kind and patriotic action which had rendered possible the provision and maintenance of so valuable an addition to the medical resources of the Army as the RWH had proved itself to be. Further, he requested that the joint committee would be good enough to convey to the staff of the hospital the thanks of the Army Council for the whole-hearted attention and devotion which they had given to the patients who had been under their care.[194]

The conduct of staff and the standard of care offered at the BWH were also positively received.[195] Dawson wrote of the facility: 'It has played an indispensable part in the medical war organisation of the country, a fact which must be a source of satisfaction to the committee and all who helped to facilitate the necessary arrangements.'[196] The military and medical establishment felt the worthiness of both the RWH and BWH. Both institutions were credited for their treatment of servicemen in the 1919 annual report of the Irish Lunacy Inspectorate.[197] As Dawson concluded: 'At all events, I think it has been shown that neither institution could easily have been disposed with, and that both in their varying degrees have deserved well of the country, and of the brave men who sacrificed so much in defending.'[198] The praise of the RWH and BWH reflected broader and even international praise of the war hospital scheme.[199] The Board of Control even described war hospitals established on asylum property as the 'best military and civil hospitals in the country.'[200]

The RWH and BWH were not, however, indisputably successful treatment facilities. Dawson deduced that a considerable number of remaining patients under treatment were 'in a terminal condition of discharge.'[201] Unless a patient's family were willing to take on responsibility for the care of the men, many of these unrecovered cases transferred to the asylum.[202] Of the 362 admissions into the RWH, thirty-one men (9 percent) were diagnosed as insane and distributed to eleven asylums throughout Ireland, with fifteen being transferred into the adjoining Richmond Asylum.[203] Before the BWH's official closure on 17 November 1919, the Richmond Asylum also received a further twenty-eight Service Patients from the facility on 16 October 1919.[204] The asylum committee resumed control of the facility on Grosvenor Road on 1 December 1919 following the closure of the BWH, although asylum patients were not retransferred to the facility.[205] Patients at the Corry-Kerr building of Belfast Workhouse, who had relocated from the old asylum to facilitate the creation of the BWH, were placed in the superior villa colony system at Purdysburn. This relocation ensured that the city's insane were within the same facility for the first time in half a century.[206]

On the closing of the RWH, Donelan advocated the continuance of 'Block 12' as an observational facility, stating: 'It would seem that, in dealing with many cases other than soldiers, some such system of preliminary uncertified treatment might be adopted with beneficial results to the community and save many from the blemish of having been certified insane.'[207] The Board of Control also wrote that a continuation of the war hospital's emphasis on early treatment and observation should continue in civilian mental health treatment in Britain.[208] Smith and Pear similarly urged: 'The medical lessons taught by the war must not be forgotten when peace comes. The civilian should be offered the facilities for a cure which have proved such a blessing to the war-stricken soldier.'[209] These suggestions were ignored in both Britain and Ireland. Instead, the asylum remained a protective barrier to segregate the dangerous lunatic from wider society.[210] Continuing the legacy of the terminology of war hospitals, even the

Board of Control's desire that asylums would be immediately reclassified as 'Mental Hospitals' to advance perceptions of the treatability of mental illness was not realised for several years. Longstanding prejudices of mental illness proved difficult to alter despite advances made as a result of the First World War.[211] The first attempt at modernisation and to adequately distinguish between those certified as insane and uncertified patients who required prior observation would not come into play in Ireland until 1932 in Northern Ireland and 1945 in the Republic of Ireland, which came two and fifteen years after the act's introduction in Britain.[212]

Kelly describes the RWH as 'an important harbinger of the much-needed reform of the Irish asylums.'[213] In opposition, Hopkins argues that that the novel approach of the war hospital scheme was matched only by the subsequent conservatism of the asylum network which was apparent in both Britain and Ireland: 'the military medical services offered, for a time at least, a more generous, compassionate and considerate regime than in the civilian asylum system. When their case became hopeless, however, the asylum claimed them as before.'[214] The reality lies somewhere between these two opposing narratives. Conservatism once again co-existed with progression in the treatment of insane Great War veterans in the inter-war asylum.

Notes

1. Reid, 'The Institutional Management of Soldiers with Shell Shock in Ireland, 1916–19', 15. The largest military hospital was installed at Dublin Castle. Its facilities, including a transformed gilded ballroom, helped to treat over 6,000 servicemen before its closure in 1919; Sylvie Kleinman, '"Scenes of gaiety now filled with Beds": Dublin Castle's Viceregal Apartments as a Red Cross Hospital, 1915–1919', *History Ireland*, 24 (2016), 6–7. For more information on the medical infrastructure established in Ireland to treat wounded servicemen during the First World War, see Durnin, *The Irish Medical Profession and the First World War*, 93–136.
2. MacPherson, *Medical Services: General History, Volume 1*, 71.
3. Brendan Kelly, *'He Lost Himself Completely': Shell Shock and Its Treatment at Dublin's Richmond War Hospital, 1916–1919* (Dublin: Liffey Press, 2014), 30.
4. Leese, *Shell-Shock*, 69; Barham, *Forgotten Lunatics of the Great War*, 45.
5. War Office, *History of the War Hospitals in England and Wales*, 68.
6. Ibid., 32.
7. HC Debates, 17 August 1916, vol. 85, cols 2045–62045; Annual Report of the Belfast District Lunatic Asylum, 1917, xvii; D. G. Thomson, 'A descriptive record of the conversion of a county asylum into a war hospital for sick and wounded soldiers in 1915', *Journal of Mental Science*, 62:256 (1916), 112; Barham, *Forgotten Lunatics of the Great War*, 45.

8   Read, *Military Psychiatry in Peace and War*, 41–2; Barham, *Forgotten Lunatics of the Great War*, 45.
9   War Office, *History of the War Hospitals in England and Wales*, 14–6, 36; Thomas Salmon, *The Care and Treatment of Mental Diseases and War Neuroses ('Shell-Shock') in the British Army* (New York: War Work Committee, 1917), 82.
10 Salmon, *The Care and Treatment of Mental Diseases and War Neuroses ('Shell-Shock') in the British Army*, 88; War Office, *History of the War Hospitals in England and Wales*, 57.
11 Salmon, *The Care and Treatment of Mental Diseases and War Neuroses ('Shell-Shock') in the British Army*, 85.
12 The uniform was made so that one size fitted all servicemen. Thus, it was not uncommon for the uniform to fit some men so poorly that they made their own alterations to the trouser legs and sleeves. Officers were not issued with the uniform and were permitted to wear personal clothing or silk pajamas with a distinctive white armband emblazoned with a red King's Crown. These stock uniforms also helped to facilitate good hygiene within military hospitals and aided administration as they were accompanied by four individually coloured armlets depending on the health of the patient. In addition, as clear identification that the wearer was a military serviceman, the outfits were believed to maintain discipline both within the hospital and when outside the facilities as well as separating patients from hospital staff and visitors; Jeffrey S. Reznick, 'The Convalescent Blues' in Frederick Cayley Robinson's 'Acts of Mercy.' [Online] Available at: http://blog.wellcomelibrary.org/2010/06/the-convalescent-blues-in-frederick-cayley-robinsons-acts-of-mercy/ [accessed 23 June 2014]; Reznick, *Healing the Nation*, 99–115.
13 The War Office were pleased with Dawson's taking up of this role writing after the war: 'In the appointment of Dr W. R. Dawson as Consultant in Mental Diseases, we were especially fortunate; this gentleman is an Inspector of lunatics under the Local Government Board, and in addition to his professional knowledge was an expert in the law resulting to Lunacy in Ireland'; NA, WO 35/179, General Headquarters Reply, Ireland, 26 January 1920.
14 Joseph Reynolds, *Grangegorman: Psychiatric Care in Dublin since 1815* (Dublin: Institute of Public Administration, 1992), 217.
15 Charles Read noted that the Richmond War Hospital provided 300 beds, a figure which was later repeated by Peter Barham; this figure is incorrect; Read, *Military Psychiatry in Peace and War*, 42; Barham, *Forgotten Lunatics of the Great War*, 45. Whilst the Crowthorne War Hospital in Berkshire was the next smallest providing forty-eight beds, the average allocation amongst converted asylums amounted to 1,193 beds; MacPherson, *Medical Services: General History, Volume 1*, 80–2.
16 Reid, 'The Institutional Management of Soldiers with Shell Shock in Ireland, 1916–19', 10.
17 Annual Report of the Inspectors of Lunatics, Ireland, 1916, xxi–xxii; Reynolds, *Grangegorman*, 217.
18 The Richmond War Hospital was also provided with a new admission and discharge register and casebooks for staff to record their clinical records. Members of the British Expeditionary Force do not appear in the Richmond Asylum's records;

Anon, 'Irish Division', *Journal of Mental Science*, 63 (1917), 299; Annual Report of the Richmond District Lunatic Asylum, 1916, 16.
19 Annual Report of the Inspectors of Lunatics, Ireland, 1919, 17.
20 Reynolds, *Grangegorman*, 217; W. R. Dawson, 'The work of the Belfast War Hospital (1917–1919)', *Journal of Mental Science*, 71:293 (1925), 219.
21 See Brian O'Shea and Jane Falvey, 'A history of the Richmond Asylum, Dublin', in German Berrios and Hugh Freeman (eds), *150 Years of British Psychiatry: Volume Two* (London: Athlone Press, 1996), 218; Reid, 'The Institutional Management of Soldiers with Shell-Shock in Ireland, 1916–19', 15.
22 Reynolds, *Grangegorman*, 217–18.
23 NAI, BR/PRIV 1223, Letter from Lieutenant Colonel Hearn, Officer in Charge, King George V Hospital, to Resident Medical Superintendent, Richmond Lunatic Asylum, 1 August 1919; RWH Admission and Discharge Register; Officer in Charge, King George V Hospital, to Resident Medical Superintendent, Richmond Lunatic Asylum, 4 August 1919.
24 Ibid., RWH, Admission Forms; RWH Admission and Discharge Register, no. 57.
25 Reid, 'The Institutional Management of Soldiers with Shell-Shock in Ireland, 1916–19', 14.
26 Malcolm, 'Ireland's crowded madhouses', 319; Annual Report of the Belfast District Lunatic Asylum, 1917, xvii.
27 PRONI, T3580/1, Printed memoir of Mr Frederick McGinley, 1900–1914.
28 As was the case with the RWH, the BWH appears to have kept its own clinical records for the facility as servicemen admitted into the BWH do not appear in Belfast District Lunatic Asylum's Admission and Discharge register; PRONI, HOS/28/1/3/1/7, Belfast Asylum, Register of Admissions, 1908–1919.
29 In a further differentiation from the RWH, the BWH also accommodated non-British Expeditionary Forces, although this equated to just over 10 percent (132 servicemen) of the overall patient profile; Dawson, 'The work of the Belfast War Hospital', 221–3; Rosaline Delargy, 'The History of the Belfast District Lunatic Asylum, 1829–1921' (PhD Thesis, University of Ulster, 2002), 229–30.
30 Annual Report of the Belfast District Lunatic Asylum, 1917, ix.
31 NAI, BR/PRIV 1223, Richmond War Hospital Admission Forms.
32 Ibid.; F. C. Purser, 'Shellshock', *Dublin Journal of Medical Science*, 144 (1917), 210.
33 Five men came from barracks, and four came from other destinations such as convalescent homes and asylums; Reid, 'The Institutional Management of Soldiers with Shell Shock in Ireland, 1916–19', 17.
34 NAI, BR/PRIV 1223, RWH, Admission Forms; RWH Admission and Discharge Register, no. 108.
35 Ibid., RWH Admission and Discharge Register, no. 144.
36 Linden and Jones, '"Shell shock" revisited', 541.
37 NAI, BR/PRIV 1223, RWH, Admission Forms; RWH, Admission and Discharge Register, no. 186.
38 Ibid., RWH, Admission and Discharge Register; Reid, 'The Institutional Management of Soldiers with Shell Shock in Ireland, 1916–19', 22; Leese, *Shell-Shock*, 85–120.

39 Leese, *Shell-Shock*, 86.
40 NAI, BR/PRIV 1223, RWH, Admission Forms; RWH, Admission and Discharge Register, no. 157.
41 Oonagh Walsh, 'The designs of providence: race, religion and Irish insanity', in Joseph Melling and Bill Forsythe (eds), *Insanity, Institutions and Society, 1800–1914* (London: Routledge, 1999), 233; NAI, BR/PRIV 1223, RWH Admission and Discharge Register.
42 Reid, 'The Institutional Management of Soldiers with Shell Shock in Ireland, 1916–19', 23–9.
43 Indeed, fifty-four patients (15 percent) were admitted without an accompanying diagnosis; NAI, BR/PRIV 1223, 'RWH Admission and Discharge Register'; W. D. Chambers, 'Mental wards with the British Expeditionary Force: a review of ten months' experience', *British Journal of Psychiatry*, 65:270 (1919), 160; Leese, *Shell-Shock*, 54; Read, *Military Psychiatry in Peace and War*, 155; E. Barton White, 'Abstract of a report on the mental division of the Welsh Metropolitan War Hospital, Whitchurch, Cardiff, September, 1917–September, 1919', *The British Journal of Psychiatry*, 66 (1920), 441; R. Eager, 'The record of admissions to the mental section of the Lord Derby War Hospital, Warrington, from June 17th to June 16th, 1917', *The British Journal of Psychiatry*, 64:266 (1918), 274; Dawson, 'The work of the Belfast War Hospital', 222.
44 Hide, *Gender and Class in English Asylums: 1890–1914*, 3, 13; Akihito Suzuki, 'Framing psychiatric subjectivity: doctor, patient and record-keeping at Bethlem in the nineteenth century', in Joseph Melling and Bill Forsythe (eds), *Insanity, Institutions and Society, 1800–1914* (London: Routledge, 1999), 116.
45 Eric Dean, *Shook Over Hell: Post-traumatic Stress, Vietnam, and the Civil War* (London: Harvard University Press, 1997), 111.
46 Caution should be applied with such information as it was volunteered by men seemingly in the midst of a psychiatric episode, and there are no guarantees that enquiries into a patient's previous mental health were made by the staff of the RWH. This caution was also noted by Dawson in his reflection upon the BWH; Dawson, 'The work of the Belfast War Hospital', 223; NAI, BR/PRIV 1223, RWH Casebook nos 74, 17, 49, 74 and 86.
47 White, 'Abstract of a report on the mental division of the Welsh Metropolitan War Hospital', 440; Eager, 'Admissions to the mental section of Lord Derby War Hospital', 281–2; Mott, *War Neuroses and Shell-Shock*, 108; William Robinson, 'The future of service patients in mental hospitals', *Journal of Mental Science*, 67:276 (1921), 43; Richmond War Hospital Casebook, 11 October 1918–11 November 1919'; Annual Report of the Inspectors of Lunatics, Ireland, 1916, x; Annual Report of the Inspectors of Lunatics, Ireland, 1917, xi; Annual Report of the Inspectors of Lunatics, Ireland, 1918, ix.
48 Anon, 'Shell-Shock', 299.
49 Purser, 'Shellshock', 202; Kelly, *'He Lost Himself Completely'*, 54.
50 Humphries and Kurchinski, 'Rest, relax and get well', 92.
51 NAI, BR/PRIV 1223, RWH Casebook, no. 1.

52 NA, PIN 26/22253, Lieutenant Harold Tronson, Royal Irish Fusiliers, Pension File.
53 Linden and Jones, '"Shell shock" revisited', 533–4.
54 Leese, *Shell-Shock*, 95, 112; Kelly, 'He Lost Himself Completely', 46.
55 NAI, BR/PRIV 1223, RWH Admission and Discharge Register.
56 Ibid., RWH Casebook, no. 43.
57 The Lord Derby and Welsh Metropolitan War Hospitals record similar instances of recovery; White, 'Abstract of a report on the mental division of the Welsh Metropolitan War Hospital', 442; Eager, 'A record of admission to the mental section of the Lord Derby War Hospital', 282.
58 Dawson, 'The work of the Belfast War Hospital', 223–4.
59 Goldwin Howland, 'Neuroses of returned soldiers', *American Medical New Series*, 12 (1917), 313–19.
60 NAI, BR/PRIV 1223, RWH Casebook. This definition aligns itself with Arthur Hurst's definition: 'The term "shell-shock" should be reserved for the condition which follows exposure to the forces generated by the explosion of powerful shells in the absence of any visible injury to the head or spine'; Arthur Hurst, *Medical Diseases of the War* (London: Arnold, 1918), 14.
61 Purser, 'Shellshock', 202; Leese, *Shell-Shock*, 109; D. Hotchkis, 'Renfrew District Asylum as a war hospital for mental invalids: some contrasts in administration. With an analysis of cases admitted during the first year', *British Journal of Psychiatry*, 63:261 (1917), 246; Dawson, 'The work of the Belfast War Hospital', 223; Eager, 'A record of admissions to the mental section of the Lord Derby War Hospital', 288.
62 NAI, BR/PRIV 1223, RWH Casebook, no. 2.
63 Ibid., no. 8.
64 Edgar Jones, Nicola Fear and Simon Wessely, 'Shell shock and mild traumatic brain injury: a historical review', *American Journal of Psychiatry*, 164:11 (2007), 1641–5.
65 Reid, 'The Institutional Management of Soldiers with Shell-Shock in Ireland, 1916–19', 27–8.
66 NAI, BR/PRIV 1223, RWH Casebook, no. 21.
67 Ibid., no. 53.
68 Ibid., no. 9.
69 Reid, 'The Institutional Management of Soldiers with Shell-Shock in Ireland, 1916–19', 28.
70 NAI, BR/PRIV 1223, RWH Casebook, no. 47.
71 Ibid., no. 44.
72 Ibid., RWH Admission and Discharge Register, no. 51.
73 The Southborough Report, 144–5.
74 Leese, *Shell-Shock*, 97–8.
75 Fiona Reid, '"His nerves gave way": Shell-shock, history and the memory of the First World War in Britain', *Endeavour*, 38:2 (2014), 53.

76 Reid, *Broken Men*, 75; Eager, 'A record of admissions to the mental section of the Lord Derby War Hospital', 284.
77 This information was only recorded in the casebook records of P. O. whose wife confided to the superintendent that the patient had falsely accused her of contemplating infidelity, which the superintendent associated with his current mental condition. Thus, it is possible that more family visitations occurred but went unrecorded; NAI, BR/PRIV 1223, RWH Casebook, no. 20.
78 The Southborough Report, 192.
79 Leese, *Shell-Shock*, 3; Shephard, *A War of Nerves*, 92; Hurst, *Medical Diseases of the War*, 15.
80 Joanna Bourke, *Fear: A Cultural History* (London: Virago Press, 2005), 125–7; Leese, *Shell-Shock*, 3.
81 Read, *Military Psychiatry in Peace and War*, 28.
82 Purser, 'Shellshock', 229.
83 Shepard, *A War of Nerves*, 64; Myers, *Shell-Shock in France*, 77; The Southborough Report, 192.
84 NAI, BR/PRIV 1223, RWH Admission and Discharge book, no. 270; RWH Casebook, no. 13.
85 Ibid., RWH Admission and Discharge book, no. 271; RWH Casebook, no. 16.
86 Ibid., RWH Casebook, no. 10.
87 Ibid., no. 91.
88 Purser, 'Shellshock', 230.
89 Hurst, *Medical Diseases of the War*, 11; R. T. Williamson, 'Treatment of neurasthenia and psychasthenia following shell-shock', *British Medical Journal*, 2:2970 (1917), 713–15.
90 Barham, *Forgotten Lunatics of the Great War*, 35–6.
91 Anon., 'Irish Division', 298.
92 NAI, BR/PRIV 1223, RWH Casebook, no. 69.
93 Ibid., no. 88.
94 Leese, *Shell-Shock*, 114.
95 NAI, BR/PRIV 1223, RWH Casebook, no. 4 and no. 33.
96 Ibid., no. 13.
97 Ibid., no. 31.
98 Suzanne Poirier, 'The Weir Mitchell rest cure: doctor and patients', *Women's Studies*, 10:1 (1983), 15–40.
99 Reid, *Broken Men*, 154; Leese, *Shell-Shock*, 62; Shephard, *A War of Nerves*, 74.
100 NAI, BR/PRIV 1223, RWH Casebook, no. 63.
101 Humphries and Kurchinski, 'Rest, relax and get well', 99.
102 Leese, *Shell-Shock*, 79; Shephard, *A War of Nerves*, 76; Reid, *Broken Men*, 38–9.
103 NAI, BR/PRIV 1223, RWH Casebook, no. 63.
104 Webb, 'Dottyville', 344; Barham, *Forgotten Lunatics of the Great War*, 86; Hotchkis, 'Renfrew District Asylum as a War Hospital for mental invalids', 238; White, 'Report on the mental division of the Welsh Metropolitan War Hospital', 445–6;

Shephard, *A War of Nerves*, 81; Leese, *Shell-Shock*, 132; NAI, BR/PRIV 1223, RWH Casebook, nos 22, 33, 45 and 59.
105 Eager, 'A record of admissions to the mental section of the Lord Derby War Hospital', 272; Webb, 'Dottyville', 343–4.
106 Catherine Cox, *Negotiating Insanity in the Southeast of Ireland, 1820–1900* (Manchester: Manchester University, 2012), 208.
107 Reynolds, *Grangegorman*, 38; Annual Report of the Richmond District Lunatic Asylum, 1914, 21; Annual Report of the Richmond District Lunatic Asylum, 1915, 13; Annual Report of the Richmond District Lunatic Asylum, 1918–1919, 46.
108 Shephard, *A War of Nerves*, 81, 85; Leese, *Shell-Shock*, 106; RWH Casebook, nos 19, 21, 33 and 39; Williamson, 'Treatment of neurasthenia', 713–15; War Office, *History of the War Hospitals in England and Wales*, 38.
109 Annual Report of the Richmond District Lunatic Asylum, 1916, 16; Reynolds, *Grangegorman*, 217–18.
110 Eager, 'A record of admissions to the mental section of the Lord Derby War Hospital', 294; Read, *Military Psychiatry in Peace and War*, 43.
111 NAI, BR/PRIV 1223, Calculated from the RWH Casebook.
112 Ibid., RWH Casebook, nos 9, 30 and 43.
113 Ibid., no. 7.
114 Patients under treatment in the Lord Derby War Hospital were noted as enjoying pass and parole, with Eager writing: 'This privilege was much appreciated, and very rarely abused'; Eager, 'A record of admissions to the mental section of the Lord Derby War Hospital', 294.
115 NAI, BR/PRIV 1223, RWH Casebook, no. 13 and no. 43.
116 The same liberty was denied to female patients; Richmond District Lunatic Asylum, 1911, 19; Richmond District Lunatic Asylum, 1914, 21; Richmond District Lunatic Asylum, 1915, 19; Richmond District Lunatic Asylum, Annual Report, 1918–1919, 46.
117 NAI, BR/PRIV 1223, RWH Casebook, no. 25.
118 Parole was similarly used as a disciplinary measure in German medical facilities; Reznick, *Healing the Nation*, 103; Stefanie Linden and Edgar Jones, 'German battle casualties: the treatment of functional somatic disorders during World War I', *Journal of the History of Medicine and Allied Sciences*, 68:4 (2013), 639.
119 NAI, BR/PRIV 1223, RWH Casebook, nos 10, 21, 23, 36, 37, 77 and 78.
120 Ibid., no. 21.
121 Ibid., RWH Admission and Discharge Register, no. 117.
122 Ibid., RWH Casebook, nos 23, 35, 44, 82 and 99.
123 Reid, *Broken Men*, 113; Barham, *Forgotten Lunatics of the Great War*, 202.
124 NAI, BR/PRIV 1223, RWH Casebook, no. 74.
125 NA, PIN 15/897, Medical Service Branch Note, 21 September 1918; WO 35/179, Appendix B – The Belfast War Hospital; Report on King George V Hospital.
126 NAI, BR/PRIV 1223, RWH Casebook, no. 25.
127 Ibid., no. 79.

128 Purser, 'Shellshock', 232.
129 Ibid., 230.
130 NAI, BR/PRIV 1223, RWH Admission and Discharge Register.
131 Ibid., RWH Casebook, no. 29; RWH Admission and Discharge Register, no. 286.
132 Ibid., RWH Casebook, no. 31.
133 Ibid., RWH Admission and Discharge Register.
134 Purser, 'Shellshock', 230.
135 RWH, Admission and Discharge Register; Brendan Kelly, 'The Aftermath, Ireland's Experience of the First World War.' [Online] Available at: www.rte.ie/radio1/the-history-show/programmes/2014/0831/638320-the-history-show-sunday-31-august-2014/ [accessed 14 April 2015].
136 Dawson, 'The work of the Belfast War Hospital', 219–21.
137 Hotchkis, 'Renfrew District Asylum as a War Hospital for mental invalids', 249.
138 NAI, BR/PRIV 1223, RWH Casebook, nos 3, 7, 14, 16, 17, 18, 40, 46, 52, 53 and 65.
139 Ibid., nos 11, 37 and 45.
140 Dawson, 'The work of the Belfast War Hospital', 221.
141 Hotchkis, 'Renfrew District Asylum as a war hospital for mental invalids', 249; White; 'Welsh Metropolitan War Hospital', 449; Eager, 'Lord Derby War Hospital', 281.
142 Reid, 'The Institutional Management of Soldiers with Shell Shock in Ireland, 1916–19', 33–40.
143 Reid, Broken Men, 24; Long, Destigmatising Mental Illness?, 4.
144 Alice Brumby, 'From "Pauper Lunatics" to "Rate-Aided Patients": Removing the Stigma of Mental Health Care, 1888–1938' (PhD Thesis, University of Huddersfield, 2015), 11.
145 Ibid., 115.
146 War Office, History of the War Hospitals in England and Wales, 60.
147 Barham, Forgotten Lunatics of the Great War, 145.
148 J. L. Crammer, 'Extraordinary deaths of asylum inpatients during the 1914–1918 war', Medical History, 36:4 (1992), 430–41.
149 Brumby, 'From "Pauper Lunatics" to "Rate-Aided Patients"', 226–83.
150 Barham, Forgotten Lunatics of the Great War, 145.
151 Portrane Asylum fell slightly below this national average at 34.5 percent; Annual Report of the Inspectors of Lunatics, Ireland, 1919, 5, 10; Dawson, 'The work of the Belfast War Hospital', 221.
152 Annual Report of the Inspectors of Lunatics, Ireland, 1919, 10.
153 Read, Military Psychiatry in Peace and War, 155.
154 Myers, Shell-Shock in France, 62.
155 G. A. Doody, A. Beveridge and E. C. Johnstone, 'Poor and mad: a study of patients admitted to the Fife and Kinross District Asylum between 1874 and 1899', Psychological Medicine, 26:5 (1996), 892.
156 RWH Admission and Discharge Book.
157 The Southborough Report, 146–7.

158 Read also surmised that some servicemen were admitted to a war hospital for psychiatric treatment by Medical Officers to prevent military punishment for unsuitable conduct. Similar instances were also cited by Barham's research into the Napsbury War Hospital; Read, *Military Psychiatry in Peace and War*, 13, 155; Barham, *Forgotten Lunatics of the Great War*, 58–9.
159 Annual Report of the Inspectors of Lunatics, Ireland, 1919, vi.
160 Brumby, 'From "Pauper Lunatics" to "Rate-Aided Patients"', 9.
161 Salmon, *The Care and Treatment of Mental Diseases and War Neuroses ('Shell-Shock') in the British Army*, 86–8.
162 Crammer, 'Extraordinary deaths of asylum inpatients during the 1914–1918 war', 440; Brumby, 'From "Pauper Lunatics" to "Rate-Aided Patients"', 112.
163 Delargy, 'The History of the Belfast District Lunatic Asylum, 1829–1921', 236; Annual Report of the Inspectors of Lunatics, Ireland, 1915, xxvi.
164 Annual Report of the Inspectors of Lunatics, Ireland, 1916, xvii; Annual Report of Inspectors of Lunatics, Ireland, 1917, ix.
165 Crammer, 'Extraordinary deaths of asylum inpatients during the 1914–1918 war', 436.
166 The replacement of butter with margarine caused great resentment with staff signing a statement that declared that they would refuse to consume the foodstuff; Belfast District Lunatic Asylum Annual Report, 1915, 18; Report of Inspectors of Lunatics, Ireland, 1915, 635; Hanora Henry, *Our Lady's Hospital, Cork: History of the Mental Hospital in Cork Spanning 200 Years* (Cork: Cork University Press, 1989), 277–8.
167 Ida Milne, *Stacking the Coffins: Influenza, War and Revolution in Ireland, 1918–1919* (Manchester: Manchester University Press, 2018), 144; Moriarty, 'Work, warfare and wages', 76; Ian Miller, *Reforming Food in Post-Famine Ireland* (Manchester: Manchester University Press, 2014), 173–97; Delargy, 'The History of the Belfast District Lunatic Asylum, 1829–1921', 228.
168 Reynolds, *Grangegorman*, 222.
169 The Cork Asylum committee were warned in May 1917 by their coal supplier that due to the 'Submarine Menace' it would be advisable to store extra provisions of coal. No such provision was undertaken; Henry, *Our Lady's Hospital*, 278; Cork Archives, Cork District Lunatic Asylum, OLH/1/5, Minutes of Proceedings of the Committee of Management, 15 May 1917.
170 Annual Report of Richmond District Lunatic Asylum, Dublin, 1917, 11–12; Annual Report of Richmond District Lunatic Asylum, Dublin, 1918–1919, 13; Henry, *Our Lady's Hospital*, 279.
171 Annual Report of the Richmond District Lunatic Asylum, 1917, 12.
172 Annual Report of Inspectors of Lunatics, Ireland, 1915, xx–xxi.
173 Annual Report of the Richmond District Lunatic Asylum, 1917, 279; the lack of finance available was repeated by the Irish Lunacy Inspectorate. See, for example, Annual Report of Inspectors of Lunatics, Ireland, 1917, 322; Annual Report of Inspectors of Lunatics, Ireland, 1919, 183.
174 Annual Report of the Inspectors of Lunatics, Ireland, 1917, xviii–xxii.

175 Annual Report of the Inspectors of Lunatics, Ireland, 1918, xviii. It is interesting to note that the inspectorate's descriptions of the condition of asylums were much more detailed in 1919 than had been offered during the war years. The more in-depth analysis provides an interesting indication that the cessation of the conflict provided an opportune moment to address the many infrastructural issues in numerous Irish asylums; Annual Report of Inspectors of Lunatics, Ireland, 1919, xix–xxiii.
176 Annual Report of Belfast District Lunatic Asylum, 1911, xi.
177 Annual Report of Belfast District Lunatic Asylum, 1912, xvii.
178 Annual Report of Belfast District Lunatic Asylum, 1913, xviii.
179 NA, WO 35/179, Medical History of the War, Appendix B – The Belfast War Hospital.
180 Annual Report of Belfast District Lunatic Asylum, 1917, xvii.
181 Annual Report of the Inspectors of Lunatics, Ireland, 1917, vi; Annual Report of the Inspectors of Lunatics, Ireland, 1919, 10.
182 Milne, *Stacking the Coffins*, 4, 148
183 Liverpool Record Office, M 614/RAI 4, Report of the Medical Superintendent, Lancaster Asylum, 24.
184 Brumby, 'From "Pauper Lunatics" to "Rate-Aided Patients"', 116–18; Liverpool Record Office, M 614/RAI 4, Report of the Medical Superintendent, Lancaster Asylum, 24.
185 War Office, *History of the War Hospitals in England and Wales*, 39.
186 Barbara Douglas, 'In the Shadow of the Asylum: Narratives of change and Stagnation, 1890–1930' (PhD Thesis, University of Exeter, 2008), 79–80.
187 Crammer, 'Extraordinary deaths of asylum inpatients during the 1914–1918 war', 440–1; Annual Report of Inspectors of Lunatics, Ireland, 1914, xxii; Annual Report of Inspectors of Lunatics, Ireland, 1915, 569; Annual Report of Inspectors of Lunatics, Ireland, 1916, 7, 9; Annual Report of Belfast District Lunatic Asylum, 1916, viii; Annual Report of Inspectors of Lunatics, Ireland, 1918, xiv.
188 Annual Report of Belfast District Lunatic Asylum, 1916, viii.
189 Douglas, 'In the Shadow of the Asylum', 225–6.
190 Salmon, *The Care and Treatment of Mental Diseases and War Neuroses ('Shell-Shock') in the British Army*, 91.
191 Crammer, 'Extraordinary deaths of asylum inpatients during the 1914–1918 war', 440.
192 Anon., 'Irish Division', 299.
193 Dawson, 'The Work of the Belfast War Hospital', 219.
194 'Richmond Asylum Committee', *Irish Times*, 20 February 1920, 7.
195 NA, WO 35/179, General Headquarters Reply, Ireland, 26 January 1920.
196 Annual Report of Belfast District Lunatic Asylum, 1919, vii.
197 Annual Report of the Inspectors of Lunatics, Ireland, 1919, ix.
198 Dawson, 'The Work of the Belfast War Hospital', 224.
199 Read, *Military Psychiatry in Peace and War*, 42; Salmon, *The Care and Treatment of Mental Diseases and War Neuroses ('Shell-Shock') in the British Army*, 90.

200 War Office, *History of the War Hospitals in England and Wales*, 1.
201 Dawson, 'The work of the Belfast War Hospital', 221.
202 Barham, *Forgotten Lunatics of the Great War*, 170.
203 Dawson, 'The work of the Belfast War Hospital', 91; RWH, Admission and Discharge Register.
204 NAI, PRIV1223/3/56, Richmond District Asylum, General Register of Admissions, 31 May 1918–25 April 1922.
205 Annual Report of the Belfast District Lunatic Asylum, 1919, vii.
206 Annual Report of the Belfast District Lunatic Asylum, 1918, vii; Annual Report of the Belfast District Lunatic Asylum, 1919, vii.
207 Kelly, 'He Lost Himself Completely', 118.
208 War Office, *History of the War Hospitals in England and Wales*, 32.
209 Smith and Pear, *Shell-Shock and its Lessons*, 25.
210 Reynolds, *Grangegorman*, 218.
211 Salmon, *The Care and Treatment of Mental Diseases and War Neuroses ('Shell-Shock') in the British Army*, 85.
212 The First World War did not solely induce these reforms as the Report of the Commission on the Relief of the Sick and Destitute Poor (1927) also strongly advocated for them; Kelly, 'He Lost Himself Completely', 119
213 Ibid., xvii.
214 Hopkins, 'Problems, Politics and Personalities', 332.

5

THE SERVICE PATIENT SCHEME IN IRELAND

A cemetery of hopeless cases?

In addition to the transferrals from RWH, Service Patients were admitted to the Richmond District Asylum from the BWH on its closure. There was a spike of 606 admissions into the Richmond Asylum between November 1918 and December 1919, which the Irish Lunacy Inspectorate recognised: 'It must be borne in mind that the closing of the Belfast War Hospital, which took place within the period under review, led to the reception of a considerable number of discharged soldiers belonging to the counties served by the asylum.'[1] The BWH's closure ensured the transferral of a further twenty-nine Service Patients to the Cork District Lunatic Asylum.[2] Of such transferrals, Dawson assessed: 'For the most part their prospects of recovery were not bright.'[3] The Ministry of Pensions echoed this assumption, regarding the asylum as a 'cemetery of hopeless cases.'[4] A closer analysis of the Service Patient scheme in the Irish asylum system helps to both verify and challenge these claims.

Patient casebook records provide an insight into the chronicity of Service Patients. M. D., transferred to the Richmond Asylum from the RWH, had received treatment in several war hospitals since December 1917. Diagnosed as a case of 'Chronic Mania', his admission records state: 'He is dull depressed sullen and morose and suffers from hallucinations of hearing. And consequent delusions of persecution. Voices say he will be brought to his depot and shot. He tells me he heard voices before going in the army. Was addicted to drink. Admits attempted suicide.' The patient remained at Richmond for over two decades with two separate updates in 1938 recording: 'Quiet depressed in appearance. Not inclined to give any information about himself except that he went stupid in France ... a dull weak-minded old man who is a good worker in the dining hall.' He died on 7 September 1941.[5] P. C. was diagnosed with 'Dementia' having also undergone treatment in several war hospitals from March 1916. His admission notes record: 'He is dull apathetic very careless and untidy in his appearance. Memory gone. He is very rambling and incoherent in his conversation. He is very violent and dangerous at times.' His final medical notes, written six months before his death in January 1929, highlight the negligible change in his condition and conduct.[6]

Long-term residencies of former soldier-patients were not exclusive to the Richmond Asylum. One driver for the Royal Field Artillery was transferred to Cork Asylum from the BWH. His patient records again underscore the acute and deteriorating nature of his mental condition:

> 20 October 1919: He is rambling and incoherent in conversation, is impulsive and makes violent homicidal attacks without warning. Delusions. Says he is eighty-seven years old.
>
> 28 October 1919: Thinks this is the year 1897.
>
> 6 May 1922: Has a tendency to make impulsive attacks on other patients ... transferred owing to his frequency to assault others, sometimes he has broken glass.
>
> 26 May 1933: Greets me with a military salute. Becomes incoherent and talks of artillery.
>
> 20 January 1935: Becoming more demented. Frequently visited but does not appear interested in his friends or himself.
>
> 19 April 1958: Demented insane laughter. Quite childish.
>
> 7 April 1961 (last entry): Subject to mental changes. Hallucinations.[7]

The discharge of a civilian patient usually occurred within two years. If held for longer than five years, however, there was a strong chance of a patient remaining under care until they died.[8] This trend was evident within the Service Patient community in the two largest institutions in the Irish Free State. Out of the seventy-two Service Patients admitted to Cork or Richmond asylum from the RWH and BWH, there were only fifteen discharges. Fourteen transferrals occurred five years after admission with the majority occurring within twelve months of entry.[9]

Discharges amongst Service Patients did occur. In the six months between September 1923 and October 1924, there were thirty-six releases in Northern Ireland and the Irish Free State.[10] By February 1922, a third of Service Patients admitted to English and Welsh asylums were also discharged, confirming that it is short-sighted to conclude the Service Patient scheme uniformly ensured a 'one-way ticket' into the asylum.[11] W. O., for example, was transferred from the RWH to the Richmond Asylum with a diagnosis of 'Confusional Insanity.' His casebook records note: 'He is very confused rambling and incoherent. He passes from one subject to another. He has vague persecutory delusions. He is very restless and untidy and is in general careless in his personal habits. Rambles much about his service as a soldier.' Such behaviour seemingly applied to the broader ex-service population; the medical superintendent wrote three years after his admittance that 'he is the typical English Tommy.' While his medical condition may have been representative of the broader ex-service asylum population, his asylum career was largely atypical. His casebook entry one year later noted: 'Quiet and well conducted. He is a little weak-minded but quite rational in conversation and expresses no delusions. He is anxious to be discharged.' He was discharged as 'recovered' ten days later. Lance Corporal T., admitted to the Cork Asylum from the BWH on 19 October 1919, was described on admission as 'childish and silly in talk and can give no sensible account of himself.' Nevertheless, his case notes for February 1920 record: 'His physical health is much better ... Much improved mentally.' He was subsequently discharged on 19 February 1920.[12]

A Service Patient's discharge was not always the consequence of a recovery. Lance-Corporal F. entered Cork Asylum with his admission notes on transfer from the BWH recording: 'Patient is very untidy. Stands muttering to himself and is frequently noisy at night.' By 1934, he was 'thin and pale ... he has no idea why he came here. His answer to most questions is "I don't know". His actions suggest auditory hallucinations ... fingers in ears and mutters to himself.' Despite his condition, he was discharged on a thirty-day trial to his brother in August who requested permission to become his carer. F.'s casebook file includes the report of a Ministry of Pensions medical staff officer who examined his subsequent living conditions:

> 14 September 1935: Visited above named today. He was sitting up fully dressed, clean, well shaven, and he has good clothes and a good bed. He is being cared for by his brother and takes him into the country for walks. Well-nourished [but] defective teeth, weakness of grip both hands, walks with a bent and shuffling gait. Very slight tremors.
>
> Mental Condition: Dull and apathetic. Rubbing hands during conversation and muttering occasionally with head turned sideways apparently listening to imaginary voices. Talks to himself. Expression vacant.
>
> Memory: Bad, poorly orientated. Is quiet, clean in habits and apparently harmless, can dress himself.

Despite the unfavourable mental condition of F., the Ministry official recommended his discharge after a decade and a half of institutionalisation to the care of his brother:

> Under the circumstances I consider he is being fairly well cared for at present. Being well nourished, clean, harmless and fair accommodation, his brother appears to be respectable and clean and he is a married man with a family. It is not considered that further institutional treatment is necessary at present.[13]

The discharge of a mentally unwell ex-serviceman was not only evidenced in the Service Patient scheme but facilitated by it. The Ministry devolved all initial authority to asylum staff who, in turn, followed pre-established lunacy procedure permitting the discharge of a patient if a friend or family member was willing to undertake responsibility for them.[14] As in the example of Lance-Corporal F., discharged ex-servicemen were not simply discarded on their families. Ex-military personnel and their families were reviewed by Ministry staff to ensure the new arrangement was manageable and suitable. This example also serves to underline the basic supervisory nature of asylum care. With Cork Asylum offering little in the form of actual medical treatment and potential recovery, domestic care was deemed suitable.

Admissions from civil society

Discharged Great War veterans admitted from civil society would join Service Patients from war hospitals.[15] There was almost a 40 percent increase in Service Patient numbers in England and Wales between early 1920 and October 1921.[16] Between 31 May 1918 and 25 April 1922, 113 Service Patients were admitted from civil society into the Richmond District Lunatic Asylum; 63 men remained in the asylum for the rest of their lives with 53 subsequently discharged. Releases occurred within five years of admission with the exception of three patients.[17] There is a clear variance between the two patient biographies that constituted the Service Patient population; those admitted from civil society were more likely to be discharged than those transferred from war hospitals. The comparative diagnostic categories of Melancholia and Dementia between the two patient populations shown in Table 8 is revealing.

The delay of over two years in implementing the Service Patient scheme in Ireland ensured a significant minority of Service Patients accumulated at the RWH and BWH before their eventual transferral into an asylum. This gathering may help to explain why transferrals of soldier-patients like P. C. suffering from 'Dementia', an irreversible genetic deterioration in brain function, were more prevalent in the war hospital transferrals in comparison to those diagnosed

Table 8 Percentage of diagnoses of dementia and melancholia in Service Patient populations.

	Dementia	Melancholia
Service Patients transferred from the RWH	40	40
Service Patients admitted from civil society	11	39

Source: NAI, PRIV1223/3/56, Richmond District Asylum, General Register of Admissions, 31 May 1918–25 April 1922.

with Melancholia, a more transient and situational diagnosis with a comparatively promising prognosis.[18] Dawson also held that many of those discharged from the RWH on its closure were so because of the agreement of the patient's family to assume care.[19] Previous research has attested to the agency of familial networks amongst the broader asylum population throughout the history of institutionalisation in Ireland.[20] With the absence of domestic caregivers apparent from the outset, those transferred from the RWH seemingly had little chance of a family member facilitating their discharge from the asylum.

Admissions from civil society appear more likely to have intrinsic links to family and friends able to facilitate their discharge. A small number of families would even use the asylum as a temporary foster facility for repeated short-term admissions. For example, J. C. was admitted into Richmond Asylum ten times until 1940; two Service Patients experienced six separate entries, and another two undertook five admissions.[21] In addition to using the asylum for respite, discharging a family member could be an act of compassion. J. M. at Londonderry Asylum, had no balance, was bed bound, and required spoon feeding. His death appeared imminent with his condition rapidly advancing. J. M.'s wife relieved him against the advice of the medical superintendent to afford her husband the dignity of dying at home rather than within the asylum.[22] The importance of the family extends beyond admission and discharge. Ministry officials at London headquarters held it was a matter of 'common knowledge' for staff that there was a reluctance amongst relatives to certify a Service Patient in Ireland via the Dangerous Lunacy Act. Many insane veterans were subsequently accommodated in domestic settings.[23] Numerous insane Great War lunatics admitted from civil society were not officially categorised as Service Patients owing to the absence of a family member to pursue an application for this status and pressure the Ministry of Pensions on behalf of their relative.[24] An Irish Service Patient's interaction with inspecting Ministry officials was often the only external contact many veterans had, foregrounding their lack of familial networks.[25]

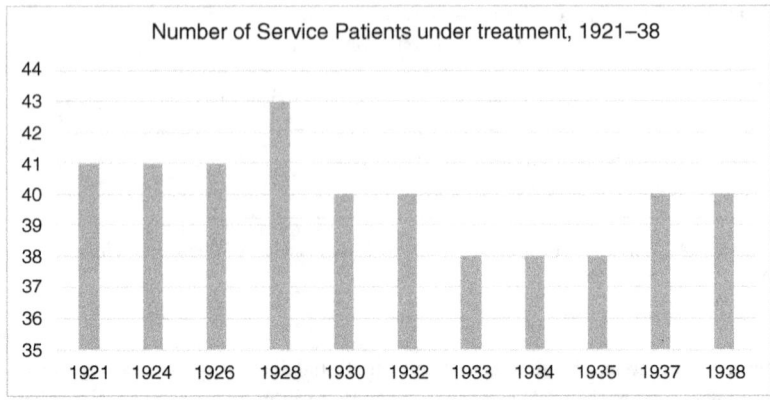

Figure 14 Number of Service Patients under treatment in Purdysburn Villa Colony, 1921–38. Calculated from Purdysburn Villa Colony Annual Reports, 1921–38; PRONI, HOS/28/1/5/9-12.

Across Britain and Ireland in 1923, 8,957 Service Patients were undergoing asylum treatment.[26] Regarding an individual case study, Ministry inspections to the Purdysburn Villa Colony, Belfast, record the relative consistency of patient populations during the inter-war period (Figure 14).

In contrast to the stable patient population numbers, admission and discharge figures fluctuated (Figure 15).

This case study exemplifies how admission and discharge statistics oscillated in tandem. The large number of admissions in 1921 denotes the number of entries and retrospective categorisation of existing asylum patients since the implementation of the Service Patient scheme in August 1919. This anomaly is unsurprising, as are the subsequent thirty discharges occurring between 1921 and 1924. They were part of the initial Service Patient population who, like their civilian counterparts, were better able to be discharged in the short term due to the transitory nature of their diagnosis and/or familial networks. Beyond 1924, however, both entries and discharges were at a premium, and a clear body of chronic and long-term patients began to predominate. By 1930, there were few improvements amongst the Service Patients at Belfast with many diagnosed with perceived chronic conditions like Dementia Praecox and Congenital Mental Deficiency.[27] By 1936, the prolongation of residencies at Omagh Asylum led Dr Forward, the Ministry inspector who reviewed Service Patients throughout Irish and British asylums, to note the recurring faces he had encountered during his previous inspections.[28]

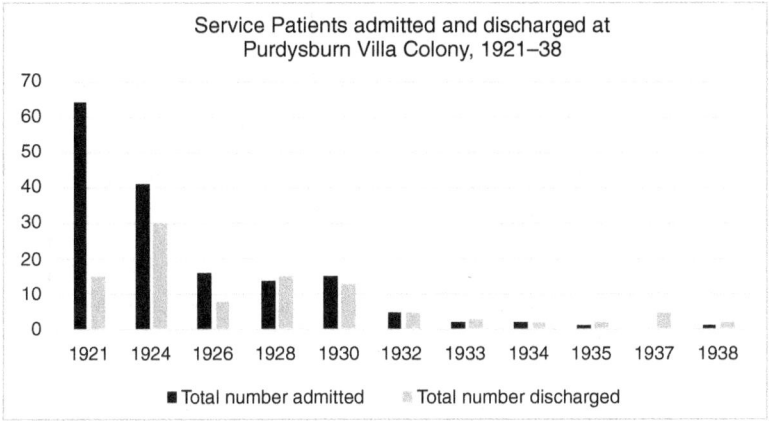

Figure 15 Number of Service Patient admissions and discharges in Purdysburn Villa Colony, 1921–38. Calculated from Purdysburn Villa Colony Annual Reports, 1921–38; PRONI, HOS/28/1/5/9-12.

Due to the aforementioned restrictions in Ministry liability and in-patient facilities, insane Service Patients in the Irish Free State quadrupled any other disabled in-patient community in the Irish Free State in 1930.[29] This phenomenon was not unique to Ireland. Despite constituting just 10 percent of disabled veterans throughout the UK suffering from the more severe war-related disabilities, insane Great War veterans were absorbing a large number of overall pension costs, constituting over 50 percent of cases requiring permanent provision.[30] Despite Major Tyron telling the House of Commons in late 1925 that 'we do not want to give up hope of curing these men', this is largely what happened.[31] C. E. Loseby MP felt that the non-asylum in-patient veteran hospitals offered by the Ministry of Pensions and ESWS were largely successful endeavours with men able to improve their mental conditions while under treatment. By contrast, he denounced the treatment afforded to Service Patients in asylums as prioritising detention before treatment.[32] This trend reflected the larger asylum population where the gathering of the chronic insane became commonplace.[33] Northern Irish mental hospitals in the early 1930s hosted approximately 4,000 patients whose outlook on treatment emphasised containment over cure.[34] Of course, we know far more today on how to treat mental illness than during the inter-war period.[35] Low recovery rates and accumulation of the insane should not be judged by contemporary standards. It is instead more conducive to assess the infrastructure and conditions of asylums shared by ex-service and civilian communities alike to consider whether recognition of war service impacted on the standards of care and lived experiences of institutionalisation.

Service Patients in Northern Ireland

Northern Ireland hosted seven public asylums during the inter-war period.[36] The distribution of Service Patients within these facilities was relatively consistent throughout the inter-war period, averaging 111 patients per year. Service Patients thus constituted less than 3 percent of the average national asylum population.[37] Accommodating over one-third of Northern Ireland's Service Patient population, Purdysburn Villa Colony housed the largest facility cohort of veterans in the country. Its Resident Medical Superintendent favourably described Purdysburn: 'beautifully situated as it is, in a fold of the hills overlooking Belfast, the Purdysburn Estate provides for the mentally ill of our city population ideal conditions for restoration of health.'[38] Forward also wrote positively of the asylum's picturesque surroundings.[39] The institution provided eleven self-contained seventy-bed villas. The villas housed patients according to their mental condition, habit and conduct. While a small number of violent and unruly Service Patients were housed with similarly afflicted civilian patients, Purdysburn House accommodated an unspecified majority of Great War veterans; this facility was the one villa designated for private patients. Reflecting the Lunacy Inspectorate's opinion, Forward commented positively on the conditions:

> The interior of the villa presented an exceptionally clean, tidy and comfortable appearance, the living rooms and dormitories being spacious bright and heated … Comfortable wicker chairs are plentifully supplied for the use of the men, and the living room presented more the appearance of a hotel lounge than the ward of an asylum.[40]

Figures 16 and 17 provide some indication of the comfortable accommodation on offer. Each self-contained villa was a separate residential home with an exclusive bathroom and kitchen where food was prepared and served.[41] The Service Patients' accommodation at Purdysburn House thus ensured segregation from pauper lunatics. The facility was also situated furthest away from the main villa colonies housing pauper lunatics. If the purpose of the Service Patient scheme was to treat insane ex-serviceman akin to private patients, then the facility largely achieved this purpose. Forward even went so far as to conclude that the accommodation was far superior to any facility he had seen in England.[42]

Segregation was not, however, absolute. Service Patients worked alongside pauper lunatics in various workshops, undertaking laundry work and assisting on the farm.[43] Medical staff stressed the importance of such activities which

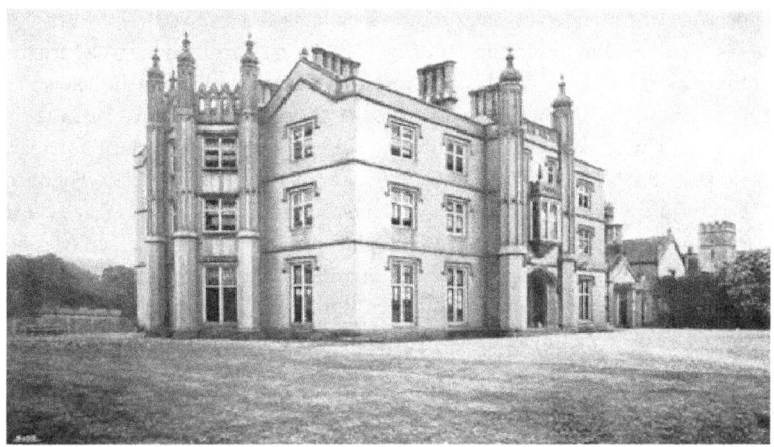

Figure 16 Purdysburn House.

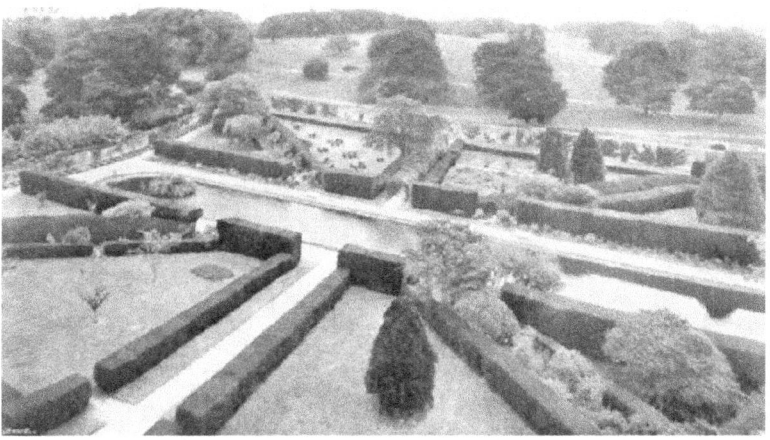

Figure 17 Pleasure grounds at Purdysburn House.

promoted self-control, discipline and productive distraction.[44] Except for patients under special observation, Service Patients enjoyed a great amount of liberty with doors and windows left unlocked. Private and non-private patients shared the Recreation Hall, which showed regular movies and provided dance recitals and concerts. The year 1922 witnessed forty-nine events in the form of dances and cinema shows with an average of 530 patients attending each event. Both communities participated in weekly football matches, and the asylum's annual sports day was attended by seven hundred patients and received a large turn-out of visitors.[45] Pocket money provided by the Ministry profited Service Patients with the extra allocation of tobacco, cigarettes and pastries. Despite the Ministry's scheme requiring the provision of tweed suits, however, ex-servicemen wore the same 'Hospital Blues' distributed to soldier-patients in military hospitals during the First World War. Nevertheless, Service Patients relayed to Forward their pleasure with their surroundings, diet and treatment despite the diet lacking variety, which was a feature in most English asylums. Ex-servicemen were in good bodily health attributed to the care afforded to them. Forward's concluding remarks heaped praise on the modern conditions describing 'the general atmosphere of contentment of the men and their appreciation of their exceptionally favourable surroundings.'[46]

This encouraging setup did not last. By Forward's second inspection in February 1924, Purdysburn House no longer hosted Service Patients. The eleven villas now segregated veterans by their conduct, mental state and requirements regarding medical care and supervision. Villa number six accomodated improving or well-conducted patients, and it housed twenty-seven Service Patients, seven were in villas where only partial supervision was needed, five were in the maximum-security observation villa, with the remaining two ex-servicemen in the adjoining hospital ward for unspecified medical reasons. Echoing the Irish Lunacy Inspectorate, the villas' order, condition, comfort and cleanliness still drew favourable reviews from Forward (Figures 18, 19 and 20).[47]

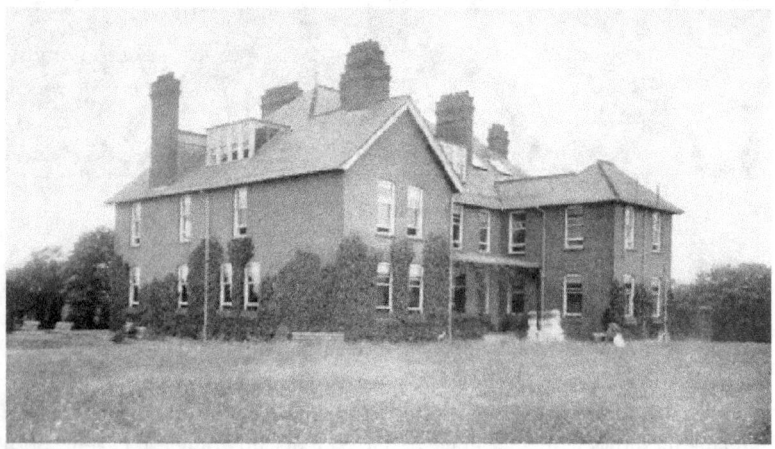

Figure 18 A regular villa.

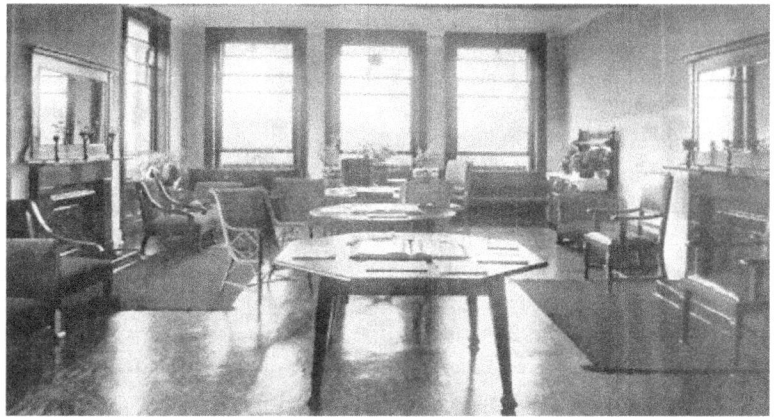

Figure 19 A villa dayroom.

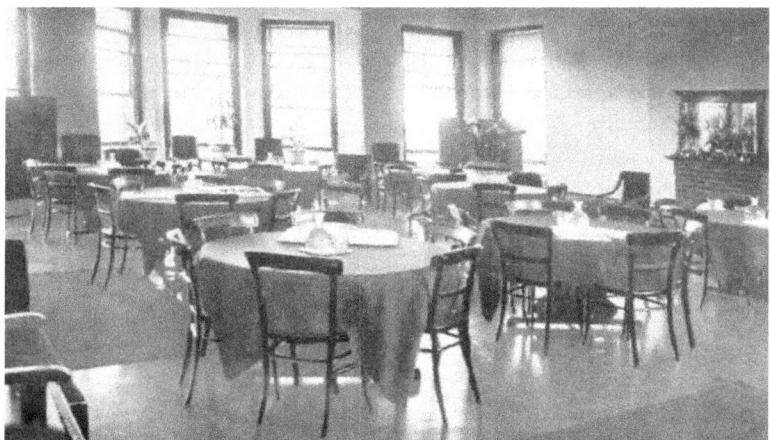

Figure 20 A villa dining hall.

The villas were a downgrade on the luxurious private accommodation afforded at Purdysburn House. Service Patients now socialised, ate, bathed and shared sanitary arrangements with non-private patients. Removed from the well-appointed Purdysburn House, the less spacious accommodation housing veterans impacted upon their daily experience as overcrowding persisted throughout the inter-war period. The overcrowding accelerated to such an extent that some dormitories accommodated patients with mattresses on the floor in 1928.[48] Villa Six was located the furthest away from Purdysburn House, providing a striking metaphor of the insane veteran's separation from private patients between 1921 and 1924. Forward's interviewees presented no complaints, articulating their contentment, comfort and humane treatment despite their downgrade in accommodation.[49]

Neither Forward nor the Lunacy Inspectorate explain the transferral. Purdysburn House continued as an exclusive facility for private patients throughout the inter-war period. Rather than being a realisation that Service Patients required specialised accommodation, their transferral appears linked to the Ministry's post-1921 austerity. The Ministry was consistently active in establishing the most economical arrangement with asylum authorities from the outset of the Service Patient scheme.[50] Not for the first time, the mentally ill Great War veteran's treatment was detrimentally affected by the increasingly austere outlook of the Ministry. The department's rigorous cost-cutting went so far as to restrict the daily lives of a tiny minority of insane Great War veterans under treatment at Purdysburn Villa Colony. Crucially, the change in villas ensured the Service Patient programme in Belfast did not treat insane ex-servicemen akin to private patients. Their segregation again emphasises the literal and metaphorical hardening in the Ministry's treatment of mentally disabled veterans.

There is a remarkable consistency in the Ministry of Pensions' and Lunacy Inspectorate's reports on Purdysburn from 1924 onwards.[51] The accommodation, care and diet drew favourable comments. The latter was held to be more substantial and diverse than what was otherwise on offer at the majority of Irish facilities. The Inspectorate's annual report reflected the narrative of the Ministry.[52] Citing 'the individual attention the patients receive and the stimulation and encouragement given to the men to keep them actively and usefully occupied', Forward wrote in 1930 that the mental condition of chronic patients had been prevented from deteriorating.[53] As was the case with Ministry in-patient facilities and the neurasthenic pensioners, a humane facility with attentive staff could, at the very least, assist in the stabilisation of Service Patient's health even if they were unable to cure it. Providing a good standard of care was prioritised at the facility. Throughout the inter-war period, the inspectorate commented favourably on the number of nurses noted as holding a Certificate of the Royal-Medico Psychological Association. By 1938, the vast majority of Purdysburn staff were fully trained and qualified, with 103 members of staff having qualified for the certificate with a further 43 currently training for it.[54] Experienced Medical Superintendents held that the experience and outlook of institutional staff dictated the atmosphere and daily running of district asylums.[55] As will be demonstrated, such high standards were not uniform across Ireland.

There were notable differences in the reports regarding clothing. The issuance of 'Hospital Blues' persisted with tweed suits only being worn from 1926.[56] Twenty-eight of the forty-three Service Patients in residence wore tweed suits by 1928. Service Patients were only given a suit if they did not exhibit slovenly and neglectful habits nor demonstrate a negligible interest in their presentation.[57] It was only in 1930 that ex-servicemen finally wore quality brown tweed suits at the expense of 'Hospital Blues.' However, when working, of which almost three-quarters of Service Patients did, all asylum patients wore working attire.[58] The differentiation of Service Patients in appearance, a supposed cornerstone of the Ministry's treatment of the insane Great War veteran, would only occur during leisure time and was not widespread until more than a decade after the Armistice.

A comparative, if less detailed, insight into the scheme at Omagh Asylum is possible via reports on the meetings of its asylum committee. An average of six Service Patients were under care at the facility between 1921 and 1936.[59] Forward again commented favourably on the clean and comfortable conditions. Omagh offered adequate heating and entertainment facilities, a diet scale superior to most other Irish asylums, a good relationship between staff and patients with Service Patients being in good bodily condition. Ministry observations repeated the view of the Lunacy Inspectorate. The committee of Omagh Asylum took great satisfaction in Forward's favourable report.[60] As was the case in Belfast, ex-servicemen were not immediately provided with personalised civil society, and they were not uniformly dressed in tweed suits until 1934.[61] An analysis of Belfast and Omagh institutions highlights the operational flaws inherent within in the Service Patient scheme. The asylum dictated an insane ex-serviceman's experience of institutionalisation rather than whether his lunacy was deemed attributable to war service. An analysis of the Free State asylum network reinforces this observation.

The Service Patient in the Irish Free State

The seventeen public mental hospitals in the Irish Free State accommodated 375 Service Patients in 1931 (Table 9). Service Patients constituted just over 2 percent of the overall mental hospital population.[62] Ex-service populations varied on an institutional basis.

As in Britain, Service Patient populations correlated with regional recruitment patterns. Richmond and Cork asylums accommodated just over half of Service

Table 9 The distribution of 375 Service Patients in Irish Free State mental hospitals, 31 December 1931.

Mental hospital	Number of Service Patients
Richmond	132
Cork	68
Ballinasloe	28
Waterford	20
Mullingar	17
Clonmel	15
Carlow	14
Castlebar	10
Portlaoighise	10
Kilkenny	10
Limerick	9
Enniscorthy	9
Letterkenny	8
Killarney	8
Monaghan	6
Sligo	6
Ennis	5

Source: NA, PIN 15/3167, Report on the Treatment of Service Patients in Mental Hospitals in the Irish Free State for the Year 1931.

Patients; these areas also accommodated the two largest ex-service populations. In contrast, in western agricultural regions, smaller asylums such as Carlow, Kilkenny and Portlaoighise experienced a lower proportion of enlistments, returning veterans and a resulting modest intake of Service Patients.[63]

Locality dictated an insane patient's daily life and experience of institutionalisation rather than the perceived origins of their lunacy and their associated status. A case study of the appalling Clonmel Asylum exemplifies this concept. In 1931, the Ministry of Pensions verified Forward's depiction of the 'dilapidated', 'antiquated' and 'unwholesome' conditions on offer at the institution. In addition to overcrowded and inadequate facilities, Forward wrote: 'The fabric of the living and sleeping quarters and the sanitary arrangements were deplorable and their condition unsuitable for patients.' He further deduced the poorly ventilated and depressing facility was not suitable to be used for the care of the mentally ill.[64] Unlike at Purdysburn, where the serene conditions were held to have stabilised and aided the institutionalised veterans' mental wellbeing, the dire conditions at Clonmel exacerbated the fifteen Service Patients' mental health: 'The type of patient at Clonmel was very low and degraded and he thought that this was to some extent attributable to the bad conditions.' Their diet lacked in variety, with few entertainments and newspapers provided for the benefit of patients. In further contrast to the infrastructure available in Purdysburn, there was a criticism of the ratio of attendants to patients for being much too low. Staff were also poorly trained and unable to benefit from training lectures to obtain certificates in mental nursing.[65] The correlation between staff qualifications and the standard of care on offer again points to the importance of the former in dictating asylum conditions during the inter-war period.

Following an inspection in 1928, one member of the committee acknowledged the Ministry's complaint regarding the old workhouse building accommodating Service Patients. Aptly titled as 'the old house', housing around 400 male patients, one committee member accepted 'it was a very depressing place where the Service Patients were accommodated … [it] was like a prison.' Another member of the committee said he had visited the building but would never do so again on account of the fact that he had been ill for days after the visit. The committee attested that those who viewed the place never wanted to see it again and it should close. Members described the facility as a 'death trap', 'a scandal' and 'a disgrace.' They also documented a total dearth of entertainments in the form of sports equipment and reading materials. An estimate calculated £2,000 for repairs and renovation of the facility, although expenditure would only meet immediate preservations. Asylum officials even suggested abandoning the building altogether due to its chronic and debilitated state.[66]

The implementation of changes and improvements proved problematic. The committee's Chairman projected the cost to ratepayers would amount to £30,000 for renovation and the erection of new buildings. One member responded that he had been barraged with objections from ratepayers against such expenditure. A compromised estimate of around £15,000 was deemed inconsequential owing to the facility's terminal condition. It was the Chairman's view that such objections would not be raised if the ratepayers were aware of the appalling conditions on offer.[67] The economic imperative held sway. Despite the Inspectorate of Mental Hospitals joining the Ministry of Pensions in advocating for the complete and immediate removal of the patients from the building, the committee continued to articulate their disgust with the building housing the majority of Service Patients five years later.[68]

Any plans to improve the facility were suspended until the economy had improved.[69] The lack of progress for male patients, including Service Patients, continued nineteenth-century policy; resistance by local ratepayers over financial interests regularly superseded initiatives to improve the treatment and care of the insane.[70] By 1938, the Inspectorate of Mental Hospitals continued to describe the poor facilities at Clonmel which British ex-servicemen shared with the broader asylum population:

> There is very considerable overcrowding in this Mental Hospital; that in the day rooms are the worst of any hospital. Owing to this there is a great deal of irritability and excitement amongst the patients ... The necessity for a central heating system is very apparent in the damp walls and floors ... The bathing accommodation is bad and insufficient. Some of the day rooms are gloomy and depressing. The sanitary accommodation is generally bad ... Many of the rooms are insufficiently furnished ... The main dining hall in the old building has a cesspool underneath it and is infested with rats. The laundry is in a shocking and dilapidated condition.[71]

As private patients whose insanity was deemed attributable war service, Service Patients' lived experience in the facility did not constitute value for money nor was it a suitable homecoming for a disabled ex-serviceman.[72]

Clothing

Clothing differentiated Service Patients in Free State asylums. Sparse research by medical historians maintains that distinct clothing effectively segregated and elevated private patients, preventing their amalgamation with pauper lunacy.[73] Forward was pleased veterans were dressed appropriately at Clonmel, with the Inspectorate of Mental Hospitals also drawing attention to the suitable attire of patients.[74] These narratives can, however, be disputed. Previous research into the Service Patient scheme in England and Wales equates the distribution of the tweed suits as a modest concession in an attempt to spare Service Patients from the shame of pauper lunacy.[75] Nowhere was the impotence of distinguishable clothing better highlighted than at Clonmel. The distribution of distinctive tweed suits appears to have taken a decade to implement. There is no explanation for this delay. It may be that asylum staff did not welcome the additional labour which came with providing individual clothing.[76] Despite numerous inspections by the Ministry, the attire of Service Patients did not improve until 1928, although only Service Patients at Limerick, Killarney and Maryborough mental hospitals required attention with a small number of Service Patients still incorrectly dressed.[77] The provision of a tweed suit depended upon the mental condition of a Service Patient. Two patients missed out at Castlebar Mental Hospital due to their 'defective habits.' One troublesome Service Patient, who had previously attempted to escape on two previous occasions, was not issued with the suit with staff fearing that it would be harder to identify him in the event of an escape attempt.[78] While working, which a decent proportion of Service Patients appear to have done, these men again wore institutional clothing alongside the non-ex-service population.[79] The distribution of segregated clothing to Service Patients in the Irish Free State was, therefore, neither prompt, consistent nor guaranteed.

Accommodation

Variable standards of accommodation existed across the Irish Free State's asylum network. The Report of the Commission on the Sick and Destitute Poor (1927) assessed that many of the dark and dank mental hospitals resembled prisons and were wholly unsuitable for providing care. Many were hot and uncomfortable during the summer; dormitory shutters were closed during daylight hours, patients changed in corridors and were able to walk around dormitories naked.[80] Forward also referenced these unbefitting conditions. Accommodation at Ennis and Killarney mental hospitals was meagre and unsuitable for the treatment of the mentally ill. One source of discontent was the inadequate and dated heating infrastructure. Accommodation at Maryborough, Enniscorthy, Mullingar and Castlebar provided inadequate sleeping arrangements with rooms described as miserable, bare and unattractive.[81] Enhancements to asylum infrastructure again depended on available investment. The lack of finances at Richmond ensured pillows and beds were worn and dated. Conditions at Tirconaill were dark and depressing, and a vast redecoration and renovation were required. The dining room at Castlebar had a pervasive odour lingering as patients ate. The majority of the institutions were also overcrowded. The Ministry of Pensions, the Inspectorate of Mental Hospitals and the Report of the Commission on the Sick and Destitute Poor all made particular reference to the severity of conditions at Castlebar, Clonmel, Ennis, Monaghan and Mullingar.[82] Overcrowding would continue into the late 1930s and had a noticeable impact on living conditions. For example, there were 239 males in excess of available accommodation at Cork with many beds being made up on the floors of dormitories. An unspecified number of beds were in corridors at Richmond.[83] At Tirconaill Mental Hospital an unspecified number of patients were treated in a separate and modern annexe of the facility where conditions were superior to those housing Service Patients.[84] Service Patients were again not afforded the best accommodation facilities available.

The congestion could prove fatal. The mortality rates for Service Patients amounted to 6 percent in 1931. Pulmonary Tuberculosis was responsible for 17 percent of the total. Mortality rates for this disease were highest at Portlaoighise and Killarney asylums. While one ex-serviceman was suffering from Pulmonary Tuberculosis in 1931, with a further two suspected of having contracted it, two patients died from the disease between 1924 and 1930 at Portlaoighise Mental Hospital. At Killarney Mental Hospital, where the walls of the facility were porous and damp, two Service Patient perished between 1924 and 1926. In April 1932, two Great War veterans died of Pulmonary Tuberculosis at Cork. Their deaths occurred despite the Ministry of Pensions previously recognising, but not acting upon, the Inspectorate of Mental Treatment's recommendation for the segregation of tubercular cases.[85] A small number of Irish veterans survived the horrors of the First World War only to be killed by a bacterial infection contracted in an overcrowded and poorly resourced district mental hospital.

Diet and recreation

The variable diet provided within the Irish Free State Mental Hospital network further highlights the subjectivity prevalent within the Service Patient scheme. The Report of the Commission on the Sick and Destitute Poor pointed out that each institution had a specific diet.[86] Forward cited the lack of variety in the meals given at Enniscorthy, Killarney, Portlaoighise, Castlebar, Monaghan, Ennis and Sligo mental hospitals. Giving an example of the frugality, breakfast at Castlebar consisted of porridge and milk on three days a week with bread, margarine and tea making up the other four. Dinner comprised of meat with vegetables or bread four days a week, soup and bread once a week, while meals on the other two days consisted of milk, potatoes and bread. In a repeat of an austere wartime policy, some institutions replaced butter with margarine. The monotonous and limited diet on offer to Service Patients in the Irish Free State led to unfavourable comparisons with English and Scottish institutions. The inferior living standards of the Irish people supposedly negated this disadvantage, with the Ministry concluding: 'One has to remember in comparing the dietary that the standard of living is much lower amongst lower classes of the Irish population who are accustomed to live principally on potatoes, stir about, eggs, soups with meat or bacon once or twice a week.'[87] Not for the first time, the Ministry's anti-Irish aspersions were outdated. Dietary standards rose in the Irish Free State during the inter-war period, especially in urban areas.[88] The Ministry's inaction also appears to be due to the lack of complaints from patients. Although it remains unclear how Service Patients were to realise their provided dietary was inferior to what was on offer in similarly isolated facilities across the Irish Sea, inspecting Ministry officials showed little inclination to disclose their inferior position.[89]

Service Patients received a 2s 6d allowance from the Ministry to improve the variety of their diet. As was the case in England, the allocation of the finance depended on asylum policy with each institution having the power to decide how to spend the grant.[90] Most facilities provided tobacco, cigarettes, sweets and fruit. The additional expenditure on tobacco in the annual accounts of Maryborough Mental Hospital was deemed attributable to its supply to Service Patients. The stipend at Cork allotted extra meal-time portions of egg, rice and milk supplementing the usual diet. Ex-servicemen had little influence how to spend the allowance.[91] It was only at Mullingar where flexibility was on offer with men able to select what their grant was spent on with staff buying goods from a local shop.[92] Barham asserts that the Service Patient scheme was nothing more than a 'lean menu of personalised options [which] made little or no difference to the treatment that was being offered.'[93] In Ireland, with one exception, the stipend was not even 'personalised.' Ex-servicemen at Mullingar were only granted the payment if their mental condition was deemed suitable to appreciate this additional expense.[94] The privilege of being allotted extra food rations was also available to the wider patient population. At Castlebar Mental Hospital, for example, working patients received extra food in the form of an egg and a pint of milk daily. Other institutions offered bread and tea to working patients.[95] It is unclear whether working Service Patients received additional portions; nevertheless, conditional access to otherwise attainable increased food rations demonstrates the allowance provided to insane veterans is less distinctive than it first appears.

All patients were offered recreational opportunities throughout the 1920s and 1930s. Onsite entertainments included walks across asylum grounds, indoor and outdoor sports, gramophone records and reading material.[96] The utilisation of associated entertainments, however, often proved problematic. Forward's reports during the 1920s attest to bands visiting asylums for patient dance recitals, travelling exhibitions and external trips to local races and football matches.[97] By 1930, due to the inadequate funding and reduction of nursing staff, most mental hospitals ceased to arrange the weekly entertainments. Ballinasloe, Enniscorthy, Clonmel, Maryborough, Cork and Killarney mental hospitals held no recreations. Opportunities for recreation inside and outside the hospital were subsequently unfavourable in comparison with British institutions, referencing a large number of idle and bored patients in these Free State facilities.[98] Entertainment for soldier-patients at the RWH continued unabated during the war even as there was a reduction in civilian opportunities. By the 1930s, however, ex-servicemen were now amalgamated within the wider austere institutional policy.

The Ministry lamented the lack of entertainment, believing such activities had a positive impact on mental wellbeing. Yet, they neither lobbied the relevant Free State authorities for their reintroduction nor subsidised such events. The department dismissed such an intervention in the Free State, explaining: 'It has to be acknowledged that the average patient met with is of a lower standard of education and intellect than those men in institutions in England and Scotland, his interests are limited and many are unable to even read or write.'[99] External inspectors of the nineteenth-century Irish workhouse also dismissed the substandard care and facilities on offer in Ireland along similarly prejudicial lines, writing: 'The poor in the West of Ireland are totally unacquainted with the ordinary conveniences of civilised life … with people in a state of ignorance as almost amount to barbarism.'[100] Like aspersions regarding diet, Ministry inaction in improving conditions in the Free State was the result of longstanding and inaccurate prejudices which were, in fact, without basis. Literacy rates and cinema visits greatly increased in inter-war Ireland. In 1913, Ireland was in a minority of countries, alongside England, France, Australia, New Zealand, Belgium and Austria, which had a literacy rate above 90 percent.[101] Prejudicial and longstanding assumptions formulated by Ministry staff attached themselves to mentally ill Irishmen who had fought in a British Army uniform both inside *and* outside of the asylum.

Privileged patients?

It is necessary to revisit the initial process which established the Service Patient system to properly evaluate its worth. The scheme aimed to distinguish the insane Great War veteran from the pauper lunatic. During initial discussions to set up the system, E. Marriot Cooke, a leading figure at the Board of Control, underlined this central aim from the outset: 'There is, as you are aware, a strong and wide feeling, shared by our board, that the stigma is one to which men who may have become insane through fighting for their country ought not to be subject, and to avoid which, every effort should be made.'[102] Austerity dictated the Ministry's thinking. The use of private asylums to cater for Service Patients, for example, was not even mentioned in the initial correspondence which discussed the implementation of the scheme in both Britain and Ireland.[103]

Being designated as a Service Patient contained undeniable benefits. Ministry officials interviewed each patient to receive feedback during their numerous inspections. The Ministry believed these interviews offered a veteran the opportunity to articulate issues they may have been reluctant to raise with asylum staff.[104] Their feedback was influential. One man's complaint at Purdysburn that his wife had not visited him resulted in the Ministry's intervening by encouraging the asylum's Medical Superintendent to contact his spouse to arrange a visit.[105] In 1921, Forward recommended that discharged Service Patients be sent to Craigavon Hospital to facilitate training in its workshops to aid employment; at least one Service Patient subsequently underwent such probation.[106] By May 1921, over 1,500 Service Patients throughout Ireland and Britain were transferred to other institutions following a Ministry inspection of district facilities.[107]

Following feedback regarding the repetitive diet on offer at Castlebar, Forward told its committee that the Service Patient's diet should be improved, suggesting an additional one ounce of butter for breakfast and supper and pudding at dinner on Wednesday and Friday. Taking this feedback on board, the Chairman of the committee agreed that the changes were justifiable as they were paying patients. Forward subsequently acknowledged an improvement in the diet in his next report.[108] In these instances, both the Ministry and the insane Great War veteran were active agents in institutional care. Regarding monetary outlay, it is also important not to dismiss the significant recompense provided. Insanity provided a 100 percent pension, ranked alongside a loss of two or more limbs, total blindness, severe facial disfigurement and paraplegia. The pension amounted to forty shillings per week, often paid to the Service Patient's family.[109]

Despite the concessions, however, the Service Patient system was fundamentally flawed. The crucial variable in explaining the lived experience of Service Patients was the condition of the asylum hosting them rather than the individual status of patients. Institutional facilities in Ireland contrasted sharply from the meagre Clonmel facility to much superior establishments like Purdysburn. For example, the Ministry of Pensions supported the Inspectorate's claim that Letterkenny Mental Hospital was the best institution in the Free State. The reports noted the outstanding order of rooms and dormitories, the suitable diet, entertainments on offer and pleasant conduct of patients and attentive nature of the staff.[110] A broad overview of Letterkenny and Purdysburn would counter Lomax's hyperbolic assertion that institutionalised veterans were consigned to 'a living death'.[111] Tellingly, Letterkenny also charged the Ministry the highest price for upkeep per Service Patient. The persistent austere outlook of the Ministry and its refusal to consider the use of superior private facilities on account of their expense appears to have had a huge impact on the daily experience of institutionalisation amongst insane Great War veterans.[112] In both suitable and unsuitable conditions, and across expensive and inexpensive facilities alike, the experience of institutionalisation in public institutions was largely shared by patients regardless of their legal status.

The Ministry recognised the corroboration of Forward's inspection of Service Patients with the Report of the Commission on the Sick and Destitute Poor's analysis of the general asylum population: 'I have compared the comments on the various Irish Mental Hospitals with the notes in Dr Forward's personal reports during the past years ... Practically all the points of criticism and praise mentioned in the Irish reports have their counterpart in Dr Forward's notes.'[113]

Both the general asylum populace and the Service Patient's experience varied on an institutional basis.[114] This phenomenon was not exclusive to the asylum. Poor Law care in the workhouse contrasted across Ireland and was highly subjective in accordance with institutional infrastructure, local economies and regional attitudes.[115] These variations are significant as the standard of care provided in an asylum could impact on the mental condition of patients. In contrast to Purdysburn, where the stabilisation of chronic patients was deemed attributable to the decent care and facilities on offer, the dire setup at Clonmel had a detrimental impact on the condition of patients. Conditions could even influence whether a Service Patient lived or died.

Provision for the insane population was generally limited in both Northern Ireland and the Irish Free State. In 1928, the Ministry recorded few advances in Ireland since their inspections carried out two years earlier. Identifying the wider social and political context, the report concluded: 'Although the need for modernising the buildings, improving the accommodation and conditions and adding to the amenities of the hospitals are fully recognised by the authorities concerned, little progress has been possible owing to the limited funds available.'[116] Northern Ireland experienced severe political and economic difficulties and anxieties throughout the 1920s and 1930s; subsequently, provisions and treatment for the mentally ill rarely featured on the government's agenda. The British Government proved unwilling to bankroll the Northern Irish Government or invest in any potential health and social reforms. The inter-war period witnessed an ever-increasing asylum population inadequately funded due to insufficient means ensuring that only rudimentary supervisory care was often possible.[117] Successive Free State governments similarly remained concerned on aspects of state and security reflecting minimal societal interest for the mentally ill. The overriding motivation centred on reducing the financial burden of ratepayers.[118] Public and voluntary hospitals received modest funding from successive governments and societal bodies, and many public hospitals were also lacking necessary medical and surgical appliances.[119]

While changes to asylum infrastructure appear glacial in pace throughout the UK, Britain's Mental Treatment Act of 1930 was reformist in the handling of mental illness. Martin Stone assesses that the shell-shock episode, and the subsequent boom in psychopathology, ushered in the introduction of the Mental Treatment Act in 1930. The legislation increased the function of out-patient treatment, enabled voluntary admissions of mentally ill patients before their condition potentially worsened and attempted to destigmatise associated language with public asylums by renaming them as 'mental hospitals.'[120] Holden went so far as to suggest that these acts equated to the 'death knell' of the old Victorian asylums.[121] With the introduction of the new act, Ministry officials urged caution to avoid voluntary veteran patients being stigmatised alongside Service Patients who, for the most part, were assumed to be long-term and chronic patients. The progressive new act underscores the stigmatised and lowly position held by the Service Patient who were otherwise assumed to be chronic, incurable and long-term residents of public institutions.[122]

The Mental Treatment Act was introduced in Northern Ireland in 1932, allowing a patient to admit themselves into a hospital voluntarily with a softening in stigmatised language. This practice matched the growing acceptance that early intervention with milder disorders could improve the mental condition of a patient. The Mental Treatment Act of 1945 was the equivalent significant step in improving mental health care in the Republic of Ireland which had replaced the erstwhile Irish Free State.[123] Although the legislation was not enforced until 1 January 1947, it had a central impact on mental health care with almost one quarter of mental hospital admissions being voluntary in its first year.[124] The legislation had a limited impact on Service Patients across Ireland. The majority of Service Patients admissions came before 1932 and 1945. The Ministry accepted that the introduction of voluntarism would have little subsequent influence on the Service Patient scheme in Northern Ireland.[125] To demonstrate its relative irrelevance, only one Service Patient would voluntarily admit himself into Purdysburn, the largest public mental health facility in Northern Ireland, under the new legislation between 1932 and the outbreak of the Second World War.[126]

'Not soldiers but lunatics'

Research into British asylums argues that the stigma of institutionalisation was so pervasive during the twentieth century that prejudices also attached themselves to patients discharged as recovered and even to mental health attendants and nurses.[127] Housing chronic, elderly and infirm patients who had little chance of recovery, previous work on the Irish workhouse argues that these facilities were also intrinsically linked to pauperism during the inter-war period.[128] British politicians and asylum superintendents similarly held that the stigma of insanity undoubtedly attached itself to Service Patients regardless of their official status and could even associate with their family members.[129] By contrast, the Chairman of the ESWS asserted that the separation of ex-servicemen from pauper lunatics helped to spare them the stigma of insanity.[130] Whether Service Patients were segregated from pauper lunacy is impossible to assess. Historians of both shell-shock and mental health care have pointed out it is extremely difficult to assess stigma and public opinion.[131] A weighing of the existing evidence suggests that the former societal viewpoint was the more persuasive.

Before the official establishment of the Service Patient scheme, correspondence amongst relevant military and medical staff discussed the potential to introduce a system to accommodate insane veterans. The Birmingham War Hospitals Committee held that asylums were unsuitable to house servicemen due to the institution's inherent association with pauper lunacy: 'The mere name of "service patients" or the amount of maintenance rate or a distinctive uniform or badge would in no way improve the patient's position.'[132] The Board of Control and pension authorities were less proactive in garnering the opinion of Irish authorities. By way of explanation, the War Pensions Committee wrote: 'In view of the fact that no differentiation is made between pauper and private patients the Statutory Committee are of the opinion that no useful purpose would be served in entering into negation as for the provision of treatment for insane sailors and soldiers in asylums in Ireland.'[133] The Ministry of Pension also noted that the Army Council made enquiries to the relevant authorities in Ireland on 1 June 1917 but did not receive a reply.[134] In August 1918, the Office of Lunatic Asylums in Dublin stated there 'was no official distinction between "private" and "pauper" patients in Irish Asylums.' They held 'that the stigma of pauperism does not attach to ordinary insane patients in this country.'[135] Pension authorities in London and the Belfast War Pensions Committee opposed this assertion. Their view was that all asylum patients in Ireland were 'branded with pauper stigma.'[136] This alternative theory appears more convincing. There was much confusion amongst the general public about mental health policy and the condition of patients owing to the various lunacy acts in existence during the earlier decades of the twentieth century. The stigma of pauper lunacy, therefore, attached itself to all those held in isolated Irish asylums.[137] It was for this reason that the Belfast War Pensions Committee opposed the placing of servicemen in Irish asylums.[138]

Smith and Pear agreed that the stigma and prejudices of institutionalisation affected an insane ex-serviceman as they did the broader lunatic population.[139] In 1920, the Board of Control wrote that many in British society 'regarded it as derogatory to a mentally disturbed soldier to be placed in a so-called pauper asylum' which was 'persistently referred in disparaging terms.'[140] Barham even contends some family members did not pursue a Service Patient application on behalf of an institutionalised relative owing to the shame and stigma of their relation's position.[141] Some observers did not even recognise the Ministry's attempt to segregate and elevate Service Patients. An article entitled *Wounded Souls: A Plea for Nerve-Strained Victims of War* (1927) complained there was no scheme in place in Britain and Ireland to aid insane Great War veterans. It was supposed that the institutionalised veteran was simply 'herded in with paupers, without any kind of special treatment.'[142] Even experienced asylum staff who had worked in district facilities during the First World War falsely broadcast that insane ex-servicemen were institutionalised alongside the pauper veteran in district asylums.[143] While these assertions are incorrect, their distribution speaks to the lack of understanding and appreciation of the Service Patient scheme outside of specialist knowledge and personal involvement. The grandchildren of one Irish veteran believed their grandfather had passed away, instead of being informed of the truth that he had been institutionalised, indicating that the stigma of asylum care was inescapable in inter-war Ireland.[144]

In the general absence of separate and exclusive asylums for private patients in public asylums, Cooke understood from the outset that many asylums would merely grant patients a few extra privileges, such as distinctive clothing and an improved diet.[145] Even when such a facility was available, Purdysburn's private facility did not accommodate Service Patients by 1924. As a leading advocate of the scheme, Cooke was well aware from the outset that a Service Patient's experience would be subjective with conditions varying widely on an institutional basis.[146] Proceeding with the scheme regardless must be contextualised with contemporary assumptions of the institutionalised veteran amongst medico-military officials. Concluding on 'The Influence of War Stress and Shell-Shock in the Production of Insanity', the Southborough Report repeated theories of degeneration and predisposition:

> A certain number belonged to the recurrent type of mental disability, and in these cases the war conditions probably played only a small, if any, part in the cause of the attack ... there is no justification for the popular belief that 'shell-shock' was a direct cause of insanity, or that the service patients still in asylums were originally cases of 'shell-shock' who have since become insane.

Many medico-military officials held a Service Patient's insanity had little to do with their war service. The committee heard the testimony of medical officials like Dr Edward Mapother, who decreed: 'Taking as insanity what would have been certifiable in a civilian, I saw few cases of insanity which seemed solely due to the stress of war.'[147] Asylum records reflect this judgement. In the admission records of Service Patients in Irish asylums, the 'stress of war' was only ever noted as being a 'secondary cause of insanity.'[148] As Reade accepted, 'stress of war' was a purposefully 'vague term.' At the very least, Reade conceded: '[war service] might possibly precipitate the onset of some smouldering psychosis.'[149] This diagnosis remains impossible to verify. As Purser, a physician in Mercer's Military Hospital in Dublin, wrote: 'How it all starts exactly is often very doubtful.'[150] Nevertheless, the flaws in the scheme are better understood with these degeneration theses in mind.

Compensatory measures within the Service Patient scheme appear to have been an attempt to appease public and political dissent. They were not, as the Ministry were keen to project, a fulfilment of a moral obligation to men they believed were mentally unwell as a result of war service. The lobbying of ex-service charities successfully linked an insane veteran's institutionalisation with war service which, in turn, shaped Ministry policy.[151] For example, in a deputation to the Prime Minister in 1920, the National Federation of Discharged and Demobilised Sailors and Soldiers in Ireland stressed the additional necessity of establishing exclusive provisions for the treatment of insane ex-servicemen:

> We consider that such ex-service men should be treated by doctors who understand their complaints, in a special institution set apart solely for ex-service men, and that they should not be treated in any asylum which is a general asylum. Their mental derangement is entirely different, or may be entirely different, and consequently, their treatment should be entirely different.[152]

The potential for a network of exclusive facilities reserved for insane veterans was, however, ruled out from the outset. Quoting the need for ten to twelve exclusive Ministry facilities to cater for the insane veteran, the Ministry held that their establishment would be too costly.[153] The British Legion also held that an insane veteran's proximity to nearby friends and family was essential to the mental condition of insane ex-servicemen, which favoured their placement in public asylums located across the UK.[154] Two Ministry of Pensions facilities were eventually set up in Britain in 1924 for insane Great War veterans of 'the hopeful type.' Established in annexed buildings on asylum grounds, these hospitals primarily operated along mental hospital lines with ex-servicemen but witnessed limited instances of recovery and discharge. The hospitals were closed in 1931 with the remaining patients subsequently transferred back to civilian hospitals. These facilities were again established to placate public dissent surrounding the incarceration of insane ex-servicemen whose mental condition offered a prospect of recovery.[155] While little information exists as to why Ireland did not establish similar amenities, the dearth of political petitioning and public lobbying on behalf of Irish veterans may have been a factor. The Ministry's desire to pacify public sentiment and to be seen as assisting the Great War veteran is demonstrated in the treatment of insane Irish Great War veterans whose medical history made them ineligible to be categorised as Service Patients.

Differences between the British and Irish experience

From the inception of the Service Patient scheme, the British Treasury agreed to facilitate around 900 insane Great War veterans as Service Patients, even when their mental illness was not deemed as attributable to war service. This compromise was not absolute as it did not extend beyond 30 September 1921, again illustrating how the British state's benevolence was drastically reduced after this year. Approaching this date, asylum committees across Ireland referred to the upcoming reversal of policy.[156] Cork asylum staff were concerned about the impending loss of £600 in maintenance revenue from the Ministry of Pensions.[157] The registrar of the Richmond Mental Hospital committee wrote to the Ministry articulating his opposition to the pending change in status, clarifying: 'My committee are becoming impatient at the numerous demands being made on them to allow the maintenance of men broken in the late war to fall on the public rates.'[158] Highlighting the lack of esteem and sympathy that Irish society attached to the disabled British veteran, Free State asylum authorities were willing to categorise these ex-servicemen veterans as 'Criminal Lunatics', despite the additional stigma attached, to exploit a legal loophole for financial gain. Even in Northern Ireland, Omagh and Londonderry institutional committees also pondered whether the impending cost of these 'non-attributable' cases would be reclassified as 'Criminal Lunatics' under the aforementioned conditions within the Lunacy (Ireland) Act, 1901, thus alleviating their expense from local rates. This eventuality did not occur.[159]

In Britain, the stripping away of these men's Service Patient status led to a resurgence in popular and political protest on behalf of the disabled veteran. The Ministry of Pensions, with the approval of the Treasury, subsequently reclassified 740 men as Service Patients.[160] Officials at the Colonial Office, the Treasury and the Ministry all attributed this measure to the public and political outrage that had arisen in the withdrawal of private status. The Treasury also held that local authorities in England had shrewdly capitalised on the ensuing public and political lobbying as a 'pretext for relieving themselves of an unwelcome, but purely normal, expense.'[161] Barham describes the reversal as 'the last gasp of the populist protest that had invigorated the People's Lunatic in 1917' which had led to the initial establishment of the scheme.[162] The annual cost of the procedure to the Ministry amounted to £32,000 in England and Wales and £4,600 in Scotland.[163]

Neither Northern Ireland nor the Irish Free State benefitted from a similar policy despite the Ministry of Finance in London believing local Irish authorities had a justifiable claim for equitable treatment. The lack of public agitation and political lobbying to extend the policy explains its omission.[164] The inactivity of ex-service associations re-emerged with no dissent from Irish departments. Many ex-service bodies in Ireland appeared unaware of the difference in policy.[165] Not for the first time, the Ministry enabled the continuation of ignorance of differences between the Irish and British experience of institutionalisation. From

September 1922, an estimated sixty men in Northern Irish mental hospitals were thus stripped of their classification as Service Patients and its associated upkeep. Their maintenance came at an estimated cost to ratepayers of around £3,400 per year.[166]

With one delegate at the Colonial Office referring to these men as 'wretched lunatics', an uncomplicated picture of the esteem in which non-attributable insane veterans emerges, despite the concessions made to them in Britain. The same official recognised Parliament might raise questions as to why ex-servicemen in Northern Ireland were being treated differently to their similarly afflicted former comrades in Britain. Given the modest outlay, the British Government considered its extension to Northern Ireland. It was, however, the fear that any such concession in Northern Ireland could set a precedent leading to its extension in the Free State which explains its continued non-application in the former.[167] The Home Office conceded in 1924 that, while accepting that the cost was relatively minor, any extension 'involves some important considerations. In principle we are in agreement with you ... If, however, this line is taken the Irish Free State may demand a similar concession, the cost of which would be considerable.'[168] Although it appeared unlikely that Free State authorities were going to make such a claim, British authorities did not consider it necessary to extend its non-attributable policy to Ireland unless insane veterans were being persecuted.[169] While unsympathetic to their plight, the Irish Free State Government did not actively discriminate against British ex-servicemen. The British Government thus consigned 'non-attributable' cases to pauper lunacy with no official recognition of their former war service in a British Army uniform. *Realpolitik* and financial concerns overrode a sense of duty to mentally ill Great War veterans.

As with neurasthenic pensioners in civil society, a recognition of the broader economic and political context and its influence on Ministry policy and remit is necessary. Since the establishment of the Irish Free State, mental hospitals were no longer legally obliged to accept Great War veterans born in the Irish Free State but who had then become insane in Britain.[170] The Colonial Office had been in contact with the Free State Government to amend this situation, but with little progress.[171] The Naval Branch suggested the Irish Free State Government refused to accept responsibility for insane ex-servicemen born in Ireland but who were undergoing treatment in Britain.[172] Free State authorities were willing to judge cases on their merits but were reluctant to provide any decisive and binding precedent on the issue. Consequently, British asylums treated an unspecified number of Irish-born Service Patients.[173] Some Service Patients were thereafter unable to be transferred across UK borders, including Belfast-born A. D. who repeatedly but unsuccessfully requested transferral to a London facility where he had lived for the past twenty-eight years.[174] Scottish medical authorities certified one Irish Service Patient, but who was then retransferred to the Armagh Asylum from an unnamed Free State Mental Hospital when officials realised his origin.[175] The post-1922 cessation of the free movement of insane ex-service patients complicated the reversal of 'non-attributable' cases. In a letter to the Colonial Office, one British official wrote: 'You remember the question of ex-service lunatics whose condition is not formally attributable to war? If we are pressed by the Irish Government to make a concession there in favour of their local authorities, we might perhaps secure this as a set off at the same time.' The letter determined: 'This is a note for possible future use; the point doesn't arise unless and until the Free State raises it.'[176] The Colonial Office wrote of the intrinsic relationship between the two statutes: 'The root of the trouble is of course that our power of removing lunatics and paupers to Ireland ... has disappeared.'[177]

During the nineteenth century, Poor Law bodies were hostile in Ireland against British authorities who, without any agreement or dialogue with Irish officials, transferred and delivered Irish pauper lunatics to district asylums. There was no preparation to facilitate transferrals the other way.[178] As one official at the Colonial Office accepted, Ireland had no authority to transfer pauper lunatics to Britain.[179] The Colonial Office thus explained:

> The establishment of the Irish Free State on the basis of a self-governing dominion has radically altered the position ... the Secretary of State regrets that he feels unable to suggest to the Government of the Irish Free State that they should assume liability for the care and maintenance of discharged naval and military lunatics born in the Irish Free State.[180]

Ultimately, any legislative agreement introduced by British authorities to transfer mentally ill patients to the Irish Free State would result in the Dáil introducing countermanding legislation relieving its mental hospitals of the responsibility. Thus, predictions arose that 'the ratepayers of Great Britain will have to shoulder the burden of maintaining large numbers of indigent Irish as part of the price we have to pay for the establishment of the Irish Free State.'[181] In the absence of any breakthrough, British Government officials held that Ireland took advantage of the migrant passages to Britain by exporting her 'indigent' and mentally ill residents to congest the English asylum. As Waterfield inferred:

> It seems to me that so long as this country continues to give free admission to casual Irish labour every harvest time, and so enables the Free State both to relieve local unemployment, and to bring home English-paid wages, we have a good case for asking that they shall not take the opportunity to dump her lunatically minded population on to us in that way.[182]

Waterfield even claimed: 'I have no information, but I suspect a good proportion of the civilian Irish lunatics in this country come from these annual migrants.'[183] Once again, the narrative of British officials continued a nineteenth-century discourse. Irish migrants, held in poor esteem by the native population, settled in vast numbers in overcrowded and poverty-ridden areas and were associated with importing disease and mental illness.[184] For example, in 1886 and 1870 local press reports in Lancashire discussed the 'Irish problem', a widely-held assumption that Irish authorities exported their mentally ill population to the north-west of England to pass the responsibility of 'ould Ireland's demented children' to local asylums.[185] Waterfield's remarks echoed and buttressed longstanding anti-Irish assumptions regarding their apparent intrinsic association with immaturity and mental illness. Such discourse attached itself to the Irish Tommy at the Front, the neurasthenic pensioner in inter-war Ireland and the insane veteran in the post-war asylum.

International and domestic comparisons

Placing the Ministry's treatment of insane veterans within a transnational context helps to underline the simultaneous liberality and miserliness of the Service Patient scheme. The comparative treatment afforded to mentally disabled veterans in France again reflects favourably on Ministry policy. Like their mentally ill ex-comrades in civil society, institutionalised veterans were detrimentally affected by their country's rehabilitative infrastructure which treated mentally ill ex-servicemen as an inferior and less-deserving veteran community. Around 4,000 insane Great War veterans were accommodated in French asylums during the inter-war period. They were unsegregated and undistinguished in poorly run and stagnant public asylums with the cost of their treatment procured from their pensions. Physically disabled pensioners in France requiring in-patient treatment were conversely afforded free health care by the state with veterans being able to choose between exclusive hospitals reserved for ex-servicemen, civil hospitals or even private institutions.[186]

In contrast, the status and treatment of the insane veteran in Australia were superior. Ex-servicemen were segregated from civilian patients, with several institutions hosting veterans in adjunct blocks on asylum grounds. Former ANZACs were afforded a better diet than the rest of the asylum population and were not required to undertake labour. The Repatriation Department, Australia's equivalent of the Ministry of Pensions, covered associated costs. On visiting one such facility in Victoria, one Ministry official noted his surprise at the 'lavish provision made for the comforts of the patients, the appointments being really suggestive of a first class hotel.'[187] Previous research contends men and their families exploited the stigma of pauperism and institutionalised mental illness, allowing them to segregate the mentally ill veteran from the wider asylum population. The subsequent stigma regarding hereditary and degenerative mental illness detached itself from the insane veteran.[188]

Closer to home, previous research has questioned the worth of private status in the inter-war English asylum, assessing that it was nothing more than a corporate deception.[189] A parallel narrative is evident in Ireland. Private patients effectively underwent treatment in the district asylum receiving little in substantial subsistence in comparison to the rest of the asylum population.[190] This infrastructure stood in contrast to the exclusive private accommodation for paying patients in the Irish Free State. With occupational therapy and recreational amenities widespread, the twelve smaller private facilities in Ireland, accommodating around 850 patients, were superior to the overcrowded and underfunded asylum hosting service and pauper patients alike.[191]

Despite its flaws, the Service Patient system bettered anything on offer to insane British Army veterans of previous wars. With regards to the Anglo-Boer War, 1899–1902, there was no special categorisation for institutionalised ex-servicemen or equitable financial compensation.[192] Despite the War Office affirming that a Service Patient's insanity was not always solely attributable to war service, the family of an institutionalised veteran still received the most financially lucrative financial compensation available.[193] There was no comparable provision available to the small number of insane Irish Civil War veterans of the Free State's National Army.[194] Bringing the attention of the Dáil to one such man in Letterkenny Mental Hospital, Major Myles queried the legislation and benefits provided to these men akin to the British Government's treatment of British First World War veterans. In response, Peter Hughes TD, Minister of Defence, said no equivalent arrangement was in place and that local rates akin to pauper lunatics paid the man's maintenance. When asked whether this was fair, Hughes responded 'it is not what I think right or Christian, but what is allowed by legislation.'[195] Wolfe raised concerns: 'I have come across cases, cruel, hard cases, that do not come within the present measure. I have come across cases, not of wounds, but worse than wounds – cases of insanity and complete loss of mental power.' He compared their treatment unfavourably with regards to equitable infrastructure afforded by the British Government: 'The British, with all their faults, have not acted in that way ... Wounds are very bad, no doubt, but to be mentally disabled, hopelessly laid aside for the rest of your life is very much worse. I think nothing could be more cruel than that.'[196] As was the case with mentally ill veterans in Free State society, societal sympathy and national memory may have been kinder to revolutionary veterans; however, the official rehabilitative policy did not reflect this lofty position and the Ministry's treatment of mentally ill Great War veterans again bettered the Free State Government's treatment of revolutionary veterans identically afflicted.

Conclusion

One of the most sensitive and complex challenges facing the Ministry of Pensions was its treatment of ex-servicemen who had lost their sanity. Attempts were made to recognise insanity as being attributable to army service and to compensate and differentiate ex-servicemen from the supposed stigma of pauper lunacy. Nevertheless, the Service Patient scheme was a failure in Ireland. Except for the initial post-war years at Purdysburn, insane veterans were not segregated from pauper patients. Further shortcomings occurred with the substantial delay in granting of tweed suits. Even then, only those whose mental condition was deemed suitable to appreciate the luxury enjoyed this benefit which, in turn, was restricted to leisure time. The same principle applied to the granting of pocket money which offered little in the way of personal control and was conditional on the Service Patient's mental state. The fundamental motivation in dictating a patient's daily experience was the condition and infrastructure of their asylum rather than their legal status within it.

If the policy was a disappointment, then it was, at the very least, a pioneering failure on behalf of a previously disregarded population. The scheme's implementation was again the result of lobbying on behalf of insane Great War veterans ensuring attempts were made to combat the stigma of mental illness. Nowhere is this motivation better exemplified than by the lack of extension of the Service Patient scheme in Ireland involving those whose insanity was not attributable to war service. This Irish case study echoes previous research that the Service Patient scheme was not the watershed moment ensuring parity of esteem of insane Great War veterans alongside their physically disabled ex-comrades. It did, however, represent a significant shift in recognition regarding trauma and mental illness, especially when considering that lunacy enabled a maximum pension akin to paraplegia and losing two or more limbs.[197] This trajectory again highlights the 'flagrant conditions [which] reflected the muddle in the Ministry of Pensions straddled between rival outlooks and between the new century and the last.'[198] We should also recognise the Ministry again continuing its duty as an 'imperial obligation' in the Irish Free State, continuing to fund and interact with Service Patients. Its assistance is magnified when remembering that Service Patients' lunacy was not generally accepted by Ministry and military officials as being attributable to war service. It is possible that the scheme's real impact may have been in influencing the mental health policy and discourse in Ireland in the longer term. The 1932 and 1945 Mental Treatment Acts introduced voluntary admission, and softened official stigmatised language, but this was too late for many of Ireland's Great War veterans.

Notes

1. Annual Report of the Richmond District Lunatic Asylum, 1918–1919, 44.
2. Cork City and County Archive, OLH/67, Cork District Lunatic Asylum Male Casebook, 9 September 1919–31, May 1920.
3. Dawson, 'The work of the Belfast War Hospital', 224.
4. Barham, *Forgotten Lunatics of the Great War*, 327.
5. NAI, PRIV1223/5/89, Richmond District Lunatic Asylum Male Casebook, 1912–1925.
6. Ibid.
7. Ibid.
8. Delargy, 'The History of the Belfast District Lunatic Asylum, 1829–1921', 242.
9. NAI, PRIV1223/3/56, Richmond District Asylum, General Register of Admissions, 31 May 1918–25 April 1922; Cork City and County Archive, OLH/67, Cork District Lunatic Asylum Male Casebook, 9 September 1919–31 May 1920.
10. NA, PIN 15/881, Ministry of Pensions, note, 6 March 1924.
11. Barham, *Forgotten Lunatics of the Great War*, 218.
12. NAI, PRIV1223/5/89, Richmond District Lunatic Asylum Male Casebook, 1912–1925.
13. Cork City and County Archive, OLH/67, Cork District Lunatic Asylum Male Casebook, 9 September 1919–31 May 1920.
14. 'Kilkenny District Mental Hospital', *Kilkenny People*, 4 March 1933, 10.
15. Research into insane Great War veterans in Australia has attested that many transferrals to the asylum were from the home; Larsson, 'Families and institutions for shell-shocked soldiers in Australia after the First World War', 103.
16. There was an increase of 879 Service Patients between 1 January 1920 and 1 January 1930 with populations increasing from 3,739 Service Patients to 4,618 Service Patients; Reid, *Broken Men*, 111; Brumby, 'From 'Pauper Lunatics' to 'Rate-Aided Patients'', 199.
17. NAI, PRIV1223/3/56, Richmond District Asylum, General Register of Admissions, 31 May 1918–25 April 1922.
18. Scull, *Madness*, 70.
19. Dawson, 'The work of the Belfast War Hospital', 221.
20. Kelly, *Hearing Voices*, 3–4; Pauline Prior, '"Where lunatics abound": A history of mental health services in Northern Ireland', in G. Berrios and H. Freeman (eds), *150 Years of British Psychiatry: Volume 2* (London: Athlone Press, 1996), 294.
21. Barham, *Forgotten Lunatics of the Great War*, 340; NAI, PRIV1223/3/56, Richmond District Asylum, General Register of Admissions, 31 May 1918–25 April 1922.
22. PRONI, HOS/17/7/8/2/11, Londonderry District Lunatic Asylum, Large files containing patient's case notes, c. 1890–1935; As in Britain, numerous Irish men

were discharged who would otherwise have remained in the asylum until their death; Barham, *Forgotten Lunatics of the Great War*, 315.
23 NA, PIN 15/3167, Report on the Treatment of Service Patients in Mental Hospitals in the Irish Free State for the year 1931.
24 Barham, *Forgotten Lunatics of the Great War*, 179.
25 PRONI, HOS/28/1/5/10, Purdysburn Villa Colony, 1930, xv.
26 Sixth Annual Report of the Ministry of Pensions, 1922–1923, 28.
27 PRONI, HOS/28/1/5/10, Purdysburn Villa Colony, 1930, xxiv.
28 'Omagh Mental Hospital', *Ulster Herald*, 18 January 1936, 3.
29 NA, PIN 15/3167, Report on the Treatment of Service Patients in Mental Hospitals in the Irish Free State for the year 1931.
30 This body of disabled veterans also included those with tuberculosis, chronic heart conditions, bronchitis and paraplegia. It is, however, worth remembering the maintenance cost of Service Patients was considerably lower than the majority of other disabled pensioners receiving in-patient treatment; Barham, *Forgotten Lunatics of the Great War*, 187, 305, 374.
31 HC Debates, 10 December 1925, vol. 189, col. 636.
32 Combat Stress Archive, Surrey, Box 7, 'Meeting held at the House of Commons to discuss the position of some Six Thousand or more Ex-Servicemen at present confined to Lunatic Asylums', 2–4.
33 PRONI, HOS/28/1/5/9, Annual Report of Belfast Mental Hospital, 1924, viii.
34 Prior, *Mental Health and Politics in Northern Ireland*, 39.
35 For example, the use of antipsychotic drugs is a relatively modern phenomenon that has developed from the mid-twentieth century. Chlorpromazine, distributed from 1954, introduced a range of anti-psychotic drugs. While such drugs do not always eradicate sensory and auditory delusions and hallucinations, they better enable sufferers to cope with their ailments with reduced anxiety and distress which, subsequently, better accommodates their reintegration into civil society; Kelly, *Hearing Voices*, ix.
36 Prior, *Mental Health and Politics in Northern Ireland*, 14.
37 PRONI, HOS/28/1/5/12, Annual Report of Belfast Mental Hospital, 1937, 46; Northern Ireland, Home Office Services Reports, 'Mental Treatment', 1938, 44.
38 PRONI, HOS/28/1/5/9, Annual Report of the Purdysburn Villa Colony, 1925, viii.
39 Ibid., Annual Report of the Purdysburn Villa Colony, 1922, xxii.
40 Ibid., Annual Report of the Purdysburn Villa Colony, 1922, xxii; Service Patients: Report on the District Asylum, Purdysburn, Belfast, by the Headquarters Medical Inspector, 1921, xx–xxv.
41 Ibid., Inspection of Service Patients in District Asylum, Purdysburn, Belfast, visited 1st February, 1924, xxv–xxvii.
42 Ibid., Service Patients: Report on the District Asylum, Purdysburn, Belfast, by the Headquarters Medical Inspector – Ministry of Pensions, 1921, xxiii.

43　Ibid., Annual Report of the Purdysburn Villa Colony, 1922, xv.
44　Ibid., Annual Report of the Purdysburn Villa Colony, 1923, xv.
45　Ibid., Service Patients: Report on the District Asylum, Purdysburn, Belfast, by the Headquarters Medical Inspector – Ministry of Pensions, 1921, xxiv–xxv; Report of the Belfast District Lunatic Asylum, 1922, xv–xxv.
46　Ibid., Service Patients: Report on the District Asylum, Purdysburn, Belfast, by the Headquarters Medical Inspector, 1921, xxv.
47　Ibid., Annual Report of the Purdysburn Villa Colony, 1922, xxii; Annual Report of the Purdysburn Villa Colony, 1925, xx; Inspection of Service Patients in District Asylum, Purdysburn, Belfast, visited 1st February, 1924, xxvi.
48　PRONI, HOS/28/1/5/9-12, Annual Report of the Purdysburn Villa Colony, 1938, 40; Annual Report of the Purdysburn Villa Colony, 1933, 29; Annual Report of the Purdysburn Villa Colony, 1932, 35; Annual Report of the Year, 1931, 34; Annual Report of the Year, 1930, 56; Annual Report of the Year, 1928, 30–1; Annual Report of the Year, 1926, 9–10; Annual Report of the Year, 1923, 9; Annual Report of the Year, 1921/22, 11.
49　PRONI, HOS/28/1/5/9, Inspection of Service Patients in District Asylum, Purdysburn, Belfast, visited 1st February, 1924, xxvi–xxvii.
50　Barham, *Forgotten Lunatics of the Great War*, 107.
51　Two reports in November 1937 and April 1938, written by two different Ministry of Pensions' officials, echo Forward's previous inspections; PRONI, HOS/28/1/5/12, Report on Inspection of Service Patients, in Belfast Mental Hospital, Purdysburn, Belfast, 1937, xxv–xxvi; Report on Inspection of Service Patients, in Belfast Mental Hospital, Purdysburn, Belfast, 1938, xxvi–xxvii.
52　PRONI, HOS/28/1/5/9, Report of the Purdysburn Villa Colony for the years 1921/22, 11; HOS/28/1/5/10, Purdysburn Villa Colony, Belfast, 20th February, 1928, xxv.
53　PRONI, HOS/28/1/5/10, Purdysburn Villa Colony, 1930, xxv.
54　NA, PIN 15/3030, Royal Medico-Psychological Association of Great Britain and Ireland; PRONI, HOS/28/1/5/9-12, Annual Report of the Purdysburn Villa Colony, 1937, 40–3; Annual Report of the Purdysburn Villa Colony, 1933, 29; Annual Report of the Purdysburn Villa Colony, 1932, 32; Annual Report of the Purdysburn Villa Colony, 1925, 10; Annual Report of the Purdysburn Villa Colony, 1923, xvi–xvii.
55　Combat Stress Archive, Surrey, Box 7, 'Meeting held at the House of Commons to discuss the position of some Six Thousand or more Ex-Servicemen at present confined to Lunatic Asylums', 9.
56　PRONI, HOS/28/1/5/9, Inspection of Service Patients in District Asylum, Purdysburn, Belfast, visited 1st February 1924, xxiii–xxvi.
57　PRONI, HOS/28/1/5/10, Purdysburn Villa Colony, Belfast, 20th February, 1928, xxv.
58　Ibid., Purdysburn Villa Colony, 1930, xxiv.

59 'Omagh District Asylum', *Ulster Herald*, 22 March 1924, 3; 'Omagh District Asylum', *Ulster Herald*, 21 April 1928, 2; 'Omagh District Asylum', *Ulster Herald*, 17 November 1934, 6; 'Omagh Mental Hospital', *Ulster Herald*, 18 January 1936, 3.
60 Annual Report of the Inspector of Mental Hospitals, 1938, 42; Annual Report of the Inspector of Mental Hospitals, 1937, 45; Annual Report of the Inspector of Mental Hospitals, 1936, 38; 'Omagh District Asylum', *Ulster Herald*, 22 March 1924, 3; 'Omagh District Asylum', *Ulster Herald*, 22 March 1924, 3; 'Omagh Mental Hospital', *Ulster Herald*, 18 January 1936, 3.
61 This 1921 inspection was commented upon in the second report in 1924, but no details were previously given; 'Omagh District Asylum', *Ulster Herald*, 22 March 1924, 3; 'Omagh District Asylum', *Ulster Herald*, 22 March 1924, 3; 'Omagh District Asylum', *Ulster Herald*, 17 November 1934, 6.
62 NA, PIN 15/3167, Report on the Treatment of Service Patients in Mental Hospitals in the Irish Free State for the year 1931.
63 Richmond was a rarity with 132 patients; only 11 asylums in England and Wales accommodated over 100 Service Patients; Barham, *Forgotten Lunatics of the Great War*, 371–3; David Fitzpatrick, 'The logic of collective sacrifice: Ireland and the British Army, 1914–1918', *The Historical Journal*, 38:4 (1995), 1020–1; Taylor, *Heroes or Traitors?*, 12.
64 NA, PIN 15/3167, Report on Mental Hospitals in the Irish Free State, 1928; Ministry of Pensions, note, 15 November 1932.
65 Ibid., Ministry of Pensions, note, 15 November 1932; Report on Mental Hospitals in the Irish Free State, 1928; Annual Report of the Inspector of Mental Hospitals, 1933.
66 'Clonmel Mental Hospital', *Nenagh Guardian*, 19 May 1928, 4.
67 A subordinate committee member countered that ratepayers would continue to protest owing to the depressed economy existing in the region; 'New Clonmel Buildings', *Nenagh Guardian*, 14 September 1929, 1.
68 Annual Report of the Inspector of Mental Hospitals, 1932, 16; 'Clonmel Mental Asylum', *Nenagh Guardian*, 18 February 1933, 7.
69 'Mental Hospital Staff', *Nenagh Guardian*, 28 July 1928, 6; 'New Clonmel Buildings', *Nenagh Guardian*, 14 September 1929, 1.
70 Finnane, *Insanity and the Insane in Post-Famine Ireland*, 103.
71 Annual Report of the Inspector of Mental Hospitals, 1938, 17.
72 Access to the records of the Clonmel Asylum was denied by the Service Manager, Carlow/Kilkenny and South Tipperary Mental Health Service, e-mail correspondence 4 November 2015.
73 Nicole Baur and Joseph Melling, 'Dressing and addressing the mental patient: the uses of clothing in the admission, care and employment of residents in English provincial mental hospitals, c. 1860-1960', *Textile History*, 45:2 (2014), 145; Hide, *Gender and Class in English Asylums*, 99–102.
74 Annual Report of the Inspector of Mental Hospitals, 1938, 17; 'Clonmel Mental Hospital', *Nenagh Guardian*, 19 May 1928, 4.

75 Barham, *Forgotten Lunatics of the Great War*, 21.
76 Paying patients at Ballinasloe Mental Hospital attired in the ordinary asylum stock caused great annoyance to their relatives. As a way of explanation, the Resident Superintendent complained that the cleaning and distribution of distinctive private clothing increased staff workload; 'Councillor Who Would have Voted against Recent Resolution', *Connacht Tribune*, 13 September 1919, 5.
77 NA, PIN 15/3167, Report on Mental Hospitals in the Irish Free State, 1928.
78 'Mayo Mental Hospital', *Connaught Telegraph*, 7 April 1928, 3.
79 This occurrence was stated in Forward's report of Castlebar Mental Hospital in 1928; 'Mayo Mental Hospital', *Connaught Telegraph*, 7 April 1928, 3.
80 The Report of the Commission on the Sick and Destitute Poor, 1927, 102. [Online] Available at: www.lenus.ie/hse/handle/10147/238535 [accessed 14 July 2015].
81 NA, PIN 15/3167, Report on Mental Hospitals in the Irish Free State, 1928; Ministry of Pensions, note, 15 November 1932; 'Careful attention in Mental Hospital', *Meath Chronicle*, 24 May 1930, 3; 'Maryborough Mental Hospital', *Leinster Express*, 15 March 1924, 3.
82 'Mayo Mental Hospital', *Connaught Telegraph*, 7 April 1928, 3; 'British Ex-Servicemen', *Ballina Herald*, 26 April 1930, 3; NA, PIN 15/3167, Report on Mental Hospitals in the Irish Free State, 1928; Report on Mental Hospitals in the Irish Free State, 1931; Annual Report of the Inspector of Mental Hospitals, 1927, 101; Annual Report of the Inspector of Mental Hospitals, 1931, 14–22; Annual Report of the Inspector of Mental Hospitals, 1938, 40.
83 NA, PIN 15/3167, Report on the Treatment of Service Patients in Mental Hospitals in the Irish Free State for the year 1931; 'Estimates for next year', *Irish Examiner*, 22 January 1936.
84 'Tirconaill Mental Hospital', *Donegal News*, 17 April 1926, 3.
85 NA, PIN 15/3167, Report on the Treatment of Service Patients in Mental Hospitals in the Irish Free State for the Year 1931.
86 The Report of the Commission on the Sick and Destitute Poor, 102; Annual Report of the Inspector of Mental Hospitals, 1931, 14–22.
87 NA, PIN 15/3167, Report on Mental Hospitals in the Irish Free State, 1928.
88 David Johnson, *The Interwar Economy in Ireland* (Dundalk: Economic and Social History Society of Ireland, 1985), 40–2.
89 NA, PIN 15/3167, Report on Mental Hospitals in the Irish Free State, 1928.
90 Brumby, 'From "Pauper Lunatic" to "Rate-Aided Patients"', 122–3.
91 NA, PIN 15/3167, Report on Mental Hospitals in the Irish Free State, 1928; 'Maryborough Mental Hospital', *Leinster Express*, 15 January 1927, 5; 'RMS's Report', *Irish Examiner*, 22 May 1928, 12; 'Inspectors Report', *Irish Examiner*, 21 May 1930, 14.
92 'Careful Attention in Mental Hospital', *Meath Chronicle*, 24 May 1930 3; 'Mullingar Mental Hospital', *Meath Chronicle*, 23 July 1932, 3.
93 Barham, *Forgotten Lunatics of the Great War*, 39.

94 'RMS's Report', *Irish Examiner*, 22 May 1928, 12; NA, PIN 15/3167, Report on Mental Hospitals in the Irish Free State, 1928.
95 'Care of the Insane', *Connaught Telegraph*, 30 March 1929, 2.
96 'Mistaken Identity Case', *Irish Examiner*, 13 April 1926, 12; 'RMS's Report', *Irish Examiner*, 22 May 1928, 12; 'Happy and Contented: Ex-Service Patients in Kilkenny Mental Hospital', *Kilkenny People*, 5 May 1928, 10; 'Kilkenny Mental Hospital', *Kilkenny People*, 1 February 1936, 5; 'Mullingar Mental Hospital', *Meath Chronicle*, 23 July 1932, 3; 'Mistaken Identity Case', *Irish Examiner*, 13 April 1926, 12; 'RMS's Report', *Irish Examiner*, 22 May 1928, 12; 'British Ex-Servicemen', *Ballina Herald*, 26 April 1930, 3; 'Mullingar Mental Hospital', *Meath Chronicle*, 23 July 1932, 3; 'Maryborough Mental Hospital', *Leinster Express*, 15 March 1924, 3; NA, PIN 15/3167, Ministry of Pensions, note, 15 November 1932.
97 'Happy and Contented: Ex-Service Patients in Kilkenny Mental Hospital', *Kilkenny People*, 5 May 1928, 10; 'Maryborough Mental Hospital', *Leinster Express*, 15 March 1924, 3.
98 PRONI, HOS/28/1/5/10, Purdysburn Villa Colony, Belfast, 20 February 1928, xxv.
99 NA, PIN 15/3167, Report on Mental Hospitals in the Irish Free State, 1928.
100 Virginia Crossman, *Poverty and the Poor Law in Ireland, 1850–1914* (Liverpool: Liverpool University Press, 2013), 17.
101 Johnson, *The Interwar Economy in Ireland*, 40–2; Ciaran O'Neill, 'Literacy and education', in Eugenio Biagini and Mary E. Daly (eds), *The Cambridge Social History of Ireland since 1740* (Cambridge: Cambridge University Press, 2016), 244–60; Eric Hobsbawm, *The Age of Empire, 1875–1914* (London: Weidenfeld and Nicolson, 1987), 345.
102 NA, PIN 15/866, Board of Control, London, note, 19 July 1916.
103 See NA, PIN 15/866, Lunacy: Arrangements with the Board of Control, 1916; PIN 15/896-899, Treatment of Lunacy (men): Ireland, 1916–1921.
104 NA, PIN 15/2601, Ministry of Pensions – Resume Concerning Constitution etc Organisation and Administration since its establishment; PIN 15/2006, Ministry of Pensions, note, 21 February 1927.
105 PRONI, HOS/28/1/5/10, Purdysburn Villa Colony, 1930, xxv.
106 Ibid., Report on Inspection of Service Patients in Belfast Mental Hospital, Purdysburn, Visited 10th February, 1926, xxii.
107 Departmental Committee of Inquiry into the Machinery of Administration of the Ministry of Pensions Report to Ian Macpherson, MP, Minister of Pensions, 1921, 104–5.
108 'County Mayo Mental Hospital'; *Connaught Telegraph*, 13 February 1928; 'Mayo Mental Hospital', *Western People*, 2 June 1928, 6; 'British Ex-Servicemen', *Ballina Herald*, 26 April 1930, 3.
109 Barham, *Forgotten Lunatics of the Great War*, 119–21; Cohen, *The War Come Home*, 195.

110 NA, PIN 15/3167, Report on the Treatment of Service Patients in Mental Hospitals in the Irish Free State for the year 1931; Annual Report of the Inspector of Mental Hospitals, 1931, 19–20.
111 Combat Stress Archive, Surrey, Box 7, 'Meeting held at the House of Commons to discuss the position of some Six Thousand or more Ex-Servicemen at present confined to Lunatic Asylums', 6.
112 NA, PIN 15/3167, Report on the Treatment of Service Patients in Mental Hospitals in the Irish Free State for the year 1931.
113 Ibid., Report on Mental Hospitals in the Irish Free State, 1928.
114 Annual Report of the Inspector of Mental Hospitals, 1931, 83–7.
115 Crossman, *Poverty and the Poor Law in Ireland*, 228; Lucey, *The End of the Irish Poor Law?*, 149.
116 NA, PIN 15/3167, Report on Mental Hospitals in the Irish Free State, 1928.
117 As Johnson points out 'the Stormont administration perpetually teetered on the edge of financial insolvency'; Johnson, *The Interwar Economy in Ireland*, 35; Prior, *Mental Health and Politics in Northern Ireland*, 10–18; Prior, 'Where lunatics abound', 29.
118 Reynolds, *Grangegorman*, 221; D. Healy, 'Irish psychiatry in the twentieth century', in G. E. Berrios and H. Freeman (eds), *150 Years of British Psychiatry: Volume 2* (London: Athlone Press, 1996), 276.
119 Mary Daly, '"An atmosphere of sturdy independence": the state and the Dublin Hospitals in the 1930s' in Elizabeth Malcolm and Greta Jones (eds), *Medicine, Disease and the State in Ireland, 1650–1940* (Cork: Cork University Press, 1999), 237.
120 Stone, 'Shell-shock and the psychologists', 242–71; Holden, *Shell-Shock*, 72; Bourke, *Dismembering the Male*, 121.
121 Holden, *Shell-Shock*, 71.
122 The files in which these issues are discussed relate only to British institutions and omit Northern Ireland and the Irish Free State; NA, PIN 15/911, Mental Treatment Act, 1930.
123 Kelly, *'He Lost Himself Completely'*, 119.
124 Kelly, *Hearing Voices*, 184–5.
125 NA, PIN 15/3167, Ministry of Pensions, note, 8 September 1933.
126 PRONI, HOS/28/1/5/11, Annual Report of the Purdysburn Villa Colony, 1934, xii.
127 Diana Gittins, *Madness in its Place: Narratives of Severalls Hospitals, 1913–1997* (London: Routeledge, 1998), 34; Long, *Destigmatising Mental Illness?*, 151–2.
128 Lucey, *The End of the Irish Poor Law?*, 150.
129 Combat Stress Archive, Surrey, Box 7, 'Meeting held at the House of Commons to discuss the position of some Six Thousand or more Ex-Servicemen at present confined to Lunatic Asylums', 2, 9.
130 Combat Stress Archive, Surrey, ESWS Chairman's Report for 1926, 8.
131 Reid, *Broken Men*, 24; Long, *Destigmatising Mental Illness?*, 4.

132 The opinion of the Birmingham War Hospitals Committee was shared by the Lancashire Asylums Board and officials at the Devon County Asylum; NA, PIN 15/866, Lunacy: arrangements with Board of Control, 1916.
133 Ibid., War Pensions and Statutory Committee Westminster to Office of Lunatic Asylums, Ireland, September 1916.
134 NA, PIN 15/897, Ministry of Pensions, note, 21 September 1918.
135 Ibid., Office of Lunatic Asylums, Dublin, note, 12 August 1918.
136 Ibid., Ministry of Pensions, note, 21 September 1918.
137 Prior, *Mental Health and Politics in Northern Ireland*, 31.
138 NA, PIN 15/897, Ministry of Pensions, note, 21 September 1918.
139 Smith and Pear, *Shell-Shock and its Lessons*, 78.
140 War Office, *History of the War Hospitals in England and Wales*, 36.
141 Barham, *Forgotten Lunatics of the Great War*, 179.
142 Philip Gibbs, 'Wounded souls: a plea for nerve-strained victims of war', *Overseas*, January 1927, 40.
143 Combat Stress Archive, Surrey, Box 7, 'Meeting held at the House of Commons to discuss the position of some Six Thousand or more Ex-Servicemen at present confined to Lunatic Asylums', 11.
144 Richardson, *A Coward if I Return, A Hero If I Fall*, 337.
145 NA, PIN 15/866, E. Marriot Cooke, Board of Control, London, to Mr Wynne, 19 July 1916; Barham, *Forgotten Lunatics of the Great War*, 39.
146 NA, PIN 15/866, E. Marriot Cooke, Board of Control, London, to Mr Wynne, 19 July 1916.
147 The Southborough Report, 146.
148 NAI, PRIV1223/3/56, Richmond District Asylum, General Register of Admissions, 31 May 1918–25 April 1922.
149 The Southborough Report, 146.
150 Purser, 'Shellshock', 228.
151 Barham, *Forgotten Lunatics of the Great War*, 270.
152 NA, LAB 2/855/ED5412/13/1921, Minutes of Proceedings: Deputation with the Prime Minister and the National Federation of Discharged and Demobilised Sailors and Soldiers, 10 Downing Street, 6 February 1920.
153 Departmental Committee of Inquiry into the Machinery of Administration of the Ministry of Pensions Report to Ian Macpherson, MP, Minister of Pensions, 1921, 105.
154 *British Legion Journal*, 2 (December, 1922), 133.
155 Alice Brumby, '"A painful and disagreeable position": rediscovering patient narratives and evaluating the difference between policy and experience for institutionalised veterans with mental disabilities, 1924–1931', *First World War Studies*, 6:1 (2014), 37–55; Brumby, 'From "Pauper Lunatics" to "Rate-Aided Patients"', 128–9.
156 Barham, *Forgotten Lunatics of the Great War*, 189; NA, PIN 67/72, Ministry of Pensions, note, 2 September 1922; 'Cork District Mental Hospital', *Irish Examiner*, 12 September 1922, 8; 'Tirconaill Mental Hospital', *Fermanagh Herald*, 23 September 1922, 8.

157 'Cork District Mental Hospital', *Irish Examiner*, 19 September 1922, 4.
158 NA, PIN 67/72, Richmond Mental Hospital to Ministry of Pensions, Dublin, 24 September 1924.
159 'Omagh District Asylum'; *Ulster Herald*, 23 September 1922; 'Derry Senator and Northern Ministry', *Fermanagh Herald*, 23 September 1922, 7; 'Ex-Service Men's Position', *Irish Examiner*, 12 June 1924, 5.
160 F. O. Roberts, *Labour and War Pensions* (London: Joint Labour Publications Dept, 1924), 3.
161 NA, T 160/214/9, The Treasury, London, to Colonial Office, London, 23 December 1924; Colonial Office, London, to the Treasury, London, 17 December 1924; T 161/1054, Ministry of Pensions, London, to the Treasury, London, 23 July 1923.
162 Barham, *Forgotten Lunatics of the Great War*, 270.
163 NA, T 160/214/9, Ministry of Finance, Belfast, to the Treasury, London, 16 October 1924.
164 Ibid.; the Government of Northern Ireland made just one claim for similar expenses to be borne out of imperial funds; Unsigned Memo, 21 October 1921.
165 Ibid., Colonial Office, London, to the Treasury, London, 23 December 1924.
166 Ibid., Ministry of Finance, Belfast, to the Treasury, London, 16 October 1924.
167 Ibid., Colonial Office, London, to the Treasury, London, 17 December 1924.
168 Ibid., Home Office, London, to Treasury, London, 18 December 1924.
169 Ibid., Unsigned Memo, 22 October 1924; Colonial Office, London, to the Treasury, London, 17 December 1924; Treasury, London, to Colonial Office, London, 23 December 1924.
170 NA, T 161/223/13, Dangerous Lunatics Discharged from Naval Forces. Question of Application of Army Act, Section 91 and Naval Enlistment Act, 1884, Section 3, 14 July 1924.
171 Ibid., Unknown Author, to Admiralty, London, 29 July 1924.
172 Ibid., Naval Branch, London, note, 12 September 1924.
173 Ibid., Colonial Office, London, to Treasury, London, 15 May 1925; Barham, *Forgotten Lunatics of the Great War*, 167.
174 PRONI, HOS/28/1/5/9, Report on Inspection of Service Patients in District Asylum, Purdysburn, Belfast, Visited 1st February, 1924.
175 'Certifying a Lunatic', *Irish Independent*, 11 May 1926, 9.
176 NA, T 160/214/9, Unsigned letter to Colonial Office, London, 10 December 1924.
177 Ibid., Colonial Office, London, to the Treasury, London, 11 October 1924.
178 Prior, *Mental Health and Politics in Northern Ireland*, 61.
179 NA, T 161/223, Colonial Office, London, to the Treasury, London, 11 October 1924.
180 NA, T 160/214/9, Colonial Office, London, to the Admiralty, London, 9 September 1924.
181 NA, T 161/223, Minute by Sir John Risely, 10 October 1923.
182 Ibid., The Treasury, London, to Colonial Office, London, 17 September 1924.

183 Ibid.
184 Cox, Marland and York, 'Itineraries and experiences of insanity', 40, 55.
185 Bernard Melling, 'Building a lunatic asylum: "a question of beer, milk and the Irish"', in Thomas Knowles and Serena Trowbridge (eds), *Insanity and the Lunatic Asylum in the Nineteenth Century* (London: Routledge, 2015), 60–3.
186 Derrien, 'Entrenched from Life', 209; Thomas, *Treating the Trauma of the Great War*, 99–109, 117.
187 NA, PIN 15/1716, Mr Gilbert's Report on his visit to Australia, 1926.
188 Larsson, 'Families and institutions for shell-shocked soldiers in Australia after the First World War', 97–114.
189 Barham, *Forgotten Lunatics of the Great War*, 106.
190 An analysis of the Service Patient scheme provides rare insight into the wider policy of private asylum care in Irish asylums. The exception here is Alice Mauger's research into nineteenth-century private institutional care. Mauger argues that while a better standard of care was on offer in private institutions, only the most affluent members of Irish society benefitted due to the cost of treatment; Alice Mauger, *The Cost of Insanity in Nineteenth Century Ireland: Public, Voluntary and Private Asylum Care* (Basingstoke: Palgrave Macmillan, 2018).
191 By 1921, there was only one private retreat available in Northern Ireland at Armagh. Unfortunately, the inspectorate's annual report does not give any indication of the facilities on offer; Prior, *Mental Health and Politics in Northern Ireland*, 22; Annual Report of the Inspector of Mental Hospitals, 1931, 26–9.
192 Indeed, when reading the patient casebooks of Irish asylums, one cannot help but be struck by significant number of insane British Army veterans of former conflicts under treatment; Jones and Wessely, 'War pensions (1900–1945)', 375.
193 The Southborough Report, 145–7.
194 Dáil Éireann, vol. 3, 13 June 1923, Army Pensions Bill 1923 – Second Stage; Dáil Éireann, vol. 7, 20 May 1924, Adjournment Debate – Position of ex-servicemen.
195 Dáil Éireann, vol. 16, 20 July 1926, Ex-members of National Army in Letterkenny Mental Hospital.
196 Orduithe An Lae, vol. 18, 25 January 1927, Orders of the day – Army Pensions (no.2) Bill, 1926.
197 Barham, *Forgotten Lunatics of the Great War*, 9, 365.
198 Ibid., 325.

CONCLUSION

The Irish experience of shell-shock does not sit seamlessly alongside existing studies into mentally disabled British Great War veterans. The lack of recognition, employment, training and treatment facilities in Ireland during the Anglo-Irish War ensured that the Ministry's initial progressive and innovative attempts to rehabilitate psychoneurotic ex-servicemen were fatally compromised. Countering long-held prejudices that Irish veterans were biologically predisposed to mental breakdown, this weakening in the Ministry's remit and function in South Ireland is evidenced in the inflated waiting lists for neurasthenic treatment in the region in 1921. The subsequent experience of mentally disabled veterans in both the Irish Free State and Northern Ireland further diversified experience. As in Britain, the Northern Irish Government provided employment and training assistance, and its society undertook philanthropic efforts to accommodate disabled ex-servicemen in both the public and private sector. Conversely, while not actively discriminating against Great War veterans, the Irish Free State Government did not prioritise disabled ex-servicemen for official employment nor did its society place much emotional currency on their sacrifice of body and nerves. This apathy, in turn, appears to have driven many ex-servicemen to the Ministry for financial relief. The Ministry's resulting expenditure in the newly formed state provided Great War veterans with an integral source of income during a time of widespread unemployment and economic depression.

With regards to institutional treatment, the war hospital scheme was innovative in the context of contemporary mental health treatment in emphasising the parity of esteem between mentally and physically wounded soldier-patients. This origination is magnified in the context of the detrimental impact the First World War had on Ireland's civilian asylum population, as the standard of care became reduced and death rates spiked. The war hospital initiative had limited impact beyond its short existence with Irish mental health care and legislation remaining relatively conservative throughout the inter-war period. An all-Ireland analysis of the various asylums and mental hospitals demonstrates the validity of previous criticisms of the Service Patient scheme. In the absence of exclusive facilities for institutionalised veterans, Service Patients shared the same premises and conditions as the wider mentally ill population. They were subsequently consigned to experience the universal dearth in medical infrastructure, with many of those veterans who were institutionalised also remaining long-term residents.

This Irish case study of mentally ill First World War veterans contributes to numerous historiographical debates. First, this study locates itself within the broader historiographical discussion of whether the First World War was a watershed moment in British and Irish society. Influential works by the likes of Paul Fussell argue that the Great War presented a distinctive break and marker between pre- and post-modernity eras in Britain.[1] Research has since countered such a thesis by emphasising the continuities evident in Britain before and after the war.[2] In addition to debates as to whether the global conflict marked a break from the past and ushered in gender equality, working-class rights and the expansion of the British electorate, a similar disagreement has occurred regarding the 'goodness' of the war for medicine in British society.[3] Shell-shock and disability features in this debate. Martin Stone, for example, contends that the First World War revolutionised the perception and treatment of mental illness, thus legitimising psychoneuroses in the mainstream of medical culture and ushering in critical progressive reforms.[4] Leading researchers of military psychiatry dispute this optimistic account. Instead, they counter that the emergence of shell-shock had little impact on post-war civilian and military psychiatry in the United Kingdom and any initial progress quickly evaporated in the aftermath of the conflict.[5] This Irish case study lies somewhere in-between these two opposing theses, foregrounding numerous instances of the Ministry's simultaneous progressiveness and conservatism.

While this disparity in the Ministry's ethos appears contradictory, these inconsistencies are not random nor unexplainable. Instead, they have been interpreted as a concept. Previous research has referenced the paradigm-shifting nature of the First World War on British society. So too, however, was there an entrenchment of Victorian and Edwardian narratives which proved hard to alter. The same paradoxical principles applied to the treatment and reception of mentally ill Irish Great War veterans with both change and continuity simultaneously evident in the aftermath of the First World War. As was the case in Barham's research into mentally ill British Great War veterans, my analysis highlights the 'flagrant conditions [which] reflected the muddle in the Ministry of Pensions straddled between rival outlooks and between the new century and the last.'[6] This conclusion bolsters the so-called 'half-way house' theses of shell-shock offered by Mathew Thomson and Tracey Loughran.[7]

This study's focus on one body of ex-servicemen, the British Army veteran, and government department, the Ministry of Pensions, exemplifies how the treatment and experiences of disabled First World War veterans depended on locality and chronology. This work hopes to contribute to the broader field of disability history by emphasising the fluidity of disability as a legal and administrative category which is often shaped to fit existing subjective socio-economic and political contexts and cultural values which, in turn, impact on the lives of disabled people.[8] With regards to the history of psychiatry, this study highlights the continuation of race-based psychiatry and its associated permutations throughout the inter-war period.⁹ Even British welfare officials charged with the after-care of disabled Irish veterans were not immune from casting such aspersions, even when it prejudiced disabled veterans whose mental illness was legally recognised as having been attributable to their former war service in a British Army uniform. Regarding analysis of veteran communities, this case study reinforces the critical variable of how post-war societies assess and value conflicts.¹⁰ The legitimacy of a war in societal consciousness shapes the post-war treatment and experiences of ex-combatants.¹¹ A study of Ireland, particularly the South and latterly defined Irish Free State, exemplifies how national memory of a conflict overrides its actual outcome. Veterans who returned to nationalist areas of Ireland were denied societal gratitude and even governmental preference by a society which placed little value on their war service despite being on the 'winning' side of the conflict.

Ultimately, this study reinforces Barham's thesis that 'the historiography of the "silent working-class soldier" has obscured much of what were actually very noisy encounters.'¹² In doing so, I hope to induce further enquiry into hitherto overlooked topics. First, more research needs to be undertaken into the legacy of the Ministry of Pensions' attempts to treat the mentally ill First World War veteran. It may be that the flawed efforts of the department were far more influential than has been previously assumed. Twenty years after its establishment, the Ministry applauded its efforts on being a 'pioneer' in the early and voluntary treatment of mentally ill citizens.¹³ Bourke similarly recognises the establishment of Ministry outpatient clinics in the aftermath of the First World War as being 'instrumental in the growth of psychiatry as a discipline.' For example, the creation of clinics such as the Tavistock Clinic founded in 1920 offered psychotherapeutic treatment to non-veteran communities.¹⁴ In 1930, the Ministry held that its remit and function in treating a wide variety of medical conditions on a wide scale had provided 'unrivalled opportunities of witnessing the progress of many types of diseases' such as neurasthenia, and had been the 'first to blaze the trail of exploration' in understanding causation and inducing a cure. The department was hopeful that its resulting extensive medical and clinical documentation could be a benefit to the progress of psychopathology.¹⁵ This study seeks to promote the Ministry of Pensions' archive. In 1931, military researchers described the department's archival collection as 'unique in character and pregnant with possibilities for research.'¹⁶ The archive's broad and detailed remit can further our understanding of a range of topics dedicated to the social history of medicine, disability history, welfare history and public policy history.

Further analysis on Ireland is now necessary. Like all ex-service and Great War veteran populations, Irish Great War veterans were not one homogenous and monolithic block.[17] The political and religious affiliation of these men requires closer scrutiny. Following a theme centred at numerous points in this book, it may be that disabled nationalist Catholics who returned to the north dissociated themselves from their war service or were discriminated against with regards to the facilities and opportunities that they should have been eligible for. Another potentially illuminating study would be the comparative treatment of Irish officers and privates which would better incorporate class and economic dimensions and their potential to shape experiences of disablement. While this thesis has analysed the First World War's impact on civilian asylum care during the war years, further research is required to assess whether the war had a similarly detrimental effect on disabled communities in other institutions such as sanatoriums and workhouses. Issues such as stigma and private mental health care during the twentieth century deserve far closer scrutiny than has thus far been offered. To date, analysis of the twentieth-century mental hospital in both Ireland and Britain lags far behind work into the nineteenth-century district asylum. An all-Ireland analysis of disabled veterans of the Second World War would also be potentially illuminating to both disability history and the history of veterans. While Northern Ireland officially participated in the second global conflict as part of the United Kingdom, the Republic of Ireland remained neutral. The comparative treatment of the two returning disabled communities will provide a unique insight into how official participation in war and national perceptions of war help to shape the post-demobilisation experiences of disabled veterans.

Incorporating both Britain and Ireland, historians have noted the necessity to address the shortage of analysis regarding the psychological impact war service had on medical personnel attached to the British Armed Forces.[18] This study has centred on how disabled Irish Great War veterans did not share the fate of their ex-comrades in Britain. This framework points the way to further transnationalism. While the post-war experiences of disabled veterans from dominions such as Canada and Australia have been produced, imperial colonies and dominions remain ignored by comparison, including India, the British West Indies and South Africa.[19] As Crouthamel claims: 'The history of mental illness is ... still a developing field, and one of the areas that begs more research is the experience of traumatised men after 1918.'[20] This study aims to be part of the journey to discover these forgotten 'madmen' of the Great War. Research into returning veterans and disabled communities in past societies should, however, also remain open to challenging conceptions of the passive and needy disabled person. Historians should acknowledge and analyse instances of success and purpose evident in disabled people's private and professional lives and recognise their agency in improving their treatment and position within society.[21]

As Gerber has previously asserted: 'By shifting the perspective toward the experience of disability may we understand the nature of the veteran's own agency in attempting to shape his relations to the state around his own conception of his needs and aspirations.'[22]

Finally, this study seeks to contribute to and advocate for a more holistic understanding of mental illness by recognising that veteran and civilian populations often shared national medical cultures and rehabilitative infrastructures. The Ministry of Pensions would recognise that the problems it faced in adequately understanding and adequately treating mental illness were repeated in domestic governments' simultaneous treatment of non-veteran populations.[23] In 1922, Percy supposed that unforeseen advances in medical science would benefit mentally ill British ex-servicemen in future conflicts: 'One hundred years hence medical science may know how to cure such men.'[24] As we approach Percy's deadline, many problems in the rehabilitation of traumatised British ex-servicemen remain unresolved.[25] It has been argued that the British medico-military and political establishment's treatment of 'shell-shock' represented the 'fundamental ambivalence' felt towards military psychiatry which persists today.[26] Indeed, contemporary problems in the treatment of the mentally ill are not restricted to ex-service personnel. The stigma surrounding mental health, underfunding of mental health resources, regional variations in available treatment facilities and high waiting lists for in-patient and out-patient treatment remain prevailing issues in contemporary Irish and British society as they did for the men discussed throughout this study.

Notes

1 Paul Fussell, *The Great War and Modern Memory* (Oxford: Oxford University Press, 1975)

2 Adrian Gregory, *The Last Great War: British Society and the First World War* (Cambridge: Cambridge University Press, 2008); Dan Todman, *The Great War: Myth and Memory* (London: Continuum, 2005).

3 Roger Cooter, 'Medicine and the goodness of war', *Canadian Bulletin of Medical History*, 7:2 (1990), 147–59.

4 Perhaps the most prominent reform was the introduction of the Mental Health Treatment Act, 1930, which allowed the mentally ill population in Britain to voluntarily admit and discharge themselves from psychiatric institutions; Stone, 'Shellshock and the psychologists', 242–71.

5 Edgar Jones and Simon Wessely, 'The impact of total war on the practice of British psychiatry', in R. Chickering and S. Förster (eds), *The Shadows of Total War: Europe, East Asia and the United States, 1919–1939* (Cambridge: Cambridge University Press, 2003), 129.

6   Barham, *Forgotten Lunatics of the Great War*, 325.
7   Loughran, *Shell-Shock and Medical Culture in First World War Britain*, 214; Thomson, *Psychological Subjects*, 185.
8   Longmore, *Why I Burned My Book and Other Essays on Disability*, 58; Stone, *The Disabled State*, 179.
9   Barham, *Forgotten Lunatics of the Great War*, 9.
10 The call for a 'new veteranology' was made by John Kinder advocating multidisciplinary research to improve understanding and the livelihoods of living veterans today; John Kinder, *Paying with their Bodies: American War and the Problem of the Disabled Veteran* (Chicago: University of Chicago Press, 2015), 298.
11 Diamant, *Embattled Glory*, 39; Grace Huxford, Ángel Alcalde, Gary Baines, Olivier Burtin and Mark Edele, 'Writing veterans' history: a conversation on the twentieth century', *War & Society*, 38:2 (2019), 126.
12 Barham, *Forgotten Lunatics of the Great War*, 315.
13 Nineteenth Annual Report of the Ministry of Pensions, 1935–1936, 19.
14 Bourke, *Dismembering the Male*, 120.
15 NA, PIN 15/65, Ministry of Pensions Ministry Sheet, 24 June 1930; Letter from Herbert Evans to M. Roberts MP, 13 August 1930; Medical Work of Ministry: general analysis.
16 Mitchell and Smith, *Medical Services*, 350.
17 Huxford et al., 'Writing veterans' history', 122–3; David Swift and Oliver Wilkinson, 'Introduction', in David Swift and Oliver Wilkinson (eds), *Veterans of the First World War: Ex-servicemen and Ex-servicewomen in Post-War Britain and Ireland* (Oxon: Routledge, 2019), 1.
18 Carol Acton and Jane Potter, *Working in a World of Hurt: Trauma and Resilience in the Narratives of Medical Personnel in Warzones* (Manchester: Manchester University Press, 2015), 32.
19 Important inroads into this field are being made. See, for example, Hilary Buxton, 'Imperial amnesia: race, trauma and Indian troops in the First World War', *Past & Present*, 241:1 (2018), 221–58.
20 Crouthamel, 'Review of *Broken Men – Shell Shock, Treatment and Recovery in Britain, 1914–1930*'.
21 David Turner and Daniel Blackie, *Disability in the Industrial Revolution: Physical Impairment in British Coalmining, 1780–1880* (Manchester: Manchester University Press, 2018), 200–2.
22 Gerber, 'Disabled veterans, the state, and the experience of disability in Western societies', 901.
23 NA, PIN 15/2601, Ministry of Pensions, Minute Sheet, 24 June 1930.
24 NA, PIN 15/1632, Lord Eustace Percy MP to Ministry of Pensions, London, 19 December 1922.
25 For example, see D. Murphy, B. Weijers, E. Palmer and W. Busuttil, 'Exploring patterns in referrals to combat stress for UK veterans with mental health difficulties between 1994 and 2014', *International Journal of Emergency Mental Health and Human Resilience*, 17:3 (2015), 562–658.
26 Jones and Wessely, *Shell-Shock to PTSD*, 47.

Select bibliography

Manuscripts

Combat Stress Archive
Annual Reports, Chairman's Annual Reports and Minute Meetings

National Archives of England and Wales
LAB 2 – Ministry of Labour Records
MH 106/2101 – Medical Sheets, Neurasthenia
PIN 15 – Ministry of Pensions Administrative Records
PIN 26 – Ministry of Pensions Individual Records
T 160–61 – British Treasury Files and Correspondence
WO 35 – Historical review of medical and sanitary work in the Irish Command during the War
WO 95 – 1st Battalion Connaught Rangers, Medical Officer's Diary

National Archives of the Republic of Ireland
BR/PRIV 1223 – Richmond War Hospital and Richmond District Lunatic Asylum Records

Public Record Office of Northern Ireland
CAB – Cabinet Secretariat Records
D4246 – British Legion Records
D989 – Southern Irish Loyalist Association Records
HOS – Northern Irish District Lunatic Asylums/Mental Hospital Records
PM – Prime Minister Department Records

Cork City and County Archive
OLH – Cork District Lunatic Asylum Records

John Rylands Library, University of Manchester
GES/2 – 'Race, Nationality and Character' (1918) by Grafton Elliot Smith

Leopardstown Hospital Archive

Admission Register – Disability Patients – 1914–18
Leopardstown Park Hospital Admission Register, 1930–36
Leopardstown Hospital Annual Report, 1938–39

Liverpool Record Office

M614 MAG/1 – Maghull Military Hospital Records

McClay Library, Queens University of Belfast, Belfast

Annual Reports on District and Private Asylums/Mental Treatment in Northern Ireland, 1921–38

Manchester City Archive

GB124.DPA/690/19 – Leslie Goodman in 'Hospital Blues'

Brotherton Special Collections, Leeds University

LIDDLE/WW1 – World War One Serviceman Transcripts

Newspapers and periodicals

American Medical New Series
Ballina Herald
British Journal of Medical Psychology
British Journal of Psychiatry
British Journal of Psychology
British Legion Journal
British Medical Journal
Connaught Telegraph
Dublin Journal of Medical Science
Fermanagh Herald
Irish Examiner
Irish Times
Journal of Mental Science
Journal of the Royal Army Medical Corps
Kilkenny People
The Lancet
Leinster Express
Meath Chronicle
Overseas
Proceedings of the Royal Society of Medicine

Reveille
The Eugenics Review
The Comrades Journal
Transactions of the Academy of Medicine in Ireland
Nenagh Guardian
Ulster Herald
War Pensions Gazette
Western People

Online UK Parliamentary Records

(https://parlipapers.proquest.com/parlipapers)
Annual Reports of the Irish Lunacy Inspectorate
Departmental Committee of Inquiry into the Machinery of Administration of the Ministry of Pensions Report to Ian Macpherson, MP, Minister of Pensions (1921)
History of the Asylum War Hospitals in England and Wales (1920)
Ministry of Pensions First to Twenty-Second Annual Reports for the period 1918 to 1939
The Report of the War Office Committee of Enquiry into Shell Shock (1922)

Lenus: the Irish health repository

(www.lenus.ie/)
Annual Reports of the Irish Lunacy Inspectorate/Inspector of Mental Hospitals
The Report of the Commission on the Sick and Destitute Poor (1927)

Houses of Parliament debates

(available online at http:/hansard.millbanksystems.com)

Dáil Éireann/ Seanad Éireann debates

(available online at http://historical-debates.oireachtas.ie/en.toc.dail.html)

Other published sources

A Voluntary Pensions Worker, *Pensioners of the Great War* (London: Robert Scott, 1922).
Culpin, Millais, *Recent Advances in the Study of the Psychoneurosis* (London: Churchill, 1931).
Eder, M. D., *War-shock. The Psycho-neuroses in War: Psychology and Treatment* (London: William Heinemann, 1917).
Fenton, Norman, *Shell-Shock and its Aftermath* (St Louis: The CV Mosby Company, 1926).
Graves, Robert, *Good-bye to All That* (Harmondsworth: Penguin, 1929).
Hogge, James, and Garside, T. H., *War Pensions and Allowances* (London: Hodder and Stoughton, 1918).

Hurst, Arthur, *Medical Diseases of the War* (London: Arnold, 1918).
Hutchinson, Woods, *The Doctor in War* (Boston: Cassel and Co, 1918).
Hutt, C. W., *The Future of the Disabled Soldier* (London: Bale & Co, 1917).
Lepine, Jean, *Mental Disorders of War* (London: University of London Press, 1919).
Llewellyn, J. L., and Jones, Arthur, *Pensions and the Principles of their Evaluation* (London: William Heinemann, 1919).
MacDonald, H. T., *What is Due to Me?: A Handy Compendium of Information on Pensions* (London: Daily Herald, 1919)
Macpherson, William, *Medical Services: General History, Volume 1* (London: HMSO, 1921).
—— *Medical Services: Diseases of the War, Volume 2* (London: HMSO, 1923).
Marr, H. C., *Psychoses of the War* (London: Hodder and Stoughton, 1919).
McMurtrie, Douglas, *The Disabled Soldier* (New York: Arno Press, 1919).
Mitchell, T. J. and Smith, G. M., *Medical Services: Casualties and Medical Statistics of the Great War* (London: H.M. Stationary Office, 1931).
Mott, Frederick, *War Neuroses and Shell-Shock* (London: Hodder & Stoughton, 1919).
Myers, Charles, *Shell Shock in France, 1914–1918: Based on a War Diary* (Cambridge: Cambridge University Press, 1940).
Parry, Edward, and Codrington, Alfred, *War Pensions: Past and Present* (London: Nisbot, 1918).
Read, Charles, *Military Psychiatry in Peace and War* (London: H. K. Lewis & Co, 1920).
Rivers, W. H. R., *Instinct and the Unconscious: A Contribution to a Biological Theory of the Psycho-neuroses* (Cambridge: Cambridge University Press, 1920).
Roberts, F. O., *Labour and War Pensions* (London: Joint Labour Publications Dept, 1924).
Roussy, G., Lhermitte, J. and Turner, William, *The Psychoneurosis of War* (London: University of London Press, 1918).
Salmon, Thomas, *The Care and Treatment of Mental Diseases and War Neuroses ('Shell-Shock') in the British Army* (New York: War Work Committee, 1917).
Sassoon, Siegfried, *Siegfried's Journey, 1916–1920* (London: White Lion, 1945).
Smith, Grafton Elliot, and Pear, Thomas, *Shell Shock and its Lessons* (Manchester: Manchester University Press, 1917).
Williams, Frankwood, *Neuropsychiatry and the War* (New York: War Work Committee, 1918).

Secondary sources

Published

Acton, Carol, and Potter, Jane, *Working in a World of Hurt: Trauma and Resilience in the Narratives of Medical Personnel in Warzones* (Manchester: Manchester University Press, 2015).
Adler, Jessica, *Burdens of War: Creating the United States Veterans Health System* (Baltimore: Johns Hopkins University Press, 2017).
Alexander, D. A., and Klein, S., 'Combat-related disorders: a persistent chimera', *Journal of the Royal Army Medical Corps*, 154:2 (2008), 96–101.

SELECT BIBLIOGRAPHY

Anderson, Julie, '"Jumpy stump": amputation and trauma in the First World War', *First World War Studies*, 6:1 (2015), 9–19.

—— *War, Disability and Rehabilitation in Britain: "Soul of a Nation"* (Manchester: Manchester University Press, 2011).

Andrews, Jonathan, 'Case notes, case histories, and the patient's experience of insanity at Gartnavel Royal Asylum, Glasgow, in the nineteenth century', *Social History of Medicine*, 11:2 (1998), 255–81.

Armstrong, David, 'The patient's view: doing medical history from below', *Social Science & Medicine*, 18:9 (1984), 737–44.

Augusteijn, Joost, *From Public Defiance to Guerrilla Warfare: The Experience of Ordinary Volunteers in the Irish War of Independence, 1916–1921* (Dublin: Irish Academic Press, 1996).

Bardon, Jonathan, *A History of Ulster* (Belfast: Blackstaff Press, 2001).

Barham, Peter, *Forgotten Lunatics of the Great War* (New Haven: Yale University Press, 2004).

Barr, Niall, *The Lion and the Poppy: British Veterans, Politics, and Society, 1921–1939* (Westport: Praeger, 2005).

Bartlett, Thomas, and Jeffery, Keith, 'An Irish military tradition?', in Thomas Bartlett and Keith Jeffery (eds), *A Military History of Ireland* (Cambridge: Cambridge University Press, 1996), 1–26.

Baur, Nicole, and Melling, Joseph, 'Dressing and addressing the mental patient: the uses of clothing in the admission, care and employment of residents in English provincial mental hospitals, c. 1860–1960', *Textile History*, 45:2 (2014), 145–70.

Beckett, Ian, *The First World War: The Essential Guide to Sources in the UK National Archives* (Surrey: Public Record Office, 2002).

Blanck, Peter, and Chen, Song, 'Civil war pensions for native and foreign-born union army veterans', in Larry Logue and Michael Barton (eds), *The Civil War Veteran: A Historical Reader* (New York: New York University Press, 2007), 221–7.

Brennan, Damien, *Irish Insanity, 1800–2000* (New York: Routledge, 2014).

Bogacz, Ted, 'War neurosis and cultural change in England, 1914–22: the work of the War Office Committee of Enquiry into "Shell-Shock"', *Journal of Contemporary History*, 24:2 (1989), 227–56.

Bourke, Joanna, *Fear: A Cultural History* (London: Virago Press, 2006).

—— '"Remembering" War', *Journal of Contemporary History*, 39:4 (2004), 473–85.

—— 'Shell-shock, psychiatry and the Irish Soldier during the First World War', in Adrian Gregory and Senia Paseta (eds), *Ireland and the Great War: 'A War To Unite Us All'?* (Manchester: Manchester University Press, 2002), 155–70.

—— 'Effeminacy, ethnicity and the end of trauma: the sufferings of 'shell-shocked' men in Great Britain and Ireland, 1914–39', *Journal of Contemporary History*, 35:1 (2000), 57–69.

—— *An Intimate History of Killing: Face to Face Killing in Twentieth Century Warfare* (London: Granta Press, 1999).

—— '"Irish Tommies": the construction of a martial manhood 1914–1918', *Bullan*, 6 (1998), 13–30.

—— *Dismembering the Male: Men's Bodies, Britain and the Great War* (London: Reaktion, 1996).

Bowman, Timothy, *Irish Regiments in the Great War: Discipline and Morale* (Manchester: Manchester University Press, 2003).

Boyce, David, '"That party politics should divide our tents': Nationalism, Unionism and the First World War", in Adrian Gregory and Senia Paseta (eds), *Ireland and the Great War: 'A War To Unite Us All'?* (Manchester: Manchester University Press, 2002), 190–217.

Bredberg, Elizabeth, 'Writing disability history: problems, perspectives and sources', *Disability & Society*, 14:2 (1999), 189–201.

Brumby, Alice, '"A painful and disagreeable position': rediscovering patient narratives and evaluating the difference between policy and experience for institutionalized veterans with mental disabilities, 1924–1931', *First World War Studies*, 6:1 (2015), 37–55.

Burke, Tom, '"Poppy day" in the Irish Free State', *Irish Quarterly Review*, 92 (2003), 349–58.

Carden-Coyne, Ana, *The Politics of Wounds: Military Patients and Medical Power in the First World War* (Oxford: Oxford University Press, 2014).

Carden-Coyne, Ana, and Anderson, Julie, 'Enabling the past: new perspectives in the history of disability', *European Review of History*, 14:4 (2007), 447–57.

Coakley, John, 'The election that made the first Dáil', in Brian Farrell (ed.), *The Creation of the Dail* (Dublin: Blackwater Press, 1994), 31–46.

Cohen, Deborah, *The War Come Home: Disabled Veterans in Britain and Germany, 1914–1939* (Berkeley: University of California Press, 2001).

Cooter, Roger, 'Medicine and the goodness of war', *Canadian Bulletin of Medical History*, 7:2 (1990), 147–59.

Cox, Catherine, Marland, Hilary, and York, Sarah, 'Emaciated, exhausted and excited: the bodies and minds of the Irish in nineteenth-century Lancashire asylums', *Journal of Social History*, 46:2 (2012), 500–24.

—— 'Itineraries and experiences of insanity: Irish migration and the management of mental illness in nineteenth century Lancashire', in Catherine Cox, Hilary Marland, and Sarah York (eds), *Migration, Health and Ethnicity in the Modern World* (Basingstoke: Palgrave Macmillan, 2013), 36–60.

Crammer, J. L., 'Extraordinary deaths of asylum inpatients during the 1914–1918 War', *Medical History*, 36:4 (1992), 430–41.

Critchlow, Donald, 'Integrating social history and the state: policy history through case studies', *The History Teacher*, 31:4 (1998), 459–66.

Crossman, Virginia, *Poverty and the Poor Law in Ireland: 1850–1914* (Liverpool: University of Liverpool Press, 2013).

Crouthamel, Jason, 'Memory as a battlefield: letters by traumatized German veterans and contested memories of the Great War', in Joan Tumlety (ed.), *Memory and History: Understanding Memory as Source and Subject* (London: Routledge, 2013), 143–60.

Crouthamel, Jason, and Leese, Peter (eds), *Psychological Trauma and the Legacies of the First World War* (Cham: Palgrave Macmillan, 2017).

Curtis, Liz, *Nothing but the Same Old Story: The Roots of Anti-Irish Racism* (Belfast: Sasta, 1984).

D'Arcy, Fergus, *Remembering the War Dead: British Commonwealth and International War Graves in Ireland since 1914* (Dublin: Stationary Office, 2007).

De Nie, Michael, *The Eternal Paddy: Irish Identity and the British Press, 1798-1882* (Wisconsin: University of Wisconsin Press, 2004).

Dean, Eric, *Shook Over Hell: Post-traumatic Stress, Vietnam, and the Civil War* (London: Harvard University Press, 1997).

Denman, Terence, 'The Catholic Irish soldier in the First World War: the "racial environment"', *Irish Historical Studies*, 27:108 (1991), 352-65.

Diamant, Neil, *Embattled Glory: Veterans, Military Families and the Politics of Patriotism in China, 1949-2007* (Lanham: Rowan & Littlefield, 2009).

Doody, G. A., Beveridge, A. and Johnstone, E. C., 'Poor and mad: a study of patients admitted to the Fife and Kinross district asylum between 1874 and 1899', *Psychological Medicine*, 26:5 (1996), 887-97.

Dungan, Myles, *They Shall Not Grow Old: Irish Soldiers of the Great War* (Dublin: Four Courts Press, 1997).

Durnin, David, *The Irish Medical Profession and the First World War* (Basingstoke: Palgrave Macmillan, 2019).

Durnin, David, and Miller, Ian (eds), *Medicine, Health and Irish Experiences of Conflict, 1914-45* (Manchester: Manchester University Press, 2016).

Dwyer, E., 'Psychiatry and race during World War II', *Journal of the History of Medicine and Allied Sciences*, 61:2 (2006), 117-43.

Eakins, Arthur, *The Somme: What Happened to the Casualties* (Belfast: Eakins Publishing, 2008).

Ellenberger, Henri, *Discovery of the Unconscious: The History and Evolution of Dynamic Psychiatry* (New York: Basic Books, 1970).

Fell, Alison, and Meyer, Jessica, 'Introduction: untold legacies of the First World War in Britain', *War and Society*, 34:2 (2015), 85-9.

Feudtner, Chris, '"Minds the dead have ravished": shell shock, history, and the ecology of disease-systems', *History of Science*, 31:4 (1993), 377-420.

Finnane, Mark, *Insanity and the Insane in Post-Famine Ireland* (London: Croon Helm, 1981).

Finnegan, Frances, *Poverty and Prejudice: A Study of Irish Immigrants in York, 1840-1875* (Cork: Cork University Press, 1982).

Fitzpatrick, David, *The Two Irelands: 1912-1939* (Oxford: Oxford University Press, 1998).

—— 'Militarism in Ireland', in Thomas Bartlett and Keith Jeffery (eds), *A Military History of Ireland* (Cambridge: Cambridge University Press, 1996), 379-409.

—— 'The logic of collective sacrifice: Ireland and the British Army, 1914-1918', *The Historical Journal*, 38:4 (1995), 1017-30.

—— *Politics and Irish Life 1913-1921: Provincial Experience of War and Revolution* (Cork: Gill and Macmillan, 1977).

Frith, Christopher, and Johnstone, Eve, *Schizophrenia: A Very Short Introduction* (Oxford: Oxford University Press, 2003).

Fussell, Paul, *The Great War and Modern Memory* (Oxford: Oxford University Press, 1975).
Gagen, Wendy Jane, 'Remastering the body, renegotiating gender: physical disability and masculinity during the First World War, the case of J. B. Middlebrook', *European Review of History*, 14:4 (2007), 525–41.
Gerber, David, 'Disabled veterans, the state, and the experience of disability in Western societies, 1914–1950', *Journal of Social History*, 36:4 (2003), 899–916.
—— *Disabled Veterans in History* (Ann Arbor: University of Michigan Press, 2000).
Grayson, Richard, *Belfast Boys: How Unionists and Nationalists Fought and Died Together in the First World War* (London: Continuum, 2009).
Gregory, Adrian, *The Last Great War: British Society and the First World War* (Cambridge: Cambridge University Press, 2008).
Gregory, Adrian, and Paseta, Senia, 'Introduction', in Adrian Gregory and Senia Paseta (eds), *Ireland and the Great War: 'A War To Unite Us All'?* (Manchester, 2002), 1–8.
Grogan, Suzie, *Shell-Shocked Britain: The First World War's legacy for Britain's Mental Health* (Barnsley: Pen & Sword, 2014).
Grossman, Dave, *On Killing: The Psychological Cost of Learning to Kill in War and Society* (Boston: Littlebrown, 2009).
Hadfield, Andrew, and McVeagh, John, *Strangers to That Land: British Perceptions of Ireland from the Reformation to the Famine* (Gerrards Cross: Colin Smythe, 1994).
Harrington, John, *The English Traveller in Ireland: Accounts of Ireland and the Irish through Five Centuries* (Dublin: Wolfhound Press, 1991).
Harrison, Mark, *The Medical War: British Military Medicine in the First World War* (Oxford: Oxford University Press, 2010).
Hart, Peter, *The IRA at War: 1916–1923* (Oxford: Oxford University Press, 2003).
—— *The I.R.A. and Its Enemies: Violence and Community in Cork, 1916–1923* (Oxford: Oxford University Press, 1998).
Henry, Hanora, *Our Lady's Hospital, Cork: History of the Mental Hospital in Cork Spanning 200 Years* (Cork: Cork University Press, 1989).
Herman, Judith, *Trauma and Recovery: The Aftermath of Violence from Domestic Abuse to Political Terror* (New York: Basic Books, 2015).
Hide, Louise, *Gender and Class in English Asylums: 1890–1914* (Basingstoke: Palgrave Macmillan, 2014).
Hobsbawm, Eric, *The Age of Empire, 1875–1914* (London: Weidenfeld & Nicolson, 1987).
Holden, Wendy, *Shell Shock: The Psychological Impact of War* (London: Channel 4 Books, 1998).
Hopkinson, Michael, *The Irish War of Independence* (Montreal: McGill University Press, 2004).
Hughes, Brian, *Defying the IRA?: Intimidation, Coercion and Communities during the Irish Revolution* (Liverpool: Liverpool University Press, 2016).
Humphreys, Margaret, *Intensely Human: The Health of the Black Soldier in the American Civil War* (Baltimore: Johns Hopkins University Press, 2008).
Humphries, Mark, 'War's long shadow: masculinity, medicine, and the gendered politics of trauma, 1914–1939', *Canadian Historical Review*, 91:3 (2010), 503–31.

Humphries, Mark, and Kurchinski, Kellen, 'Rest, relax and get well: a re-conceptualisation of Great War shell shock treatment', *War & Society*, 27:2 (2008), 89–110.

Huxford, Grace, Alcalde, Ángel, Baines, Gary, Burtin, Olivier and Edele, Mark, 'Writing veterans' history: a conversation on the twentieth century', *War & Society*, 38:2 (2019), 115–38.

Jefferson, Robert, "Enabled courage': race, disability, and black World War II veterans in postwar America', *The Historian*, 65:2 (2003), 1102–24.

Johnson, David, *The Interwar Economy in Ireland* (Dundalk: Economic and Social History Society of Ireland, 1985).

—— 'The Northern Ireland economy, 1914–39', in Liam Kennedy and Phillip Ollerenshaw (eds), *An Economic History of Ulster* (Manchester: Manchester University Press, 1985), 184–223.

Johnstone, Tom, *Orange, Green and Khaki: The Story of the Irish Regiments in the Great War, 1914–18* (Dublin: Gill and Macmillan, 1992).

Jones, Edgar, 'Shell shock at Maghull and the Maudsley: models of psychological medicine in the UK', *Journal of the History of Medicine and Allied Sciences*, 65:3 (2010), 368–95.

Jones, Edgar, and Wessely, Simon, 'Battle for the mind: World War 1 and the birth of military psychiatry', *The Lancet*, 384:9955 (2014), 1708–14.

—— *Shell Shock to PTSD: Military Psychiatry from 1900 to the Gulf War* (Hove: Psychology Press, 2005).

—— 'The impact of total war on the practice of British psychiatry', in R. Chickering and S. Förster (eds), *The Shadows of Total War: Europe, East Asia and the United States, 1919–1939* (Cambridge: Cambridge University Press, 2003), 129–50.

—— 'War Pensions (1900–1945): Changing models of psychological understanding', *The British Journal of Psychiatry*, 180 (2002), 374–9.

Jones, Edgar, Fear, Nicola, and Wessely, Simon, 'Shell shock and mild traumatic brain injury: a historical review', *American Journal of Psychiatry*, 164:11 (2007), 1641–5.

Kearns, Kevin, *Dublin Tenement Life: An Oral History* (Dublin: Gill and Macmillan, 2006).

Keegan, John, *The Face of Battle* (London: Pimlico, 1976).

Kelly, Brendan, *Hearing Voices: The History of Psychiatry in Ireland* (Kildare: Irish Academic Press, 2016).

—— *'He Lost Himself Completely': Shell Shock and Its Treatment at Dublin's Richmond War Hospital, 1916–1919* (Dublin: Liffey Press, 2014).

—— 'The Mental Treatment Act 1945 in Ireland: an historical enquiry', *History of Psychiatry*, 19:1 (2008), 47–67.

Kinder, John, *Paying With Their Bodies: American War and the Problem of the Disabled Veteran* (Chicago: University of Chicago Press, 2015).

Kinsella, Eoin, *Leopardstown Park Hospital, 1917–2017: A Home For Wounded Soldiers* (Dublin: Heritage, 2017).

Kleinman, Arthur, *Writing at the Margin: Discourse between Anthropology and Medicine* (California: University of California Press, 1997).

Kowalsky, Meaghan, "This honourable obligation': the King's National Roll Scheme for disabled ex-servicemen 1915–1944', *European Review of History*, 14:4 (2007), 567–84.

Laffan, Michael, *Judging W. T. Cosgrave* (Dublin: Royal Irish Academy, 2014).
Larsson, Marina, *Shattered Anzacs: Living with the Scars of War* (Sydney: UNSW, 2009).
—— 'Families and institutions for shell-shocked soldiers in Australia after the First World War', *Social History of Medicine*, 22:1 (2008), 97–114.
Leed, Eric, *No Man's Land: Combat and Identity in World War I* (Cambridge: Cambridge University Press, 1979).
Leese, Peter, *Shell-Shock: Traumatic Neurosis and the British Soldiers of the First World War* (Basingstoke: Palgrave Macmillan, 2002).
—— 'Problems returning home: the British psychological casualties of the Great War', *Historical Journal*, 40:4 (1997), 1055–67.
Lengel, Edward, *The Irish through British Eyes: Perceptions of Ireland in the Famine Era* (Westport: Wolfhound Press, 1991).
Leonard, Jane, 'Survivors', in John Horne (ed.), *Our War: Ireland and the Great War* (Dublin: Royal Irish Academy, 2008), 209–23.
—— '"Facing the finger of scorn": veteran's memories of Ireland after the Great War', in Martin Evans and Ken Lunn (eds), *War and Memory in the Twentieth Century* (Oxford: Berg, 1997), 209–24.
—— 'The twinge of memory: Armistice Day and Remembrance Day Sunday in Dublin since 1919', in R. English and G. Walker (eds), *Unionism in Modern Ireland* (Basingstoke: Macmillan, 1996), 99–114.
—— 'Getting them at last: The IRA and ex-servicemen', in David Fitzpatrick (ed.), *Revolution? Ireland, 1917–1923* (Dublin: Trinity History Workshop, 1990), 118–29.
Linden, Stefanie, and Jones, Edgar, '"Shell shock" revisited: an examination of the case records of the National Hospital in London', *Medical History*, 58:4 (2014), 519–45.
—— 'German battle casualties: the treatment of functional somatic disorders during World War I', *Journal of the History of Medicine and Allied Sciences*, 68:4 (2013), 627–58.
Long, Vicky, *Destigmatising Mental Illness?: Professional Politics and Public Education in Britain 1870–1970* (Manchester: Manchester University Press, 2014).
Longmore, Paul, *Why I Burned My Book and Other Essays on Disability* (Philadelphia: Temple University Press, 2003).
Loughran, Tracey, *Shell-Shock and Medical Culture in First World War Britain* (Cambridge: Cambridge University Press, 2016).
—— 'Shell-shock, trauma, and the First World War: the making of a diagnosis and its histories', *Journal of the History of Medicine and Allied Sciences*, 67:1 (2012), 94–119.
—— 'Hysteria and neurasthenia in pre-1914 British medical discourse and in histories of shell-shock', *History of Psychiatry*, 19:1 (2008), 25–46.
Lucey, Seán Donnacha, *The End of the Irish Poor Law?: Welfare and healthcare reform in revolutionary and independent Ireland* (Manchester: Manchester University Press, 2015).
Mahone, Sloan, 'The psychology of rebellion: colonial medical responses to dissent in British East Africa', *The Journal of African History*, 47:2 (2006), 241–58.
Malcolm, Elizabeth, '"A most miserable looking object" – The Irish in English asylums, 1851–1901: migration, poverty and prejudice', in John Belchem and Klaus Tenfelde

(eds), *Irish and Polish Migration in Comparative Perspective* (Essen: Klartext Verlag, 2003), 115–26.

—— '"Ireland's crowded madhouses": the institutional confinement of the insane in nineteenth- and twentieth-century Ireland', in Roy Porter and David Wright (eds), *The Confinement of the Insane: International Perspectives, 1800–1965* (Cambridge: Cambridge University Press, 2003), 315–34.

—— '"The house of strident shadows": the asylum, the family, and emigration in post-famine rural Ireland', in Greta Jones and Elizabeth Malcolm (eds), *Medicine, Disease and the State in Ireland, 1650–1940* (Cork: Cork University Press, 1999), 177–87.

Mantin, Mike, 'Coalmining and the national scheme for disabled ex-servicemen after the First World War', *Social History*, 41:2 (2016), 155–70.

Mauger, Alice, *The Cost of Insanity in Nineteenth Century Ireland: Public, Voluntary and Private Asylum Care* (Basingstoke: Palgrave Macmillan, 2018).

McDermott, Jim, *Northern Divisions: The Old IRA and the Belfast Pogroms, 1920–1922* (Belfast: Beyond the Pale, 2001).

McGaughey, Jane, *Ulster's Men: Protestant Unionist Masculinities and Militarization in the North of Ireland, 1912–1923* (Montréal: McGill Queens University Press, 2012).

Mcnally, Richard, and Frueh, Bartley, 'Why are Iraq and Afghanistan war veterans seeking PTSD disability compensation at unprecedented rates?', *Journal of Anxiety Disorders*, 27:5 (2013), 520–6.

Melling, Bernard, 'Building a lunatic asylum: "a question of beer, milk and the Irish"', in Thomas Knowles and Serena Trowbridge (eds), *Insanity and the Lunatic Asylum in the Nineteenth Century* (London: Routledge, 2015), 57–71.

Mercer, Eric 'For King, country and a shilling a day: Belfast recruiting patterns in the Great War', *History Ireland*, 11 (2003), 29–33.

Meyer, Jessica, *Men of War: Masculinity and the First World War in Britain* (Basingstoke: Palgrave Macmillan, 2009).

—— 'Separating the men from the boys: masculinity and maturity in understandings of shell shock in Britain', *Twentieth Century British History*, 20:1 (2008), 1–22.

Micale, Mark, *Approaching Hysteria: Disease and Its Interpretations* (Princeton: Princeton University Press, 1995).

Micale, Mark, and Lerner, Paul, *Traumatic Pasts: History, Psychiatry, and Trauma in the Modern Age, 1870–1930* (Cambridge: Cambridge University Press, 2001).

Miller, Martin, 'The concept of revolutionary insanity in Russian history', in Angela Brintlinger and Ilya Vinitsky (eds), *Madness and the Mad in Russian Culture* (Toronto: University of Toronto Press, 2007), 105–16.

Milne, Ida, *Stacking the Coffins: Influenza, War and Revolution in Ireland, 1918–1919* (Manchester: Manchester University Press, 2018).

Moriarty, Theresa, 'Work, warfare and wages: industrial controls and Irish trade unionism in the First World War', in Adrian Gregory and Senia Paseta (eds), *Ireland and the Great War: 'A War To Unite Us All'?* (Manchester: Manchester University Press, 2002), 73–94.

Morris, David, *The Evil Hours: A Biography of Post-Traumatic Stress Disorder* (Boston: Houghton Mifflin Harcourt Publishing, 2015).

Mosse, George, 'Shell-shock as a social disease', *Journal of Contemporary History*, 35:1 (2000), 101–18.
Murphy, D. Weijers, B., Palmer, E. and Busuttil, W., 'Exploring patterns in referrals to combat stress for UK veterans with mental health difficulties between 1994 and 2014', *International Journal of Emergency Mental Health and Human Resilience*, 17:3 (2015), 652–8.
Myers, Jason, *The Great War and Memory in Irish Culture, 1918–2010* (California: Academica Press, 2013).
O'Day, Alan, 'Varieties of anti-Irish behaviour, 1846–1922', in P. Panayi (ed.) *Racial Violence in Britain in the Nineteenth and Twentieth centuries* (Leicester: Leicester University Press, 1996), 26–43.
O'Halpin, Eunan, 'Problematic killing during the War of Independence and its aftermath: civilian spies and informers', in James Kelly and Mary Ann Lyons (eds), *Death and Dying in Ireland, Britain and Europe: Historical Perspectives* (Dublin, Irish Academic Press, 2013), 141–58.
O'Shea, Brian and Falvey, Jane, 'A history of the Richmond Asylum, Dublin', in German Berrios and Hugh Freeman (eds), *150 Years of British Psychiatry: Volume Two* (London: Athlone Press, 1996), 407–33.
Oram, Gerard, *Worthless Men: Race, Eugenics and the Death Penalty in the British Army during the First World War* (London: Francis Boutle, 1998).
Perry, Heather, *Recycling the Disabled: Army, Medicine and Modernity in World War One Germany* (Manchester: Manchester University Press, 2014).
Perry, Nicholas, 'Maintaining regimental identity in the Great War: the case of the Irish infantry regiments', *Stand To: The Journal of the Western Front Association*, 52 (1998), 5–11.
—— 'Nationality in the Irish regiments in the First World War', *War and Society*, 12:1 (1994), 65–95.
Poirier, Suzanne, 'The Weir Mitchell rest cure: doctor and patients', *Women's Studies*, 10:1 (1983), 15–40.
Porter, Roy, 'The patient's view', *Theory and Society*, 14:2 (1985), 175–98.
Prior, Pauline, 'Mental health law on the island of Ireland, 1800–2010', in Pauline Prior (ed.), *Asylums, Mental Health Care and the Irish 1800–2010* (Dublin: Irish Academic Press, 2012), 316–34.
—— 'Overseeing the Irish asylums: the Inspectorate in Lunacy, 1845–1921', in Pauline Prior (ed.), *Asylums, Mental Health Care and the Irish 1800–2010* (Dublin: Irish Academic Press, 2012), 221–45.
—— '"Where lunatics abound": A history of mental health services in Northern Ireland', in G. Berrios and H. Freeman (eds), *150 Years of British Psychiatry: Volume 2* (London: Athlone Press, 1996), 292–308.
Ralls, Walter, 'The Papal aggression of 1850: a study in Victorian anti-Catholicism', *Church History*, 43:2 (1974), 242–56.
Reid, Fiona, *Medicine in the First World War: Soldiers, Medics, Pacifists* (London: Bloomsbury, 2017).

—— '"His nerves gave way": shell shock, history and the memory of the First World War in Britain', *Endeavour*, 38:2 (2014), 91–100.
—— *Broken Men: Shell Shock, Treatment and Recovery in Britain, 1914–1930* (London: Continuum, 2010).
—— 'Distinguishing between shell-shocked veterans and pauper lunatics: the ex-services' welfare society and mentally wounded veterans after the Great War', *War in History*, 14:3 (2007), 347–71.
Reynolds, Joseph, *Grangegorman: Psychiatric Care in Dublin since 1815* (Dublin: Institute of Public Administration, 1992).
Reznick, Jeffrey, *Healing the Nation: Soldiers and the Culture of Caregiving in Britain during the Great War* (Manchester: Manchester University Press, 2004).
Richardson, Neil, *A Coward If I Return, a Hero If I Fall: Stories of Irish Soldiers in World War I* (Dublin: O'Brien Press, 2010).
Robinson, Michael, '"Nobody's children"?: the Ministry of Pensions and the treatment of disabled Great War veterans in the Irish Free State, 1921–1939', *Irish Studies Review*, 25:3 (2017), 316–35.
—— 'Perceptions of the mentally ill Irish population during the nineteenth and early twentieth centuries', *Études Irlandaises*, 42:2 (2017), 59–71.
Scull, Andrew, *Madness: A Very Short Introduction* (Oxford: Oxford University Press, 2011).
Shay, Jonathan, *Odysseus in America: Combat Trauma and the Trials of Homecoming* (New York: Scribner, 2002).
Shephard, Ben, *A War of Nerves: Soldiers and Psychiatrists in the Twentieth Century* (London: Jonathan Cape, 2000).
Showalter, Elaine, *The Female Malady: Women, Madness, and English Culture, 1830–1980* (London: Virago, 1985).
Skocpol, Theda, *Protecting Soldiers and Mothers: The Political Origins of Social Policy in the United States* (Cambridge MA: Harvard University Press, 1992).
Stone, Deborah, *The Disabled State* (Basingstoke: Macmillan, 1984).
Stone, Martin, 'Shellshock and the psychologists', in Roy Porter, W. F. Bynum and Michael Shepherd (eds), *The Anatomy of Madness: Essays in the History of Psychiatry, Volume 1: People and Ideas* (London: Tavistock, 1988), 242–71.
Suzuki, Akihito, 'Framing psychiatric subjectivity: doctor, patient and record-keeping at Bethlem in the nineteenth century', in Joseph Melling and Bill Forsythe (eds), *Insanity, Institutions and Society, 1800–1914* (London: Routledge, 1999), 115–37.
Swift, David, and Wilkinson, Oliver (eds), *Veterans of the First World War: Ex-servicemen and Ex-servicewomen in Post-War Britain and Ireland* (Oxon: Routledge, 2019).
Swift, Roger, 'Crime and the Irish in nineteenth century Britain, 1871–1921', in Roger Swift and Sheridan Gilley (eds), *The Irish in Britain, 1815–1939* (London: Pinter, 1989), 163–83.
Switzer, Catherine, *Unionists and Great War Commemoration in the North of Ireland 1914–1918* (Dublin: Irish Academic Press, 2007).

Taylor, Paul, *Heroes Or Traitors?: Experiences of Southern Irish Soldiers Returning from the Great War, 1919–1939* (Liverpool: University of Liverpool Press, 2015).

Thomas, Gregory, *Treating the Trauma of the Great War: Soldiers, Civilians, and Psychiatry in France, 1914–1940* (Louisiana: Louisiana University Press, 2009).

Thomson, Mathew, *Psychological Subjects: Identity, Culture and Health in Twentieth Century Britain* (Oxford: Oxford University Press, 2006).

Todman, Dan, *The Great War: Myth and Memory* (London: Continuum, 2005).

Townsend, Charles, *The Republic: The Fight for Irish Independence, 1918–1923* (London: Penguin, 2013).

Turton, Jaqueline, 'Mayhew's Irish: the Irish poor in mid nineteenth-century London', in Roger Swift and Sheridan Gilley (eds), *The Irish in Victorian Britain: The Local Dimension* (Dublin: Four Courts Press, 1999), 122–55.

Van Der Kolk, Bessel, *The Body Keeps the Score: Mind, Brain and Body in the Transformation of Trauma* (London: Penguin, 2015).

Walsh, Dermot, 'Did the Great Irish Potato Famine increase schizophrenia?', *Irish Journal of Psychological Medicine*, 29:1 (2012), 7–15.

Walsh, Oonagh, 'The designs of providence: race, religion and Irish insanity', in Joseph Melling and Bill Forsythe (eds), *Insanity, Institutions and Society, 1800–1914* (London: Routledge, 1999), 223–42.

Wanke, Paul, *Russian/Soviet Military Psychiatry, 1904–1945* (London: Frank Cass, 2005).

Webb, T. E. F., '"Dottyville": Craiglockhart War Hospital and shell-shock treatment in the First World War', *Journal of the Royal Society of Medicine*, 99:7 (2006), 342–6.

Wilson, Tim, *Frontiers of Violence: Conflict and Identity in Ulster and Upper Silesia, 1918–1922* (Oxford: Oxford University Press, 2010).

Winter, Jay, *War Beyond Words: Languages of Remembrance from the Great War to the Present* (Cambridge: Cambridge University, 2017).

—— 'Families', in Jay Winter (ed.), *The Cambridge History of the First World War: Volume 3: Civil Society* (Cambridge: Cambridge University Press, 2014), 46–68.

—— *Remembering War: The Great War between Memory and History in the Twentieth Century* (New Haven: Yale University Press, 2006).

—— 'Shell-shock and the cultural history of the Great War', *Journal of Contemporary History*, 35:1 (2000), 7–11.

Wootton, Graham, *The Official History of the British Legion* (London: Macdonald and Evans, 1956).

Unpublished

Bettinson, Helen, '"Lost Souls in the House of Restoration"?: British Ex-Servicemen and War Disability Pensions, 1914–1930', PhD Thesis (University of East Anglia, 2002).

Brumby, Alice, 'From "Pauper Lunatics" to "Rate-Aided Patients": Removing the Stigma of Mental Health Care, 1888–1938', PhD Thesis (University of Huddersfield, 2015).

Delargy, Rosaline, 'The History of the Belfast District Lunatic Asylum, 1829–1921', PhD Thesis (University of Ulster, 2002).

Diver, Luke, 'Ireland and the South African War, 1899–1902', PhD Thesis (Maynooth University, 2014).

Douglas, Barbara, 'In the Shadow of the Asylum: Narratives of Change and Stagnation, 1890–1930', PhD Thesis (University of Exeter, 2008).

Hopkins, John, 'Problems, Politics and Personalities in the Treatment of Mental and Nervous Casualties in the British Army, 1914–1918', PhD Thesis (University of Leicester, 2002).

Kowalsky, Meaghan, 'Enabling the Great War: Ex-Servicemen, the Mixed Economy of Welfare and the Social Construction of Disability, 1899–1930', PhD Thesis (University of Leeds, 2007).

Latcham, Andrew, 'Journey's End: Ex-servicemen and the State during and after the Great War', PhD Thesis (University of Oxford, 1996).

Loughran, Tracey, 'Shell-Shock in First World War Britain: An Intellectual and Medical History, 1860–1920', PhD Thesis (Queen Mary, University of London, 2006).

Louis, Diana, 'Peculiar Institutions: Representations of Nineteenth-Century Black Women's Madness and Confinement in Slavery and Asylums', PhD Thesis (Emory University, 2014).

Redmond, Paul, 'Denis Kilbride M.P. 1848–1924', MA Thesis (University of Maynooth, 2003).

Reid, Peter, 'The Institutional Management of Soldiers with Shell Shock in Ireland, 1916–19', MA Thesis (University College, Dublin, 2014).

Stone, Martin, 'The Military and Industrial Roots of Clinical Psychology in Britain, 1900–1945', PhD Thesis (London School of Economics, 1985).

Interviews

Interview with Ann O'Ryan and John O'Ryan in Ann O'Ryan's home in Saint Helens on 23 February 2019.

Index

abreaction therapy 23, 41–2
age distribution of asylum patients 165–6
American Civil War veterans 106
Anderson, Julie 9
anti-Irish prejudice 11, 15–16, 25–9, 51, 71, 82, 90, 104, 202, 204, 214, 227
Armstrong, David 10
Arnold, J. B. 8, 30–3, 39–40, 69–73, 79–80, 102, 118, 125
artificial legs 39
Ashurst War Hospital 71
asylums
    accommodation available in 201–2
    containment emphasised over cure 191
    death rates 165, 169–72, 201–2
    reclassified as mental hospitals 174, 206
    supervisory nature of 188
Australia 214

Baldie, A. 63, 66, 90
Ballinasloe Asylum 168
Barham, Peter 4, 11, 42, 109, 124–5, 203, 208, 211, 228–9
Barker, Pat 3
Barnes, G. 48–9, 65
bed space 148, 153, 168, 201
Belfast Asylum 10, 151–2
Belfast War Hospital (BWH) 23, 149–52, 156, 162, 165, 168–9, 173, 185–8
Birmingham War Hospitals Committee 208
'Black and Tan' forces 69, 84
Blackrock Hospital, Meath 39, 112
Boer War (1899–1902) 215

Bourke, Joanna 4, 89–90, 229
Boyce, D. G. 5
British Legion 35, 39, 75, 106, 114, 128–9, 133–4, 210
Brown, William 104
Buckinghamshire County Asylum 165
burial alive 156
Burtchaell, Charles 65
Byrne, A. 126

Campbell, Gordon 84
Carruthers, D. A. 101
Castlebar Asylum (later Mental Hospital) 168, 200–5
Catholic communities 83, 88–9
causation of mental illness 154–8
charities providing for ex-servicemen 8, 35, 127–8, 210
Chelsea Hospital 30
childlike behaviour 21, 26–8
Chrystal, George 109
civil disobedience 69
class divisions 26, 230
Clonmel Asylum 198–201, 205–6
clothing for patients 200–1
    see also 'hospital blues'; tweed suits issued to some patients
coal shortages 168
Cognitive Behavioural Therapy (CBT) 41
Collie, Sir John 24
Collins, Michael 101
colonial conflicts, veterans of 6
colonial narratives 15
Colonial Office 212–13
combat neurosis 10, 21, 24–5, 103, 132
    see also war neuroses
Commission on the Sick and Destitute Poor 201–2

Committee on the Claims of
    Ex-Servicemen 128
conscription 30
Cooke, E. Marriot 204, 209
Corden-Coyne, Ana 25
Cork Asylum 168, 186, 188, 197–8, 201,
    203, 211
Cosgrave, William 103, 126
cowardice 104
Cox, John 42
Craig, James 48, 116
Craigavon Hospital 44, 48, 50, 72, 88,
    112, 121–2, 204
Craiglockhart War Hospital, Edinburgh
    23–4
Crammer, J. L. 165, 172
'Criminal Lunatics', treatment of 38–9, 211
Crouthamel, Jason 88, 230
Cunningham, Michael 83

Dáil Éireann 82, 100, 126, 213
The Daily Telegraph 28
Dale, Henry 80–1
Danesfort, Lord John 124
Dangerous Lunacy Act (1838) 73, 189
Dawson, W. R. 36–7, 78, 149–56,
    172–3, 185, 189
delusions 157–8
dementia 188–9
depression as a medical condition 156
Deputy Commissioners of Medical
    Services (DCMS) conference
    (London, 1921) 63, 65
de Valera, Éamon 101
Devine, E. T. 35
diagnosis 40, 209
Diamant, Neil 86
dietary standards 202, 205
disability and disabled people 13, 15, 68
discharges from hospital 163, 186–8
discrimination 12, 25, 79, 82–3
    against war veterans 113–18, 227
Donelan, Dr 151, 164, 172–3

Draper, Thomas 26
dreams 158–9
Dunning, Gertrude 45, 112

Easter Rising (1916) 4, 81
electric shock treatment 23, 160
emotionality 21, 26–8
employability of disabled ex-servicemen
    108–9, 116
enlisted men, numbers of 30
Ennis Mental Hospital 114, 201
Enniskillen bombing (1987) 5
entertainments for patients 161, 168,
    203
Esplin, W. D. 119
ESWS see Ex-Services Welfare Society
    (ESWS)
Ewell War Hospital 71
exclusive medical facilities for veterans
    210, 227
Ex-Services Welfare Society (ESWS) 4,
    35, 37, 106, 109, 119, 129–31,
    191, 207

facilities, shortage of 71–4, 89, 105
Fallon, W. G. 101, 125
familial networks 127, 189–90
Federation of Discharged and
    Demobilised Sailors and
    Soldiers 35, 78, 81–2, 84, 210
Fielding, Rowland 29
Final Awards 107
financial control 33
First World War 4–5, 15–16, 22, 30–1,
    49, 90, 228
Fitzpatrick, Peter 37, 68, 107, 121–3
Forde, M. J. 51, 157, 161, 172
Forward, E.L. 67, 71–5, 78–81, 87,
    190–205
'forward psychiatry' 23
France 125, 214
Freud, Sigmund 43
funding for hospitals 206

further research, need for 229–30
Fussell, Paul 3, 15, 228

Gagen, Wendy Jane 7
'Geddes axe' 13, 105
gender divisions 26
general practitioners 105
Gerber, David 231
Germany 126
Good Friday Agreement (1998) 5
Graham, William 171
Graves, Robert 3
Grayson, Richard 82–3
Great War *see* First World War

hallucinations 157–8
Hart, Peter 85
Hebb, John Harry 44, 66, 76–8, 109
Herman, Judith 86
Holden, Wendy 3, 206
Home Office 212
Hopkins, John 174
'Hospital Blues' (clothing) 149–50, 194, 197
hospital types 148
Hughes, Brian 86
Hughes, Peter 215

imperialism 27–8
influenza 169
insanity associated with military service 216
institutional treatment 9–13, 37–45
institutionalisation 188–9, 192, 197–9, 205–11, 215
Irish Free State 5, 12, 90, 100–3, 113, 118, 124–5, 133–5, 206–7, 211–16, 229
 Service Patients in 197–200
Irish neutrality 12
'Irish problem' 214
Irish Republican Army (IRA) 5, 12, 69–70, 82–5, 89, 101–2

The Irish Times 48, 100, 116, 134
Islandbridge 134

Johnstone, Tom 3
Journal of the American Medical Association 29
Jung, Carl 43

Kay, A. G. 1
Kelly, Brendan 174
Kilbride, Denis 28
Killarney Mental Hospital 201–2
Kilmainham Hospital, Dublin 30
King George V Hospital, Dublin 23, 87–8, 149–53, 160–1
King's National Roll 35, 84–5, 116–17, 134
Kipling, Rudyard 29
Knox, Robert 26

Land War (1879) 28
Lawson, Jack 123
Leed, Eric 3
Leese, Peter 3–4, 24
Lemass, Seán 115
length of military service of wounded men, and of their medical treatment 153, 167
Leonard, Jane 5, 85
Leopardstown Hospital 8, 71, 44–8, 88, 102, 105, 109–13, 135
Letterkenny Mental Hospital 205
literacy rates 204
Lloyd George, David 81
Lomax, Montagu 165, 205
Loseby, C. E. 191
Loughran, Tracey 4, 26, 228
Louis, Diana 27
Lunacy Act (1890) 22
Lunacy (Ireland) Act (1901) 211

McDonagh, Michael 29
McDougall, William 28–9
McGauly, Michael 24

McGrath, William 70
McLeod, J. K. 29
Macpherson, Ian 101
Maghull *see* Red Cross Military Hospital
Mapother, Edward 209
Maryborough Mental Hospital 203
Mayo, Earl of 102
medical advances 1
medical personnel attached to British armed forces 167, 230
medication 159–60
melancholia 153, 156, 188–9
mental casualties and physical injuries, differential treatment of 148–9
  see also parity of esteem between mental and physical disability
mental illness
  discharges as a result of 11
  history of 230
  holistic understanding of 231
  racial connotations of 29
  treatability of 14, 174
Mental Treatment Acts 206–7, 216–17
Meyer, Jessica 26
Mills, T. H. 119
Milner, Frederick 38
Ministry of Labour 34–5, 79–84, 101, 116
Ministry of Pensions 2–3, 6–14, 30–5, 38–46, 49, 51, 63, 67–84, 87–90, 100–1, 105–14, 122–8, 135, 186, 189–91, 196–9, 202–11, 214–16, 227–31
  archives of 6–7, 10, 229
  attitude shown to mentally ill veterans 122
  austerity policies imposed by 196, 204–5
  district committees 34
  establishment of 30–1
  'hardening' policy 109
  hospitals operated in Ireland 109–10

internal records 7–8
regional offices 33–4
Mooney, Paddy 131–2
Mooney, Stephen 132
The Morning Chronicle 28
Morrison, John 24–5
Mosse, George 30
Mott, Frederick 155
Mulcahy, Daniel 118
Mullingar Mental Hospital 203
Mushatt, Harry 132
Myers, Charles 1–2, 66, 165

National Hospital for Paralysed and Epileptic, Queen Square, London 23
nationalism 27
nationality, definition of 65
neurasthenia 1–2, 13, 15, 36–7, 40, 43–5, 49, 63–90, 101–2, 106–9, 113, 119–26, 129–34, 158, 229
  far-reaching and ill-defined nature of 36
  pensions for 37
  symptoms of 36
nightmares 158–9
Nixon, Richard 86
Northern Ireland 4–5, 12–13, 90, 115–16, 129, 134, 206–7, 211–12, 227, 230
  Service Patients in 192–7
No. 4 London General Hospital 23
No. 26 General Hospital, near Etaples 22

observation wards 162
occupational therapy 43, 160
O'Connor, Steven 69
O'Halpin, Eunan 85
O'Higgins, Kevin 134
Omagh Asylum 190, 197
O'Ryan, Ann 120
O'Ryan, Patrick John 1, 7–9, 25, 37, 87, 119–23, 127–8, 131, 135

O'Sullivan, George 133
overcrowding 168, 195–6, 201
Ozzard, Harold 119

paramilitary activity 69
parity of esteem between mental and
    physical disability 216, 227
parole system 161–2
pauperism 38, 204, 207–8, 215
Pear, Thomas 26, 41, 43, 45, 118, 173, 208
pension payments 1, 9, 30–2, 37, 123–4
Percy, Eustace 120, 122–3, 231
'PIE' system 23
Pierce, Bedford 45
pocket money 216
politicisation 4
Poor Law 206, 213
Portlaoighise Mental Hospital 201–2
post-mortem examinations 171
Post-Traumatic Stress Disorder (PTSD)
    10–11, 45, 67, 86, 89
post-war societies 229
Prestwich Asylum 165
private patients 215
psychiatry, history of 228–9
psychoanalysis 45, 159
psychoneurosis 1–2, 11–12, 22–4, 36,
    40, 49, 119–20, 126–7, 228
    see also neurasthenia
Pulmonary Tuberculosis 38, 201–2
Purdysburn House and Villa Colony
    168–9, 173, 190–8, 204–9, 216
'purification rights' 133
Purser, F. 25, 156, 159, 162–4, 209

qualifications of staff 199

racial stereotyping 25
Read, Charles 158–9
'reconstruction' philosophy 31, 44, 46
recovery rates 165
Red Cross 68, 130
Red Cross Military Hospital, Maghull
    23–4, 40–3, 107–8, 164–5

Regan, Patrick 114
rehabilitation 3, 9, 11–13, 31, 40, 51,
    67–8, 103, 215–16, 227, 231
Reid, Fiona 4
remembrance ceremonies 133–4
republicanism 4, 28
resettlement allowances 31–2
respite care 189
Rhodes, Wilfred 80
Richmond District Asylum, Dublin 74,
    149–51, 161–2, 166–8, 172–3,
    185–9, 197–8, 201
Richmond War Hospital (RWH) 9,
    13–14, 23, 149–65, 168, 172–3,
    188–9, 203, 211
Rivers, W. H. R. 23, 42, 158
Rows, R. G. 23, 40–2, 164–5
Royal Victoria Military Hospital, Netley
    22–3
Russia 126

Sandham Jeudwine, Sir Hugh 103
Sassoon, Siegfried 3
sectarianism 12, 83, 88
Service Patient scheme 2, 9–10, 14,
    38–9, 73–4, 87, 89, 149, 162–3,
    173, 185–217
    admissions from civil society 188–9
    aims of 204
    benefits to patients 204
    criticisms of 205, 227
    in the Irish Free State 197–200
    in Northern Ireland 192–7
    subjectivity in 202
Shay, Jonathan 86
shell-shock 3, 15, 22–6, 30–1, 43, 90,
    106, 122, 153, 209, 227–8, 231
    definition of 2
    early uses of the term 1–2, 66
    'half-way house' theses of 228
    Irish experience of 26
    responses to 23–4
    'wounded' and 'sick' categories of 2
Shephard, Ben 42

Shotley Bridge Hospital 72
Showalter, Elaine 26
Sim, C. A. 71
Sinn Féin 4, 69–70, 73, 80–3
Smith, Grafton Elliot 26–7, 41, 43, 45, 63–5, 173, 208
Smith, William 24
social construction of disability 66
social prejudice 30
  see also anti-Irish prejudice
societal concern for disabled veterans 106
Southborough Report (1922) 103–5, 209
Southern Irish Loyalists Association (SILA) 78–9, 102, 114, 123, 128–30, 135
Soviet Union 126
specialist treatment 164
Spender, W. B. 88
stereotyping 25, 27
stigma
  attached to mental illness 6, 8, 11–12, 51, 65–8, 79, 83, 87, 89, 103, 113, 119, 122, 135, 149, 206–9, 214–16, 231
  attached to service in the British Army 6, 81, 83, 87–90, 100, 135, 204
  conveyed by official language 216–17
Stone, Martin 206, 228
Sugars, Harold 34, 46, 69–78, 105, 109
suicide 132–3

targeting of British ex-servicemen 85–7
Tavistock Clinic 229
Taylor, Paul 5, 85, 113
Taylor, Pritchard 104
Thomson, Mathew 228
time-limits for decisions about long-term care 149
Tirconaill Mental Hospital 201
training for disabled ex-soldiers 83–5, 101

transfer of power to the Irish government 100–1
traumatisation 5, 86
treatment allowances 74–8
treatment capacity, effectiveness of increases in 79
triggering of psychosis 156
Tronson, Harold 155
the Troubles 5
tweed suits issued to some patients 197, 200–1, 216
Tyron, G. C. 112, 191

United Irish rebellion (1798) 28

Vietnam War veterans 45, 89
vocational therapy 46, 108
voluntarism 48, 207

waiting lists for treatment 11–12, 45, 51, 63–4, 71–8, 90, 227, 231
Wallis, S. J. 28
war hospitals
  establishment of 166–7
  use of the term 149
war neuroses 11, 26, 104, 127
  see also combat neurosis
War Office 12–13, 103, 215
War Pensions Acts 31, 75–6, 106–7
War Pensions Committee 208
War Pensions Gazette 43
Webb, Sir Arthur Lisle 36
Webb, Thomas 24
Weir–Mitchell treatment 23, 160
Whelan, Thomas 110–12
Whitman, Elizabeth 128
Winter, Jay 10, 127, 132
Wolfe, G. 114
Wolfe, H. 83, 215
work, benefits of 66–7, 77
workhouses 207

Yealland, L. R. 23
Young, Allan 67

EU authorised representative for GPSR:
Easy Access System Europe, Mustamäe tee 50,
10621 Tallinn, Estonia
gpsr.requests@easproject.com

www.ingramcontent.com/pod-product-compliance
Lightning Source LLC
Chambersburg PA
CBHW070236240426
43673CB00044B/1818